THE PROCESS OF COMMUNITY HEALTH EDUCATION AND PROMOTION

Third Edition

THE PROCESS OF COMMUNITY HEALTH EDUCATION AND PROMOTION

Third Edition

Eva I. Doyle
Baylor University

Susan E. Ward
Texas A&M University

Jody Early
University of Washington Bothell

WAVELAND

PRESS, INC.

Long Grove, Illinois

For information about this book, contact:
Waveland Press, Inc.
4180 IL Route 83, Suite 101
Long Grove, IL 60047-9580
(847) 634-0081
info@waveland.com
www.waveland.com

10-digit ISBN 1-4786-3664-5
13-digit ISBN 978-1-4786-3664-9

Printed in the United States of America

7 6 5 4 3 2 1

We dedicate this book to our families and students,
and to the communities we serve.
You are our source of encouragement and inspiration.

Contents

PART 1
HEALTH AND COMMUNITY PERSPECTIVES

---

3 Epidemiological Considerations   53

PART II
THE PROCESS OF HEALTH PROGRAMMING

PART III
COMMUNICATING NEEDS AND MANAGING RESOURCES

13   Resource Access and Management · 317

14   Trends in the Global Community · 349

Preface

This textbook provides an introductory overview of information, perspectives, and competencies needed to effectively promote health and quality of life in community health education and health promotion, public health, and health care settings. Our discussions in chapters 1 and 2 about the socio-ecological factors that influence health and quality of life and the powerful impact of interprofessional and community partnerships, are indicative of our philosophy and intended audience for this book. We invite all who are interested in the health and quality of life of individuals and whole communities to engage in the experiential learning approach that lies at the heart of this textbook.

A Recommended Learning Perspective

This book was written by three individuals who view learning as a journey rather than a destination. In fact, we confess that we actually *enjoy* the learning process. This is probably because life experience has taught us that change is inevitable and constant, and that we all learn through this ongoing change process whether we like it or not. We use the word *enjoy* loosely because experiences in which true learning occurs are often as demanding and exhausting as they are exhilarating. That is the experience we wish for our readers. We are by no means implying that merely reading this book will demand, exhaust, and exhilarate. We are, however, suggesting that its application in the real world of community health promotion can contribute to your lifelong learning experience in ways that can be significant and worth the effort.

We invite you to view this book as more than a required reading assignment in a college course. If you only read it to memorize facts to regurgitate on an exam, you will have missed its intent. Instead, we encourage you to think of it as a tool for action. Because people learn by doing (more so than by reading, listening, or taking notes), we encourage you to consider the following recommendations as you read this book.

1. *Ask "so what?"* When you read a passage, ask yourself why you would need to know that information. Think about how that knowledge or developed skill could be of value to you in your current or future practice as a health professional. There is a rationale and intended use for each chapter section. Reading with the intention of discovering this practical use can enhance your learning and application.

2. ***Seek second opinions.***   Don't just take our word for it. Though we have worked to present accurate and current information and to discuss issues from differing viewpoints, we encourage you to further explore alternative perspectives. Learning from varying perspectives can broaden and enrich your understanding of the profession.

3. ***Apply it and customize it.***   Test the textbook information and recommended approaches in the real world at every opportunity. (See "Textbook Highlights" for suggestions.) Your experimentation will breathe life into your learning experience and will help you master the ability to adapt textbook content for a variety of situations and uses.

About Professional Paradigms and Interprofessional Collaboration

Chapter 1 contains a brief description of emerging professional paradigms and a rationale for forging partnerships across health disciplines. We encourage you to use the exercise described in *For Your Application* to explore your own perspectives and philosophies.

The chapter also contains information about the socio-ecological factors that influence population health and the *Core Competencies of Interprofessional Collaboration*. As you read these sections, we encourage you to consider ways in which cross-disciplinary teams may be more effective than those professionals from a single health discipline to effectively address the complexities of public health problems and their influencing factors.

We urge you to become actively involved in professional organizations, seek and maintain professional certifications, remain abreast of evolving frameworks throughout your professional career, and become a champion of interprofessional collaborative efforts to promote health and quality of life.

Stronger Emphasis on Health Equity

Chapter 4 in our previous editions was designed to equip you with an understanding of the evolving and diverse "faces of America" and the need for cultural humility as a health professional. Though we continue with that goal in this edition, we strengthened our focus on health disparities and health equity in chapter 4. We also replaced information that focused on cultural norms of selected groups (which may have inadvertently contributed to stereotypes) with descriptions of some specific health issues for certain population groups within the context of social determinants, socio-ecological influences, and health equity. We followed this section with a discussion about essential elements for promoting health equity. We hope you will *enjoy* our new approach and find it useful.

Textbook Highlights

Each chapter of this textbook is designed to engage you in thought, discussion, and action. Where possible, we use examples about real people, illustrations that relate to common elements of life, practical questions, a conversational tone, and even a little humor to engage you in a personal way. We also include special features to help you explore ideas, test recommended approaches, and develop knowledge and competencies that will inform your health promotion efforts. We highlight these features below and provide more in-depth information for the course instructor in an accompanying Instructor's Guide.

FOR YOUR INFORMATION

Every chapter contains *For Your Information* (FYI) boxed features that provide nutshell descriptions, how-to guidelines, checklists, and examples that complement and expand on chapter content. In some cases, the FYI material serves as a prompt for or example of information you can use in a course project (see "Course Project") or as a self-directed learning activity.

FOR YOUR APPLICATION

You will find the *For Your Application* (FYA) feature at the end of each chapter. The FYAs contain instructions for recommended activities that can be undertaken on your own if they aren't assigned by the instructor. Some FYA activities can occur totally within the confines of a classroom. Others may require you to visit a local neighborhood or community organization for a stronger real-world experience. Moreover, some FYA activities can reinforce your work on a course project if one is assigned (see "Course Project") or further develop your professional résumé or portfolio. In all cases, FYA activities are designed to engage you in discussion and application of the knowledge and competencies described in that chapter.

COURSE PROJECT

One of the most basic responsibilities for those working in community health is to assess the actual and perceived needs of communities. Therefore, the *Community Assessment Project* described in Appendix A can serve as a major project for a course. Steps in the assessment process are outlined succinctly in chapter 6. You will find that many of the FYA activities throughout each chapter can serve as components of this project and/or stand-alone learning activities.

LEARNING OBJECTIVES AND REVIEW QUESTIONS

The learning objectives at the beginning of each chapter and the review questions at the end will help you highlight and organize your reading and notes around targeted learning concepts. The chapter content that addresses each objective/question not only provides key definitions and concepts but is designed to help you understand those concepts as they are applied in real-world settings.

To the Instructor

We believe the accompanying Instructor's Guide, found on the book's Web page at www.waveland.com, will be a valuable resource as you design and teach your course. It offers a wealth of materials and the flexibility to adapt them to various teaching styles and preferences. In the guide, you will find teaching tips linked to specific features of this text; a test bank and answer key; chapter-specific PowerPoints; and electronic versions of the following four appendices that you can adapt for your course needs: *Community Assessment Project Guide* (Appendix A), *Community Health Professional E-Portfolio Guide* (B), *Planning a Social Media Strategy for Advocacy* (C), and *Creating a Resource Inventory for Community Health* (D).

Acknowledgments

The concept that "it takes a village" could be applied to this project. We thank the multitude of students and community partners whose input identified the need for and shaped the content of this book. We also thank a variety of colleagues whose encouragement and honest critique helped us reach our goal. We would like to especially acknowledge the assistance of Ms. Taylor Caulk, a graduate student in nursing at the University of Washington, who helped us organize some of the PowerPoints for the Instructor's Guide; Amanda Espinosa, an instructor at Texas Woman's University, who helped us update our ancillary materials, including quizzes and Web resources; and Gabe Benavidez, a graduate student in public health at Baylor University, who helped us check and organize our references. In addition, we thank our families who supported us throughout this process and exhibited understanding when writing this took us away from them. We also extend our gratitude to those instructors and students who have used our text and have sent us feedback. We welcome comments, suggestions, and personal stories about applying these concepts in the field; your insights will help us keep future editions of this textbook current and meaningful.

PART I

HEALTH AND COMMUNITY PERSPECTIVES

1

Health, Quality of Life, and Emerging Professional Perspectives

The elderly woman leans back in her chair and absentmindedly pushes her glasses back up on her nose. She gives you a knowing, tolerant look and says, "Honey, I ain't never had a need for that before. Don't see why I should start now." She's talking about the low-fat diet you just described to her. You knew before you started that it would be a tough sell—in some ways tougher than explaining the complexities of her diabetic condition. She continues, "And, you're telling me to buy fresh vegetables. Now, where am I gonna get the money for that?! Heck, they don't even SELL fresh vegetables at the corner store where I walk to buy stuff, and I ain't got no car!" This person has already overcome more of life's challenges than you may ever face. Yet, you are asking her to change life-long eating habits and somehow find a way to overcome complex financial and environmental obstacles. How do you convince her that such a drastic lifestyle change could make a difference in her health and quality of life? And, what can you do when lack of resources is a significant barrier?

Chapter Objectives

1. Describe varying perspectives on and definitions of health and quality of life.
2. Recount the historical development of professional concepts related to health, wellness, and quality of life.
3. Name immediate and global factors that influence health and quality of life.
4. Analyze the reciprocal relationships between social conditions, health, and quality of life.
5. Explain the basic concepts of the socio-ecological approach.
6. Describe emerging professional paradigms and approaches in health care, public health, and health education.
7. Define and explain the benefits of interprofessional collaborative partnerships.

≣ Health and Quality of Life

Imagine yourself as a talk-show host who goes out on the street to conduct an informal survey. Your quest is to capture the "average" person on national television with a microphone in his face as he tries to think of intelligent answers. Your first question seems harmless enough: "How do you define health?" Your victim scratches his head and blurts out an answer. You look knowingly into the camera, repeat his answer, and try not to laugh. Then you ask with a smug look on your face, "What is quality of life?" Now he's really stumped. He stammers as he tries to form a coherent response. You grin and the camera cuts back to the studio.

Few health professionals would ever intentionally interview someone in the condescending manner just described. Yet, experienced health professionals sometimes feel like the talk-show host who can't believe what she is hearing. The overarching goal of most health professionals is to enhance the health and quality of life of individuals and communities. But they often find it difficult to accomplish this goal given the imprecise array of health-related definitions and perspectives among clients, community leaders, and even other professionals. If you want to accomplish your professional goal of promoting healthy lifestyles, you have to know how people define health. To gain a clear understanding of your goals as a developing health professional, we invite you to examine some diverse and evolving perspectives about health and quality of life.

Common Viewpoints about Health

Take a moment to jot down words or concepts that come to mind when you think of the word *health*. Try to avoid textbook or professional definitions. Instead, think of your childhood experiences and how your family, friends, and others shaped your ideas about what it means to be healthy. Think of older adults that you know who are approaching the later stages of life, or think of someone who is challenged with a disability, and imagine how that person may define health.

The point of this exercise is to help you remember that the definition of what it means to be healthy can differ from person to person, and that some individuals you will encounter as a health professional have no clear understanding of the professional definitions presented in this textbook. These differing health views can significantly impact a person's life and your ability to help. The woman in this chapter's introductory story is a diabetic patient. A change in her eating habits and other behaviors could mean the difference between a life of relative wellness and one racked with health complications. Her calm rejection of a healthier diet could be driven by the belief that she is "healthy enough"—a viewpoint that could eventually cost her dearly.

To develop a better understanding of common views about health, we interviewed 393 children, parents, and elementary school teachers in a local community to learn how they defined *health*. Listed below are responses from a few of our participants:

- "Health is seeing the dentist and doctor regularly and particularly if you are sick." (Kyle, age 13)
- "It's not feeling sick, not having a cold." (Mary, age 7)
- "Health is how you feel. How your body works and how your systems work. The way you eat—not eating too much junk food. What activities you do, like swimming and running." (Katie, age 9)

Like Kyle and Mary, many of our participants thought health was related to illness. Some, like Katie, thought health had something to do with the actions we take or the activities in which we participate. Several elementary school teachers added dimensions beyond physical well-being such as "coordination of mind and body;" "skills to perform effectively in life—socially, emotionally, and academically;" "mind, body, and spirit;" and "keeping safe, avoiding anything damaging, feeling good about self, and [having] socialization skills." One said, "Health is a whole host of things from exercise to religion." Despite these few holistic perspectives, the majority confined their health definition to a physical state marked by the absence of disease. These findings serve as a sobering reminder that despite gains in health education and promotion, health professionals have more work to do to promote health awareness in all of its dimensions.

Evolving Professional Concepts

It's not surprising that people hold different views about health: Even health professionals can't agree on a single definition, and literally hundreds of definitions and descriptions of health can be found in the professional literature. These differing professional views may be partially due to the natural evolution of information and concepts that occurs in most professions. Newly discovered health information and technologies, shifting population demographics, evolving cultures, historical events at global and local levels, and a host of other factors have contributed to an ongoing demand for health professionals to adapt to a changing world.

To remain abreast of these constant changes, students enrolled in university degree programs are often encouraged to continue to attend professional conferences, read journals, and stay connected to the profession long after they graduate. It is also important for students and their instructors to examine the prevailing professional philosophies and approaches of the present within the context of the past; in other words, how those philosophies and approaches evolved. Mastering this historical perspective will help you effectively integrate proven approaches and further refine them in the future. Without a sense of your chosen profession's history, you could inadvertently repeat mistakes of the past or contribute to a complacent acceptance that "we now know all there is to know." A good place to begin developing this historical perspective is with some of the early definitions of health used by recognized health organizations and leaders.

In 1947, the World Health Organization (WHO, 1947) told the world that **health** is "a state of complete physical, mental, and social well-being, and not merely the absence of disease and infirmity" (pp. 1–2). That declaration may not seem like earth-shattering news as you read it now. But prior to 1947, the prevailing view of health among many health leaders had mirrored what we learned through our recent survey of students, parents, and teachers: Health had been largely viewed as the absence of infectious diseases.

There were good reasons for a focus on infectious diseases at that time in history. The classic story of smallpox eradication (Henderson, 2006) illustrates this point. In the early 1900s, smallpox was a widespread killer in the United States. Though outbreaks of its severest form had declined by 1929, a 1947 outbreak in New York City resulted in the immunization of 6 million city residents. Smallpox continued to claim lives around the globe for decades, but a declaration by the World Health Assembly in 1958 led to the launching in 1967 of a global WHO campaign to eradicate smallpox. That goal was finally achieved in 1980. Thus, a definition of health as the absence of smallpox resulted in millions of lives saved.

The need for vigilance over infectious diseases is still an important component of public health. Emerging and re-emerging diseases, including growing rates of antibiotic-resistant illnesses, currently demand the attention of many health professionals (Centers for Disease Control and Prevention [CDC], 2016c; National Institute of Allergy and Infectious Diseases [NIAID], 2014; NIAID, 2015). However, from a historical perspective, emerging health issues of a more chronic nature, such as cancer and heart disease, have become a critical focus.

By 1970, the U.S. Communicable Disease Center had changed its name to the Centers for Disease Control (currently, the Centers for Disease Control and Prevention) to reflect a broader scope that included chronic disease control and health promotion (Keck, 2006). During this time, the traditional epidemiology model (agent, host, and environment) gave way to an early version of the **social-ecological model** (Morris, 1975; Figure 1.1) because the latter included social and behavioral factors as well as the environment as part of the complex web surrounding chronic health issues. Similarly, the Canadian Ministry of Health and Welfare's **health field concept** (Lalonde, 1974) encompassed the four areas or types of factors that contribute to health: human biology (bodily systems, genetics, maturation, etc.), environment (climate, economics, community structure, social norms, etc.), lifestyle (controllable choices and behaviors), and the health care system (factors related to health care delivery).

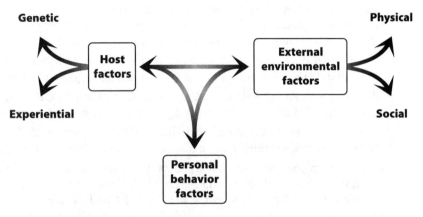

Figure 1.1   The social-ecological model (early version).

From *Uses of Epidemiology*, 3rd ed., by J. N. Morris, 1975, Edinburgh: Churchill Livingstone.

By the early 1980s, the U.S. government had embraced a massive undertaking that changed the course of how health is viewed and addressed by health professionals. The effort was launched by the publication of two landmark reports. In the first report, *Healthy People: The Surgeon General's Report on Health Promotion and Disease Prevention* (U.S. Public Health Service, 1979), the surgeon general described the health status of Americans and announced national goals for preventing premature deaths and promoting healthy lifestyles. A follow-up report in 1980, *Promoting Health/Preventing Disease: Objectives for the Nation*, contained more than 200 targeted health objectives designed to help Americans achieve the *Healthy People* goals by 1990 (U.S. Department of Health and Human Services [USDHHS], 1980). The U.S. government has been tracking and reporting *Healthy People* achievements related to those goals and objectives since 1980, and updated goals and objectives are announced at the beginning of each new decade. (See chapter 2 for more information about current community-based *Healthy People* goals and activities.)

We can examine the evolution of the *Healthy People* initiative to illustrate how views about health have changed over the past several decades. The initial 1979 and 1980 reports marked a significant shift from a traditional **medical model** perspective (Friedson, 1988), which emphasized "fixing a problem" through diagnosis and treatment, to a **wellness** perspective that focused on moving toward a positive state of health and well-being. This shift in perspective compelled health professionals to learn more about what wellness can mean for a person who is not currently ill and to devise programs to help people achieve wellness. By the mid- to late-1990s, it was generally accepted that wellness is influenced by the multidimensional interplay of physical, emotional, spiritual, environmental, social, and interpersonal factors (Insel & Roth, 1994). Five commonly accepted dimensions of personal wellness include:

- *Physical wellness.* A physical state that enables a person to perform daily activities that lower the risk of preventable disease and are conducive to high levels of wellness in the other four dimensions, and to carry out such activities at levels that are personally satisfying.

- *Intellectual wellness.* A cognitive state that enables a person to apply sound critical-thinking processes when gathering information, forming opinions, making decisions, solving problems, and communicating with others.

- *Emotional wellness.* An emotional state that enables a person to recognize and understand, and effectively manage and express, feelings and emotions.

- *Social wellness.* An interactive state that enables a person to interrelate with others in ways that are mutually satisfying, supportive, and/or productive.

- *Spiritual wellness.* A communal state that enables a person to develop a sense of life purpose and meaning and/or a sense of connectedness with a higher power.

A sixth dimension, occupational wellness, is included in the Six Dimensions of Wellness (Hettler, 1976) of the National Wellness Institute. We discuss this dimension as a community setting in chapter 2 (see *Work Setting*).

Total wellness describes an integrated or holistic combination of all dimensions of personal wellness. As illustrated in the illness-wellness continuum (Figure 1.2), total wellness is dynamic in that it can fluctuate back and forth along a range from premature death to high-level wellness (Insel & Roth, 2000).

| Low level of wellness | Physical, mental, emotional symptoms | Change and growth | High level of wellness |

Malaise   Vital, meaningful life

Figure 1.2   The illness-wellness continuum.
Personal wellness is composed of five interrelated dimensions, all of which must be developed in order to achieve total wellness.

Adapted from *Core Concepts in Health,* by P. M. Insel and W. T. Roth. © 2000. Used with permission of the McGraw-Hill Companies.

The concepts of wellness and equality were addressed jointly in *Healthy People 2000* (USDHHS, 1990), which advanced the goals of increasing life spans, reducing health disparities, and increasing access to preventive services for all Americans. The national data generated through earlier *Healthy People* efforts had demonstrated that all Americans were *not* equal in terms of health status and service access. That meant that health professionals needed to work with others to address a wide variety of environmental factors (e.g., social, financial, political, cultural, physical) that contribute to imbalances across groups.

By the time the *Healthy People 2010* goals (USDHHS, 2000) were announced in 2000, yet another important health-related concept had emerged, quality of life (WHO, 2005, *The World*). The hard work of health professionals throughout the country had resulted in the good news that many Americans were living longer than previous generations. However, it had also become evident that living longer did not necessarily mean that Americans were living healthy and well throughout their life span. And though important progress had been made to address health disparities, some groups in America continued to suffer at disproportionate levels. For these reasons, the two overarching goals for *Healthy People 2010*, "to increase quality and years of healthy life" (p. 8) and "to eliminate health disparities," (p. 11) were used to establish quality of life as a critical component of health and to focus efforts on marginalized groups.

In *Healthy People 2020* (USDHHS, 2014, *Healthy*), quality of life was further emphasized in one of the overarching goals ("promote quality of life, healthy development, and health behaviors across all life stages") and became one of the four foundation health measures for that initiative. Though many people agree that quality of life is an important health-related consideration, the need to precisely define and measure quality of life presents some challenges. According to the Centers for Disease Control (CDC, 2016d), **quality of life** is a "broad multidimensional concept that usually includes subjective evaluations of both positive and negative aspects of life" (para. 2). Those "aspects of life" include several domains (e.g., housing, employment, neighborhoods) in addition to health. The term **health-related quality of life** (HRQoL) emerged through efforts to better understand the relationships between health and overall quality of life. The following description of HRQoL provides further detail about what it means and how it connects with well-being.

> Health-related quality of life (HRQoL) is a multi-dimensional concept that includes domains related to physical, mental, emotional and social functioning. It goes beyond direct measures of population health, life expectancy and causes of death, and focuses on the impact health status has on quality of life. A related concept of HRQoL is well-being, which assesses the positive aspects of a person's life, such as positive emotions and life satisfaction. (USDHHS, 2017c, para. 1)

In the *Healthy People 2020* initiative, HRQoL was measured within the context of three domains: self-rated physical and mental health, overall well-being, and participation in society.

As you can see, the evolution of health perspectives since 1947 has followed an interesting path. The traditional emphasis on disease-causing agents for infection control gave way to a new focus on chronic health problems and a wide spectrum of influences. Medical model perspectives were overshadowed by a more positive orientation toward wellness and prevention. Quality of life became the motivator for making healthy choices and the benchmark for comparing health status across individuals and whole communities. The prevailing viewpoint about health, shared by health professionals from a wide array of subdisciplines, is that the health of individuals can only be effectively understood within the context of entire communities and broader environments, meaning that efforts to promote health and quality of life must encompass both individual and community-wide strategies.

≡ Personal Wellness, Quality of Life, and Broad Social Issues

The visual in Figure 1.3 was designed to illustrate the reciprocal interplay between personal wellness, quality of life, and broader social and environmental issues. We represent these three areas of concern as separate wheels (center of diagram) because that is how some professional efforts address them—as separate entities. Two examples of these isolated approaches include health care treatments that

Figure 1.3   Wellness, quality of life, and broad social issues.
Wellness, quality of life, and broad social issues are connected through reciprocal relationships. Both immediate concerns and global factors influence all three directly or indirectly through their influence on any one component.

are designed to promote personal wellness without consideration of the patient's real or perceived quality of life and political efforts to combat crime (a social issue) without consideration of how quality of life issues may contribute to violent behavior. We placed cogs on the wheels and arrows around them to symbolize how a change in any one area, either positive or negative, can impact conditions in the other two areas. This mutually influencing relationship is referred to by Bandura (1977) as **reciprocal determinism**.

In the black boxes linked to each wheel, we provide dimensions or factors that would commonly be addressed within that area of concern. The close proximity of the wheels representing quality of life and personal wellness illustrates the connections between these two entities on an individual basis. In the sections that follow we describe some immediate factors than can influence a person's level of wellness and quality of life. We then turn to the third wheel of the diagram, broad social issues and global factors of influence.

Immediate Factors of Influence

The list of immediate factors in Figure 1.3 includes those that can directly impact individuals and members of their immediate groups (e.g., families, neighbors, local churches, social or work groups). Individual behavior is a strong determinant of health and quality of life. It is often influenced by individual thoughts (knowledge, attitudes, beliefs, values) and the thoughts and behaviors of significant people in one's life (cultural norms and group dynamics). **Noncontrollable risk factors,** such as age, gender, and genetics, can impact the type and severity of health and quality of life issues.

Quality health care can immediately improve a person's health and quality of life; conversely, the lack of quality care can destroy both. But the presence of skilled health professionals and up-to-date facilities is no guarantee that all eligible clients know how to access and fully benefit from these services. Complex systems, confusing forms, medical jargon, and rushed appointments are a few of the factors that can confuse and discourage those in need of care. **Health literacy** is a term often used to describe knowledge and skill levels needed to navigate the health care system and obtain quality care. It is technically defined as "the capacity of an individual to obtain, interpret, and understand basic health information and services and the competence to use such information and services in ways that are health enhancing" (Gold & Miner, 2002, p. 6). Being health literate and having access to health care are thus important determinants of your personal wellness and quality of life.

Social Issues and Global Influences

The United Nations (UN, 2012b) tracks the developmental status of countries around the globe through social indicators (see FYI 1.1). **Social indicators** are "statistics, statistical series, and all other forms of evidence that enable us to assess where we stand and are going with respect to our values and goals, and to evaluate specific programs and determine their impact" (Bauer, 1967, p. 1). A social indicator can be a partial measure of the physical environment in which people live, such as the degree to which safe and adequate housing, drinking water, and sanitation are available.

FYI

Social indicators are statistical measures of environmental factors (physical and social) that serve as evidence of a community's health and well-being.

POPULATION	**Population size**	• Population, total and by sex • Sex ratio (women/100 men)
	Composition of the population	• Percentage of total population under 15 years • Percentage of total population aged 60 years and above, by sex • Sex ratio in 60+ age group (men/100 women)
	Population growth and distribution	• Annual population growth rate • Percentage urban population • Sex ratio (women/100 men) of international migrants
HEALTH	**Life expectancy**	• Life expectancy at birth, by sex • Life expectancy at age 60, by sex
	Maternal mortality and infant mortality	• Maternal mortality ratio • Infant mortality rate • Under 5 mortality rate
	Child-bearing	• Adolescent fertility rate • Total fertility rate
	Contraceptive prevalence	• Contraceptive prevalence among married women of childbearing age
	HIV/AIDS	• Estimated number of adults living with HIV/AIDS • Women's share of adults living with HIV/AIDS
HOUSING	**Persons per room**	• Average number of persons per room by urban/rural area
	Human settlements	• Population distribution (%) by urban/rural area • Annual rate of population change (%) by urban/rural area
	Water supply and sanitation	• Improved Drinking Water Coverage (%) by urban/rural area • Improved Sanitation Coverage (%) by urban/rural area
EDUCATION	**Literacy**	• Adult (15+) literacy rate, by sex • Youth (15–24) literacy rate, by sex
	Primary education	• Primary net enrolment ratio, by sex • Girls' share of primary enrolment
	Secondary education	• Secondary net enrolment ratio, by sex • Girls' share of secondary enrolment
	Tertiary education	• Tertiary gross enrolment ratio, by sex • Women's share of tertiary enrolment
	School life expectancy	• School life expectancy (primary to tertiary education) by sex
WORK	**Income and economic activity**	• Adult (15+) economic activity rate, by sex • Per capita GDP (US dollars)
	Part-time employment	• Percentage of adult employment that is part-time, by sex • Women's share of part-time employment
	Distribution of labor force by status in employment	• Percentage employees, by sex • Percentage employers, by sex • Percentage own-account workers, by sex • Percentage contributing family workers, by sex
	Adult unemployment	• Unemployment rate, by sex

Adapted from *Social Indicators*, United Nations, 2012, Geneva, Switzerland: Author. Retrieved from https://unstats.un.org/unsd/demographic/products/socind/

Other social indicators can measure the social environment (for example, childbirth rates, crime, and education).

In some instances, these environmental factors have a direct and readily detectable impact on health. For example, in a 2014 report on climate change, UN leaders (Smith et al., 2014) noted the effects of extreme heat waves and increased flooding on mortality (heat strokes and drowning) and food- and vector-borne diseases.

Though many direct links between the environment and health exist, physical and social elements also impact the health of individuals and communities through indirect routes that are not always obvious. In Figure 1.3 we included global factors that indirectly influence personal wellness and quality of life through their effect on social conditions. For instance, political decisions and other historical events like financial recessions and natural disasters have, through time, contributed to unemployment rates and poverty throughout the world. Widespread poverty and lack of community resources in turn force individuals to live in crowded, substandard housing where exposure to infectious diseases and environmental hazards is high. The inability to afford health care and limited access to healthy foods can in turn lead to long-term health complications. Poor education and few opportunities for personal development can impact quality of life and contribute to poor behavioral choices, high birth rates, and crime. It is easy to see how these consequences of unemployment and poverty can become part of the vicious cycle that sends some societies into a downward spiral. In contrast, strong political and professional efforts to bring about positive changes in the social and physical environment can promote high levels of wellness and quality of life for individuals and communities.

Picture trying to put out a raging house fire with a single glass of water, or imagine painting a gigantic mural on the side of an office building using only a Q-tip. With these images in mind, you can begin to grasp the difficulty of bringing about meaningful change in a society that is beset by the complex web of factors we have described. To approach public health promotion on this scale, we need a model that incorporates the immediate and the far-reaching effects of people's social and physical environments. One such model is illustrated in Figure 1.4. The **socio-ecological model** (McLeroy, Bibeau, Steckler, & Glanz, 1988) provides a visual conceptualization of the broad approach needed to truly impact health and quality of life for individuals within the context of their environments. This model helps health professionals and community partners visualize how health and quality of life are impacted by ever-widening layers of influence. These factors or levels of influence include interpersonal groups such as friends and family, organizations or institutions that provide needed support, community organizations and social groups, and public policies that influence the availability and quality of health services and other needed resources. We will discuss in chapter 2 some concepts and processes of community health promotion as they relate to the socio-ecological approach. We will also address in chapter 4 how social factors and other determinants of health impact the health and well-being of specific populations. Before you read those discussions, it may be useful to consider some related perspectives and approaches that shape how health and quality of life are addressed by health professionals.

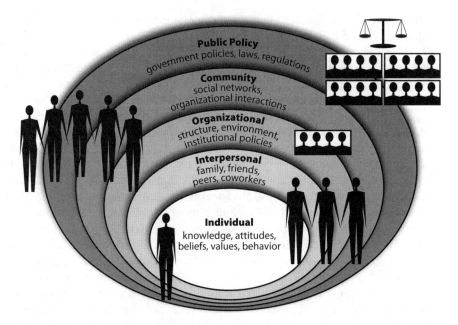

Figure 1.4   The socio-ecological model.
The socio-ecological model provides a tool for conceptualizing how the health and quality of life of individuals are impacted by ever-widening layers of influence from interpersonal groups, individual organizations or institutions, community networks, and public policies.

Source: "An Ecological Perspective on Health Promotion Programs," by K. R. McLeroy, D. Bibeau, A. Steckler, and K. Glanz, 1988, *Health Education Quarterly* 15(4): 351–377.

Emerging Professional Perspectives

To complete our discussion in this chapter about health and quality of life concepts, we have included here a brief description of some evolving professional paradigms within the health professions. We define a **professional paradigm** as the philosophical or theoretical framework and related practices of a profession. A professional paradigm contains the rationale for *why* and *how* members of that profession use certain approaches in their work. Professional paradigms are usually evident in a profession's stated mission and goals, theoretical constructs and evidence-based methods, and professional competencies and skills taught and used in that profession. Evolving professional paradigms in health care, public health, and health education can have a profound impact on the health and quality of life of the individuals and communities served by these professions. That is why we have included a brief description of differences and connections across these professions.

Health Care Paradigms

The health care professions play a critical role in health and quality of life issues for reasons that are probably obvious. The diabetic woman in our introductory story would be less likely to have known she was diabetic had it not been for the health care professionals who diagnosed her condition, and the interventions offered to manage her diabetes can make a huge difference in her quality of life.

The health care profession saves lives because of a commitment to quality diagnosis and treatment within its professional paradigm. However, philosophies among health care professionals have been evolving, and individual diagnosis and treatment are no longer considered sufficient for addressing the health needs of our society (Navarro et al., 2007; WHO, 2006b). The leaders of such major health organizations as the World Health Organization, National Academy of Medicine (formerly the Institute of Medicine [IOM]), Centers for Disease Control and Prevention, and the U.S. Department of Health and Human Services have called for a more collaborative, community-wide approach that combines health care, humanitarian actions, and the promotion of healthy lifestyles (CDC, 2007a; Graffunder & Sakurada, 2016; IOM, 2002, 2003, 2012; Mattessich & Rausch, 2014; Partnership for Prevention, 2008; USDHHS, 2000; WHO, 2006b). There is also a growing emphasis in health care on empowering patients and their families to become active partners in their care (IOM, 2013).

In a landmark report called *Who Will Keep the Public Healthy?* (IOM, 2003), leaders of the Institute of Medicine recommended that medical and nursing schools include public health training as part of their curriculum and that health care professionals become part of collaborative teams to address the health of entire communities. In a follow-up study mandated by the U.S. Congress, the IOM (2007) recommended an integrated approach that would prepare *all* physicians (through medical schools and professional development programs) to some degree to work with whole populations (the public health approach) while providing specialty training in public health to those who choose to become public health physicians. This movement in the medical field toward population-based health care (in contrast to traditional individual practice) is a primary reason for the growing focus on the professional paradigm of public health.

Public Health Paradigms

For an interesting and interactive way to learn about public health, we invite you to visit a website called *Discover: What Is Public Health?* (Association of Schools and Programs of Public Health [ASPPH], 2017a). This site contains the "Public health is. . ." information provided in FYI 1.2. The public health paradigm focuses on the protection and improvement of community health with a primary goal of preventing health problems (rather than treating illnesses). This goal calls for a multidisciplinary approach to public health services.

Traditionally, public health professionals were expected to possess a basic understanding of five core areas of study (biostatistics, environmental health sciences, epidemiology, health policy and management, and social and behavioral sciences) and most completed public health degrees with specialization in one of the five traditional areas of study (Council on Education for Public Health [CEPH], 2011). However, the public health profession has adapted to a changing world and emerging needs for additional and, in some ways, different competencies. Examples of new or adapted competency areas that have emerged include communication, leadership skills, and the ability to perform on interprofessional teams; specific processes related to systems thinking, program planning and management, and policy and organizational partnership development; and the development and use of evidence-based approaches to public health (ASPPH, 2017b; CEPH, 2016a). You can learn more about current and evolving competencies and specializations on the websites of the Council on Education for Public Health and the Association of Schools and Programs of Public Health.

The National Board of Public Health Examiners (NBPHE, 2016) established in 2008 a certification exam for public health professionals to become **certified in public health** (CPH). This certification is based on competencies related to the core areas of public health and related competencies. Visit the NBPHE website for more information about this certification and its related competencies.

Many professionals from the health care and public health traditions have embraced the emerging trend of working in collaborative partnerships to improve human conditions. They understand that, to impact the health and quality of life of individuals and communities, they must develop perspectives and skills that allow them to connect and work with partners from a broad array of perspectives, experiences, and professional disciplines. The professional paradigms and workplace settings that once distinguished health care from public health are beginning to blur in ways that could positively influence the health and quality of life of individuals and communities.

Health Education and Health Promotion Paradigms

The professional paradigm of health education is framed by a broad mission: to promote healthy lifestyles and environments that enhance health, wellness, and quality of life for individuals and communities. We include *health* and *wellness* in this mission statement because of the tendency for some to think of health as merely the absence of disease. Though disease prevention is often one of the targeted outcomes of health education, it is not the primary focus. Health education is "a discipline of applied social-behavioral sciences" (Woodhouse, Auld, Livingood, & Mulligan, 2006, p. 260) that is well-grounded in research related to the psychosocial aspects of health behavior. This research points to quality of life goals as a primary incentive for adopting healthy lifestyles and improving environments among individuals, organizations, and communities. We present a detailed discussion of evidence-based theories and models needed for this work in chapter 5. In our discussion here, we want to stress that health and wellness are considered means of achieving quality of life goals and are not just measures of success in disease prevention.

You probably noticed that health educators, now referred to as *health education specialists* (Doyle et al., 2012), were listed in the previous section as part of the public health workforce. So, you probably would not be surprised to learn that the professional paradigms of health education and public health share some common elements. The socio-ecological model and multidisciplinary approaches to community-based health promotion are valued in both paradigms. In fact, the processes of health promotion and health education have received considerable attention as key elements of collaborative health initiatives (National Prevention Council, 2011; Navarro et al., 2007). The Joint Committee on Terminology for Health Education and Promotion (2012) provided the following definitions for these two processes:

> **Health promotion:** Any planned combination of educational, political, environmental, regulatory, or organizational mechanisms that support actions and conditions of living conducive to the health of individuals, groups, and communities (p. 14, para. 1).

> **Health education:** Any combination of planned learning experiences using evidence-based practices and/or sound theories that provide the opportunity to acquire knowledge, attitudes, and skills to adopt and maintain healthy behaviors (p. 12, para. 5).

Health education and promotion are valued components of the socio-ecological approach to promoting health and quality of life in communities and populations (IOM, 2000, 2003; Liburd & Sniezek, 2007; Navarro et al., 2007). Health education is a recognized component of the traditional public health core in behavioral sciences (ASPPH, 2017c), and community health education is a recognized area of specialization in public health settings (CEPH, 2016b; Woodhouse et al., 2006).

One way to learn more about the role of health education specialists is to consult the *Occupational Outlook Handbook* of the Bureau of Labor Statistics (BLS, 2018). Information about "health educators" and "community health workers" are listed together in this online handbook, which confuses the perspective a bit because these two professional groups adhere to distinctly different sets of required credentials and trainings. However, the list of duties provided in the handbook and included below about what health educators do can be useful.

Health educators typically do the following:

- Assess the health needs of the people and communities they serve
- Develop programs and events to teach people about health topics

- Teach people how to manage existing health conditions
- Evaluate the effectiveness of programs and educational materials
- Help people find health services or information
- Provide training programs for community health workers or other health professionals
- Supervise staff who implement health education programs
- Collect and analyze data to learn about a particular community and improve programs and services
- Advocate for improved health resources and policies that promote health (BLS, 2018, *What they do*, para. 2).

As is the case for the public health profession described in a previous section, health education specialists work in a wide variety of settings that include public health agencies, nongovernmental organizations (NGOs), health care facilities, private businesses, universities, and schools (BLS, 2018). The common denominator of health education work across these settings lies in the application of specific professional competencies that have been clearly defined by the health education profession.

We previously indicated that a professional paradigm contains the rationale for the *why* and *how* of the methods they use. Professional competencies are also part of a professional paradigm because they represent *what* members of that profession should be able to do. A **professional competency** is a measure of ability or a standard of performance in a specific skill area that is needed to effectively practice in a profession. Professional competencies often serve as a guide for developing education and training programs, certification and licensure exams, performance standards, and job descriptions and hiring practices in a profession.

An example of how competencies are linked to professional paradigms can be illustrated using the concept of total wellness. In the professional paradigm of health education, total wellness is considered an important conceptual framework and motivational tool for helping individuals and communities reach their health and quality of life goals. The ability to effectively use evidence-based techniques and strategies to promote total wellness is part of the professional competencies of the health education profession.

If you have completed, or are near completion of, a degree that focuses on health education competencies, you may be eligible to take a national exam to become a **certified health education specialist** (CHES). There is also an advanced certification opportunity for qualified professionals to become a **master certified health education specialist** (MCHES). You can learn more about these certifications through the website of the National Commission for Health Education Credentialing (NCHEC).

You will also find on that website a list of the most current competencies, framed within **seven areas of responsibility**, of a health education specialist. This competency framework is used in university degree programs, CHES and MCHES certification, and professional development efforts for health education specialists. This framework is periodically validated and updated based on input from practicing health education specialists. However, the general focus of each area of responsibility has remained relatively consistent through each update. In general, these competency areas encompass assessment, planning, implementation, evaluation and research; administration and management; serving as a resource; and communicating, promoting, and advocating for health, health education/promotion, and the profession (NCHEC, n.d.). We encourage you to go to the NCHEC website and download a copy of the most current framework so that you can gain familiarity with the exact area labels and the specific competencies and sub-competencies linked to each area.

Interprofessional Education and Collaboration

The diabetic woman in our introductory scenario faced daunting obstacles that included some entrenched and unhealthy eating habits and attitudes, along with low access to healthy foods. A cross-disciplinary approach to addressing these issues could include providing culturally-tailored information about healthful eating that could be more palatable, connecting her to a non-profit organization that provides fresh fruits and vegetables to those who cannot afford them or do not have access, and creating a collaborative and supportive health care approach to help her monitor and manage her diabetes.

Diabetes is a complex health issue. When a single health profession attempts to address complex health issues on its own, the result can be similar to trying to use that one glass of water to put out the house fire previously mentioned. It has become increasingly clear that cross-disciplinary teams of health professionals and community partners are needed to develop effective solutions.

The call for a professionally unified approach began as early as 1972 when leaders from medicine, nursing, dentistry, pharmacy, and other health professions met to discuss interrelationships among their professional preparation programs. The host of this event was the Institute of Medicine (now called the National Academy of Medicine). In the resulting IOM report, *Educating for the Health Team* (IOM, 1972), these professional leaders recommended that members of the health professions learn and work as cooperative teams. This group concluded that professional training in all health professions should include the social and behavioral sciences and opportunities to learn as an interdisciplinary team working in clinical settings. These teams should also engage patients, families, and whole communities as partners to provide effective health care.

This teamwork concept may appear to be a very logical and simple solution. However, if you have ever worked on teams to accomplish a task, you probably know that "teamwork" is sometimes more easily stated than accomplished. Many health professions and their respective paradigms have been in place for a very long time. Even when these professionals value the teamwork approach, the process of working together can be confusing and time-consuming. The outcomes of that effort can include mixed results.

D'Amour and Oandasan (2005) used the term *interprofessionality* to recommend a needed paradigm shift among health professionals that could lead to effective cross-disciplinary teamwork. They defined **interprofessionality** as "the process by which professionals reflect on and develop ways of practicing that provides an integrated and cohesive answer to the needs of the client/family/population" (p. 9). This new interprofessional paradigm would need to be deliberately and methodically forged by training professionals from multiple health disciplines to continually inter-act, share knowledge, explore a variety of education and care approaches, and engage the patient as a team member.

WHO developed a framework for integrating this needed paradigm shift into how health professionals are trained and practice (WHO, 2010). This **Framework for Action on Interprofessional Education and Collaborative Practice** (WHO, 2010), was designed to encourage policy-makers to integrate the new paradigm into profes-sional training and health service delivery. The following terms were developed for the framework.

> **Interprofessional education (IPE)**: "When students from two or more professions learn about, from and with each other to enable effective collaboration and improve health outcomes" (WHO, 2010, p. 13).

> **Interprofessional collaborative practice (ICP):** "When multiple health workers from different professional backgrounds work together with patients, families, careers, and communities to deliver the highest quality of care across settings" (WHO, 2010, p. 13).

The six national associations of schools and colleges listed below responded to the IPE challenge by jointly creating an Interprofessional Education Collaborative Expert Panel (IECEP, 2011).

American Association of Colleges of Nursing

American Association of Colleges of Osteopathic Medicine

American Association of Colleges of Pharmacy

American Dental Education Association

Association of American Medical Colleges

Association of Schools of Public Health

This multidisciplinary panel determined that the primary goal of IPE programs should be to "prepare all health professions students for deliberatively working together with the common goal of building a safer and better patient-centered and community/population oriented U.S. health care system" (IECEP, 2011, p. 3). The panel identified four competency domains for interprofessional collaborative practice. For each domain, they also created a general competency statement and specific com-petencies to be used in IPE programs to prepare health professionals to work in teams.

This initial work helped launch a growing movement toward interprofessional collaboration. By 2016, an additional nine institutional members had joined the IPEC and the original model for interprofessional collaborative practice had been updated to reflect a single domain called *interprofessional collaboration* that contained four core competencies and related sub-competencies (Interprofessional Education Collabora-tive, 2016). Figure 1.5 depicts the four core competencies of Interprofessional Collab-oration Competency Domain. FYI 1.3 (on p. 22) includes the full statements for each of the four core competencies.

You may have noticed that these competency statements do not include skills and knowledge unique to only one or two health professions. These interprofessional competencies are not intended to replace profession-specific competencies needed to

Interprofessional Collaborative Practice Domains

The Learning Continuum pre-licensure through practice trajectory

Figure 1.5   Interprofessional Collaboration Competency Domain.
These four core competencies for interprofessional collaboration were developed for training health professionals from diverse disciplines to work together. Team members should be equipped to understand shared values, ethics, and commitments; appreciate how differing professional roles and responsibilities complement each other; and effectively communicate with each other, patients, families, and communities.

From *Core Competencies for Interprofessional Collaborative Practice: 2016 Update,* Interprofessional Education Collaborative, 2016, Washington, DC: Author.

practice in each health profession. Instead, the interprofessional competencies focus on skills needed to effectively work on interdisciplinary teams that also include patients and community members.

For example, in a team-based approach, a physician, nurse, and health education specialist can combine their professional knowledge and skills to accurately and effectively diagnose, monitor treatment, and equip a patient and his/her family to effectively manage a chronic illness. However, for the approach to be a true team effort, each professional must value what other professionals and the patient can contribute to the effort. Maintaining a climate of mutual respect and shared efforts, rather than one of competition or a hierarchy of professional importance, is an essential component of competencies one (values/ethics) and two (roles and responsibilities). Consistent and thorough communication (competency three) and applying

1.3 Core Competencies of Interprofessional Collaboration	
Core Competency	**Competency Statement**
1. Values/Ethics for Inter-professional Practice	Work with individuals of other professions to maintain a climate of mutual respect and shared values.
2. Roles/Responsibilities	Use the knowledge of one's own role and those of other professions to appropriately assess and address the health care needs of patients and to promote and advance the health of populations.
3. Interprofessional Communication	Communicate with patients, families, communities, and professionals in health and other fields in a responsive and responsible manner that supports a team approach to the promotion and maintenance of health and the prevention and treatment of disease.
4. Teams and Teamwork	Apply relationship-building values and the principles of team dynamics to perform effectively in different team roles to plan, deliver, and evaluate patient/population centered care and population health programs and policies that are safe, timely, efficient, effective, and equitable.

Adapted from *Core Competencies for Interprofessional Collaborative Practice: 2016 Update,* Interprofessional Education Collaborative, 2016, Washington, DC: Author.

principles of team dynamics and relationship-building (competency four) among all professionals on the team and with the patient and his/her family can positively impact patient well-being.

In IPE programs, students from multiple health disciplines have engaged in team-building and experiential learning exercises in community- and clinic-based settings (Bridges et al., 2011). An increasing number of professional teams (e.g., family physicians, nurse practitioners, physician assistants, and certified nurse midwives) are working together in practice settings (Peterson et al., 2013). In these training and practice settings, team members are learning to maintain a strong professional identity linked to their own discipline while also learning to understand and value the role of professionals from other disciplines on the team.

Though more time is needed to fully determine the degree to which IPE training impacts the quality of health care and health promotion in real-world settings, positive outcomes have been detected in:

> diabetes care, emergency department culture and patient satisfaction; collaborative team behaviour and reduction of clinical error rates for emergency department teams; collaborative team behaviour in operating rooms; management of care delivered in cases of domestic violence; and mental health practitioner competencies related to the delivery of patient care. (Reeves, et al., 2013, p. 2).

We strongly encourage you to seek interprofessional training and experience to enhance your ability to effectively work within emerging cross-disciplinary approaches.

≡ In Conclusion

Promoting health and quality of life for individuals and communities can be a challenge, especially when your clients and professional and community partners think differently about what those concepts mean and how to promote them. The socio-ecological perspective, emphasizing the interplay between health and wellness, quality of life, and broad social issues, can help you better prepare for your role as a health professional.

We encourage you to engage in interprofessional collaborative practice to more effectively impact the lives of those you serve. You *cannot* know everything and, despite what some may tell you, you cannot find all the answers within your chosen profession. Exciting and innovative ideas can be generated when people push themselves outside the boundaries of their professional comfort zones.

Guiding principles for effective interprofessional collaboration include work that is patient/family centered, community/population oriented, relationship focused, and process oriented (IECEP, 2011). The information and processes described in this textbook are built upon these guiding principles. This book can be useful to all members of your current and future collaborative teams as you work together to promote health and quality of life in communities and populations.

REVIEW QUESTIONS

1. Define health and quality of life.

2. Describe the dimensions of wellness and the illness-wellness continuum.

3. Explain how general professional concepts about health have changed through the years as they relate to the medical model, total wellness, and the socio-ecological approach.

4. List some social indicators and explain how they are connected to health.

5. Explain the reciprocal relationships between health, wellness, and broad social issues; and name some factors that influence these relationships.

6. Describe the professional paradigms of health care, public health, and health education.

7. Describe concepts, principles, and competencies of interprofessional education and interprofessional collaborative practice.

FOR YOUR APPLICATION

Mapping Your Philosophy

Examine your personal philosophy about health through this cognitive mapping exercise. You'll need 1–2 sheets of paper, a pencil, and small, self-adhesive sticky notes (if available). In the middle of one sheet of paper write the word *health*. Draw a small circle around it. Ask yourself: *What factors can affect a person's health?* Write every factor you can think of in the space surrounding your *health circle* (or write each factor on a separate sticky note and place it on the paper.) Work quickly and generate as many factors as possible. When finished, look for patterns in the factors you generated. Group them by categories (connect similar factors with lines or cluster sticky notes). Example categories include behaviors (hand-washing, smoking), attitudes (sense of humor, hate physical activity), people (supportive family, stressful employer), circumstances (educational opportunities, unemployment), environments (social connectedness, air pollution), and services/programs (high quality, nonexistent). Were you more likely to name factors people can control (attitudes, behaviors) or factors not easily controlled (the economy)? Did you name more illness-causing (stress) or wellness-promoting (physical activity) factors? Based on this exercise, what would you say is your personal philosophy about health and wellness? What can be done to promote health and quality of life? Write your observations on a second piece of paper and use them to create your professional philosophy for inclusion in your professional portfolio. You can also adapt and use this exercise to interview members of a community to learn more about their health perspectives and philosophies.

2

Community and Partnership Concepts

You didn't mean to take that wrong turn back there. This part of town can be a little dangerous after dark. The shabby buildings with bars on the windows make you feel a little uneasy. Is that a person lying over there next to the garbage can? A block later, a ball bounces out of nowhere into the street and you slam on your brakes—just missing the little girl who ran after it and the teenager who ran after the little girl. The teenager scoops up the girl and the ball and turns toward an apartment building where an elderly woman stands waiting for them with her hands on her hips. This neighborhood looks weary—the people, the buildings, the dirty streets. You feel guilty for being glad you don't have to wake up to this every morning. But what about the people who do?

Chapter Objectives

1. Describe the characteristics and actions of a healthy community.
2. Explain how social determinants of health impact the health and well-being of individuals and whole communities.
3. Describe the components of community structure and capacity.
4. Explain the connections between Maslow's hierarchy of needs, heritage consistency, and social connectedness.
5. Describe concepts and recommended approaches to community capacity building and partnership development.
6. Discuss the differences between and usefulness of cultural competence and cultural humility in partnership building.
7. Describe partnership concepts and approaches in school, work place, health care, and community settings.

Healthy People in Healthy Communities

If you have ever lived or visited the kind of neighborhood described in this chapter's opening scenario, you probably do not need to be further convinced that people are impacted by where they live. Communities can create momentum to "make healthy living easier where people live, learn, work, and play" (CDC, 2016a, para 1). But, did you also realize that the health of individuals can, in turn, impact the health and well-being of a whole community? Leaders of the now historical *Healthy People 2010* (USDHHS, 2000) explained this reciprocal relationship in the following statement.

> Over the years, it has become clear that individual health is closely linked to community health—the health of the community and environment in which individuals live, work, and play. Likewise, community health is profoundly affected by the collective beliefs, attitudes, and behaviors of everyone who lives in the community. Indeed, the underlying premise of *Healthy People 2010* is that the health of the individual is almost inseparable from the health of the larger community and that the health of every community in every state and territory determines the overall

health status of the Nation. That is why the vision for *Healthy People 2010* is "Healthy People in Healthy Communities." (USDHHS, 2000, p. 3)

Efforts to promote health and quality of life must encompass both individual and community-wide strategies (Minkler, 2012).

Now that we have established the connection between the health of individuals and communities, the next logical step is to gain an understanding of what it means to be healthy as an individual and as a community. The discussions about health, wellness, and quality of life in chapter 1 provide a firm foundation for conceptual understanding. In the chapters that follow, we provide details about the processes and resources used to assess and promote individual and community health. But what standards will you use to work, and motivate others to work with you, toward the goal of healthy individuals in healthy communities? In other words, how will you know when an individual or a community is healthy?

Healthy Individuals

The U.S. Department of Health and Human Services (2014d) has identified 26 *Healthy People 2020* **leading health indicators** to measure the health of the nation (Figure 2.1 on the next page). These indicators, categorized into 12 topics, were selected because they represent factors (for example, lack of physical activity) that contribute in significant ways to the health of individuals and whole populations. They serve as a guide for developing *Healthy People* goals and objectives, strategies for health promotion, and standards for measuring success in those efforts. They also serve as a guide for targeting risky health-related behaviors that are tracked through the CDC's Behavioral Risk Factor Surveillance System (CDC, 2017c).

A number of quality resources exist for health professionals and individuals who are interested in learning more about individual health, how it is measured, and the steps a person can take to improve it. We recommend you start by visiting the CDC's website to take advantage of the wide array of information provided there about healthy living and other health topics. For the purposes of our discussion here about healthy individuals in healthy communities, we point out that the 10 leading health indicators for individuals and communities are influenced by both individual choices and community resources and support for healthy living.

Healthy Communities

A **healthy community** is one that "continuously creates and improves both its physical and social environments, helping people to support one another in aspects of daily life and to develop to their fullest potential" (CDC, 2014a, para. 1). As illustrated in Figure 2.1, a community's leading health indicators are shaped by information access, behavioral choices, and living conditions which, in turn, compel a community to provide quality treatment and prevention services, healthy and safe environments, and healthy infrastructures. Healthy infrastructures provide community members with opportunities to pursue education, work, and recreation within safe environments, and also motivate residents to help maintain those environments. The following description of what a health community can do for its members is provided by the Massachusetts Department of Public Health.

A Healthy Community is where people come together to make their community better for themselves, their family, their friends, their neighbors, and others. A Healthy Community creates ongoing dialogue, generates leadership opportunities for all, embraces diversity, connects people and resources, fosters a sense of community, and shapes its future. (Massachusetts Department of Public Health, 2018, para. 1)

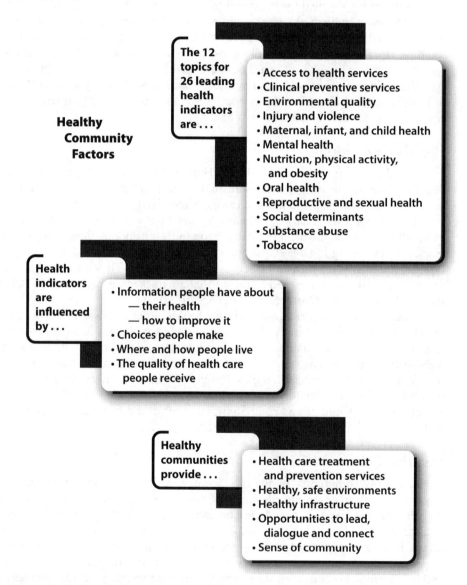

Figure 2.1   Healthy community factors.

Sources: *Healthy People 2020: Leading Health Indicators*, USDHHS, 2014d, September 1; *Healthy Communities Program*, Centers for Disease Control and Prevention, 2013, October 25; *What Is a Healthy Community?* Massachusetts Department of Public Health, Office of Healthy Communities, 2013.

With the ultimate goal of fostering healthy individuals and healthy communities in mind, we can now turn to a more specific description of factors that impact the health status of individuals and communities. The following section contains a framework used in public health to identify these factors.

Social Determinants of Health

"A world that is greatly out of balance in matters of health is neither stable nor secure" (WHO, 2012b, p. VII). Those were the words of Dr. Margaret Chan, Director-General of the World Health Organization, in a report of the 2011 World Conference on Social Determinants of Health (WHO, 2012b). She was talking about inequities within and between countries around the world—how differences in income levels, living conditions, opportunities, power, and access to care impact the health of populations.

Dr. Chan's words may resonate more strongly if we consider some examples of these differences. Differences between countries can be illustrated by a WHO (2017c) comparison of infant mortality rates in Iceland (2 deaths per 1,000 live births) and Mozambique (over 120 per 1,000), and a comparison of the lifetime risk of maternal death during or shortly after pregnancy in Sweden (1 in 17,400) to that of Afghanistan (1 in 8). Differences among groups within a single country can be illustrated by the finding that, in Bolivia, infants born to mothers with no formal education were 2.5 times more likely to die as infants born to mothers with at least a secondary education (WHO, 2017c). Differences within a single city can be illustrated by what is now referred to as the *Glasgow effect*, in which the life expectancy at birth for men living in one low-income neighborhood of Glasgow, Scotland, was 28 years lower than the rate of men living in an affluent neighborhood just 12 kilometers away (Reid, 2011).

What contributes to these drastic health differences between countries, populations within a country, and even residents of the same city? In most instances, the answer to that question can be at least partially addressed through use of a conceptual framework known as the social determinants for health. The World Health Organization (2017, *Social*) refers to **social determinants of health** as "the circumstances in which people are born, grow up, live, work and age, and the systems put in place to deal with illness. These circumstances are in turn shaped by a wider set of forces: economics, social policies, and politics" (para. 6). The Centers for Disease Control and Prevention (CDC) defines these determinants as follows.

> The complex, integrated, and overlapping social structures and economic systems that are responsible for most health inequities. These social structures and economic systems include the social environment, physical environment, health services, and structural and societal factors. Social determinants of health are shaped by the distribution of money, power, and resources throughout local communities, nations, and the world. (CDC, 2014d, *Social determinants of health*)

These two definitions can serve as a reminder that virtually every aspect of a person's environment and life circumstances can influence one's health status and quality of life. The challenge lies in developing a concise framework through which we can examine and address the long list of factors that fall within the realm of a social determinant.

Leaders of the *Healthy People 2020* initiative have created a framework of social determinants that contains five key areas: economic stability, education, social and community context, health and health care, and neighborhood and built environment. They have also identified some critical components (or key issues) relevant to each of the five areas. These five key areas and their critical components are illustrated in Figure 2.2.

One of these five key areas, economic stability, is a critical social determinant for a number of reasons. As we indicted in chapter 1, insufficient economic resources impact access to other resources and opportunities such as the ability to pay for a college education, healthy foods, adequate housing, safe neighborhoods, preventive health care, and quality medical treatment. The resulting poor health can make it difficult to maintain a job, continue one's education, and engage in other activities that could prevent on-going poverty.

Your consideration of these and other social determinants is so essential to promoting health and well-being that we continue to discuss these factors in various ways throughout this textbook. (For example, in chapter 4 we describe and provide examples of the impact of social determinants on health equity.) However, in sections that follow within this chapter, we wish to continue our discussion about communities: how they are structured, how we can build a community's capacity to address health issues, and the importance of community-based partnerships in these efforts.

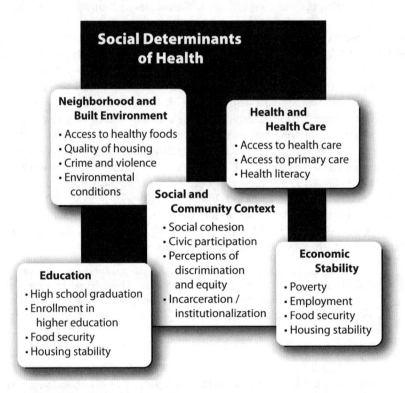

Figure 2.2   Social determinants of health.

Adapted from *Healthy People 2020: Approach to Social Determinants of Health*, USDHHS, 2018, May 18, Washington, DC: U.S. Government Printing Office. Retrieved from http://www.healthypeople.gov/2020/topics-objectives/topic/social-determinants-health

Community Structure and Capacity

When you hear the word *community*, what comes to mind? If you picture a small midwestern town where neighbors are friendly and most children grow up in one place, you can probably understand why the term seems to have lost its meaning in some parts of America. In some communities, low-income apartment buildings stand next to factories while, blocks away, high-income apartments are built near business districts. In the suburbs, residents may commute long hours to work or school, and life moves at a fast pace. For these and other reasons, communities aren't necessarily well-defined by geographic boundaries alone.

Instead, we invite you to think of communities in terms of their structure and capacity. In using the word *structure*, we aren't necessarily referring to the physical buildings of a community, though physical structures do partially define a community. But a community's structure can also be defined in terms of social, cultural, and even political networks that bond individual community members into unified groups. These bonds can be viewed as assets that shape a community's capacity to be a healthy community.

People in Communities

Communities are usually defined by what people have in common. The common link may be structural, as in a shared neighborhood, workplace, or school. Or it may reflect common values, interests, or incomes. Age, ethnicity, and sexual orientation can bond individuals into a community. Followers of a particular religion or spiritual belief may function as a community. Even members of the same civic organization or social club can function as a community when goals and activities are shared. Regardless of the common link, people are the heart of a community.

People interact with one another for many reasons. You may, for example, interact with university professors to meet a desired career goal or with family members to satisfy needs for emotional or financial support. Abraham Maslow (1954), a well-known American psychologist, would argue that people are motivated to act (and we would add "to interact with others") based on five levels of human needs that are often referred to as **Maslow's hierarchy of needs** (Figure 2.3). We believe this hierarchy explains why individuals bond into communities.

According to Maslow's hierarchy, physiological needs (food, water, oxygen) and the need for physical safety are the most basic and influential motivators of human behavior. You may never have experienced an intense physiological or safety crisis that led to desperate action. Yet you can likely understand why a starving person would resort to stealing food or an abused teenager would choose to live on the streets. When safety and physiological needs are at stake, nothing else seems to matter. That's why it is sometimes necessary for community health efforts to address these basic needs first before attempting to tackle less crisis-oriented health issues.

On a higher level of Maslow's hierarchy, the need for love, acceptance, appreciation, and respect can motivate people to join formally structured groups (churches, clubs, etc.) and informal social networks (friends from work, neighbors, etc.). Though gang membership and other negative relationships can result from this need, positive connections can help an individual advance to the highest level of the hierarchy.

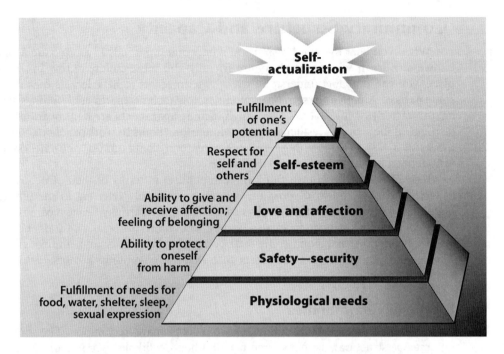

Figure 2.3   Maslow's hierarchy of needs.
Maslow reminds us that a community's basic physiological and safety needs must be met before efforts can focus on higher level needs such as self-actualization.

Adapted from *Motivation and Personality*, by A. Maslow, 1954, New York: Harper & Row.

Self-actualization is characterized by emotional and spiritual health in which a person accepts oneself and others, optimizes personal capabilities, and possesses a keen sense of fulfillment and purpose in life. Individuals at this level may become active in community organizations, work on college degrees, or choose a specific profession or interest area because these challenges provide opportunities for self-improvement and the chance to make a difference to society.

Maslow's hierarchy explains why, within any given community, you will likely find smaller subgroups of individuals bound together by need. At lower hierarchy levels, individuals may join support groups to deal with addictions, disease, or other problems. Some community volunteers working in these programs may do so because they have been personally touched by the problem and wish to make a difference for someone else. At higher hierarchy levels, individual community members who seek to connect with others and to perhaps pursue self-actualization may become valuable partners in your effort to promote community health.

Cultural Connections

Our previous discussion about the human need for acceptance sets the stage for an examination of how culture and ethnicity shape communities. Though culture and ethnicity share some common elements, these concepts represent different and equally important characteristics of a community. To clarify these differences, we will describe the concept of heritage consistency, which represents the degree to which a person's lifestyle reflects his or her traditional culture or cultural roots (Spector, 2013). This is an important concept because individual members of a cultural group or ethnic community may adhere to different levels of heritage consistency, which impacts the depth and nature of community connections.

Spector (2013) proposed a model of heritage consistency in which a person's worldview is shaped by three intrinsically linked elements—culture, ethnicity, and religion. **Culture** encompasses the knowledge, beliefs, practices, values, customs, and norms of a group of people that are passed from one generation to the next. It is learned from family and community members and shaped by traditional religion, the environment, and historical events. Culture can serve as the framework that bonds individuals within a close-knit community. It is a powerful shaper of human behavior and often dictates how people interact. **Ethnicity** is distinguished from culture in this model as the degree to which a person deliberately chooses to identify with and embrace the practices and beliefs of an ethnic group. This distinction allows for the possibility that individuals may be shaped by their cultural roots without openly embracing an ethnic identity.

Religion, the third component of the model, is defined as "a set of beliefs, values, and practices based on the teachings of a spiritual leader" (Office of Minority Health, 2001, p. 132). Despite shifting patterns in religious beliefs and practices in the United States, religion remains a powerful predictor of ethnicity (Abramson, 1980; Eck, 2001; Spector, 2013). Religious teachings often provide the framework for ethnicity-specific values and norms, and are particularly influential in shaping ethics, purpose, and life meaning. These religious teachings and other bonds of heritage consistency can positively impact a community's environment.

Community Environments

As we stated in chapter 1, the socio-ecological model reminds us that individuals, groups, and whole communities are impacted by a variety of environmental factors. **Environmental health** is a core area of public health and is particularly relevant in terms of the health risks associated with the physical environment. Economic, political, and social environments are also important components of a community's structure and capacity. A clear understanding of these environmental dimensions is essential to your ability to promote community health.

The Ministry of Social Development of New Zealand (MSD, 2008) described the **physical environment** as "land, air, water, plants and animals, buildings and other infrastructure, and all of the natural resources that provide our basic needs and opportunities for social and economic development" (*Introduction*, para. 1). Common environmental health issues around the world include the provision of safe drinking water, clean air, and protection from toxic elements. The physical environment is central to the emergence of **healthy community design**, "the process of planning and designing communities that make it easier for people to live healthy lives" (National Center for Environmental Health, 2008, para. 2).

A community's **economic environment** undeniably impacts its health. Low-income communities struggle with unemployment and low wages, poor housing conditions and insufficient infrastructure, limited access to quality health care, and numerous other challenges to quality of life that are intertwined with complex social issues. A community's **political environment** plays a significant role in the extent to which leaders can obtain needed assistance; for example, becoming a designated **medically underserved area** (MUA) or **medically underserved population** (MUP) qualifies the community to receive government assistance (U.S. Health Resources and Services Administration, n.d.). Political leaders impact community health through decisions related to water quality, wastewater treatment, landfills, industry zoning laws, and support of police and fire departments. The availability and quality of city parks and recreational areas, schools and libraries, and community centers also affect health because they offer opportunities to exercise mind and body, develop social skills, and enhance quality of life.

The state of a community's **social environment** is often measured by such indicators as literacy rates, housing quality, and other factors that draw attention to community shortcomings (see FYI 1.1). The term *social connectedness* "refers to the relationships people have with others and the benefits these relationships can bring to the individual as well as to society" (MSD, 2016, *Introduction*, para. 1). When social connectedness is high in a community, members enjoy positive social roles and relationships that help them "feel they belong and have a part to play in society. People who feel socially connected also contribute towards building communities and society" (MSD, 2016, *Introduction*, para. 3). Social connectedness fulfills a need for acceptance, enhances health and well-being, and compels people to think of others. Communities with high levels of social connectedness are usually healthier communities.

Community Capacity

A community's ability to take action on its own behalf is an essential characteristic of a healthy community. For you to be able to promote a community's ability to take action, you must first be able to measure the community's capacity to do that. In the health promotion profession, **community capacity** is often defined as "the characteristics of communities that affect their ability to identify, mobilize, and address social and public health problems" (Goodman et al., 1998, p. 259). So, what *are* those capacity characteristics? A multidisciplinary team from sociology, urban planning, psychology, and social work created a conceptual framework for understanding community capacity (Chaskin, Brown, Venkatesh, & Vidal, 2001). According to this framework (Chaskin et al., 2001), the four characteristics of community capacity are:

- a sense of community (connectedness among members and recognition of mutual circumstances),
- commitment to the community among its members (assumed responsibility and a willingness to act),
- an ability to solve problems (to translate commitment into action), and
- access to resources (economic, human, physical, and political within and beyond the community. (p. 16)

Community capacity "is what makes well-functioning communities function well" (Chaskin et al., 2001, p. 7). It is built through the interaction of human capital (leadership, skills, etc.), organizational resources, and social capital.

The concept of social capital has emerged as an important concept in community health education. Putnam (1995) defined **social capital** as "the relationships and structures within a community, such as civic participation, networks, norms of reciprocity, and trust, that promote cooperation of mutual benefit" (p. 66). Leaders at the Centers for Disease Control and Prevention (CDC, 2013b) provided the following description of the concept.

> The fabric of a community and the community pool of human resources available to it is often called its "social capital." This term refers to the individual and communal time and energy that is available for such things as community improvement, social networking, civic engagement, personal recreation, and other activities that create social bonds between individuals and groups. (para. 1)

World Bank researchers (Grootaert, Narayan, Jones, & Woolcock, 2004) measured social capital in five dimensions: the existence of supportive groups and networks; a cohesive sense of trust and solidarity; collective action and cooperation for working together; social inclusion in collective action, decision making, and access to services; and communication that promotes access to information. When social capital is combined with human capital, needed resources, and effective organization, a community's capacity for action increases.

≡ Capacity-Building Concepts

A number of communities in the United States and other parts of the world possess at least some characteristics of a healthy community. But others could hardly be defined as *communities* in terms of social connectedness, social capital, and other capacity elements. In most areas, some form of capacity building is needed.

Concept Model for Capacity Building

Figure 2.4 illustrates how some elements of capacity described in the previous section fit within the concept of capacity building. Social connectedness, social capital, and community action share common elements that often take root in the beginning stages of capacity building. The sequence in Figure 2.4 illustrates a snowball effect with growth in each component contributing to the development of other components. For example, social connectedness, which begins with shared needs, interests, and/or heritage consistency, can develop into stronger connections of trust and social cohesion (social capital dimensions). As these connections deepen, stronger networks are developed and enable the community to communicate and work cohesively on a common cause that can include political or social actions (other social capital dimensions). This developed social capital, which combines relationship links with a capacity for organized effort, can launch the kinds of community action described in Figure 2.1 that result in healthy communities: quality health care treatment and prevention services; healthy environments; healthy infrastructures; opportu-

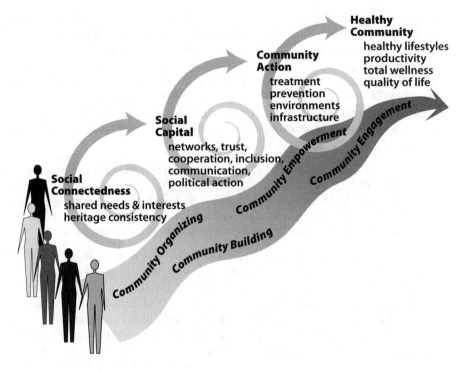

Figure 2.4   Capacity building for a healthy community.

Sources: *Healthy People in Healthy Communities*, U.S. Department of Health and Human Services, 2001, February, Washington, DC: U.S. Government Printing Office; *Overview: Social Capital*, World Bank, 2008, Washington, DC: Author. Retrieved from http://go.worldbank.org/C0QTRW4QF0

nities to lead, dialogue, and connect; and a sense of community. The ultimate goal of this effort is to establish a community that enables its members to live healthy and productive lives and enhances their well-being and quality of life.

Community Building, Empowerment, and Engagement

Has anyone ever "helped" you in a way that wasn't really helpful? In some communities, your offer to help may be welcomed by some and viewed suspiciously by others. Though they may trust your sincerity, they may be skeptical about your ability to maintain long-range commitments; or they may simply be uncomfortable with the idea of *needing* help. As noted public health educator Dr. Larry Green explained, "Many communities have grown weary . . . with yet another . . . initiative seeking to point out their needs, which usually translate as deficiencies embarrassingly catalogued and publicized, often without solution" (Gilmore & Campbell, 2005, p. vii).

We encourage you to consider the meaning of the word *help* within the context of three terms often used when discussing community capacity building. The challenge in describing these terms is that varying definitions and uses have sometimes blurred their distinctions. To avoid confusion, we urge you to consult the discussion of these concepts by Wallerstein, Minkler, Carter-Edwards, Avila, and Sanchez (2015); Minkler (2012); and Chaskin et al. (2001). Meanwhile, we have provided some basic information that begins with operational descriptions from Wallerstein et al. (2015):

> **Community organizing:** The process by which communities are helped to identify common problems or change targets, mobilize resources, and develop and implement strategies to reach their collective goals. (p. 277)

> **Community building:** An orientation to community that engages and collectively builds capacity in the process. (p. 278)

> **Community empowerment:** A social action process by which individuals, communities, and organizations gain mastery over their lives in the context of changing their social and political environment to improve equity and quality of life. (p. 285)

Notice that community organizing and empowerment are described above as *processes* while community building is called an *orientation to community* (a perspective or way of thinking about a community).

Community organizing (or community organization) has evolved since the late 1800s into a broad approach to helping communities achieve goals. Multiple models have been developed to focus on the processes and/or tasks needed to help communities solve problems (Wallerstein et al., 2015). However, this original emphasis on community collaboration to address deficiencies is viewed by some as being too outsider- and problem-focused to foster real community leadership toward achieving positive goals (Chaskin et al., 2001; Wallerstein et al., 2015; Minkler, 2012).

We certainly are *not* suggesting that you should hesitate to help a community get organized and accomplish needed processes and tasks. Community organizing efforts can help identify common problems and mobilize key individuals and groups to address them. As illustrated in Figure 2.4, this process can contribute to social connectedness and social capital. However, we *are* encouraging you to embrace the concepts of community building and empowerment as the primary guides for how you view and work with communities. In contrast to the traditional problem-focused orientation of community organizing, the community-building approach focuses on community assets and strengths and blends community identity and autonomy with the dimensions of community planning and community action (Wallerstein et al., 2015). And, instead of the outsider/organizer-led work of some community-organizing efforts, community empowerment fosters *community-led* initiatives to reach *community-defined* goals. Thus, the community building and empowerment perspectives contribute to capacity building by shifting the focus from *doing for* the community to *working with* the community in partnerships that enable the community to *do for itself.* Wallerstein et al. (2015) couched this principle under the conceptual umbrella of *community engagement*, a broad term they use to encompass concepts and principles of capacity building, empowerment, community participation, and the need to recognize health inequities.

Leaders within the World Bank (2017) have developed an approach to working with communities based upon this partnership principle. In the following quote from their program website, note their discovery about the observed abilities of low-income populations when capacity-building partnerships were in place.

Community-driven development (CDD) programs operate on the principles of local empowerment, participatory governance, demand-responsiveness, administrative autonomy, greater downward accountability, and enhanced local capacity. Experience has shown that when given clear explanations of the process, access to information and appropriate capacity and financial support, poor men and women can effectively organize to identify community priorities and address local problems by working in partnership with local governments and other supportive institutions. (World Bank, 2017, para. 1–2)

We encourage you to visit their website and learn more about their success using this approach.

A healthy community can emerge when community members develop social capital and invest it in health-promoting actions (see Figure 2.4). We use these concepts throughout this textbook to talk about such processes as assets mapping (chapter 6), coalition building (chapter 7), and community-based participatory research (chapter 9).

Partnership Development

Capacity building that is based on the principles of community building and empowerment necessitates the development of strong community-based partnerships. Your partnership-building objective should be to nurture a shared vision that connects community goals to the services and actions you can help develop. The strategies for partner development listed in FYI 2.1 may help you achieve your objective.

A true community-based partnership is evident when the community commits to identifying its own needs, creating community-based goals, and using its own strengths to achieve those goals. Though we understand that your role in the partner-

2.1   Strategies for Partnership Development

Community-Based Goals: Emphasize community goals rather than agency objectives. Clearly state agency objectives and activities but frame them as partnership contributions toward community goals.

Strength-Focused Discussions: Focus on community strengths, assets, and capacities rather than shortcomings.

Shared Power: Involve community members as true partners. Share decision-making power, responsibilities, and credit. Whenever possible, be flexible and follow their lead.

Realistic Expectations: Be cautious and realistic about promised contributions, planned activities, and expected outcomes. Establish clear understandings about roles, limitations, and expectations for all partners. Be consistent and follow through.

Celebrate Accomplishments: Celebrate every stage of accomplishment. Be willing to adapt to changing needs and capacities over time.

Sources: *Community Capacity and Capacity Building*, by R. J. Chaskin, P. Brown, S. Venkatesh, and A. Vidal, 2001, Hawthorne, NY: Aldine; *Health Behavior and Health Education: Theory, Research, and Practice*, 5th ed., by K. Glanz, B. K. Rimer, and K. Viswanath (Eds.), 2015, San Francisco: Jossey-Bass; *Community Organizing and Community Building for Health*, 3rd ed., by M. Minkler (Ed.), 2012, New Brunswick, NJ: Rutgers University Press.

ship must in some way match the goals of your work setting, these goals should be presented to the community as a guide for how *you* can partner with *them* to achieve *their* goals. Discussions that emphasize community strengths and capacities can help avoid the unintended implication that the community needs to be rescued by you. Identifying community assets can facilitate a shared power approach that engages community members as true partners in decisions and responsibilities.

All partners engaged in the effort must maintain realistic expectations. One way to accomplish this is through clear communication about the expected roles of each partner. Open discussions about expectations, progress, and anticipated outcomes will help avoid misunderstandings. You will likely find that a sincere, ongoing effort to be true to your word and to follow through may strengthen the community's trust in you; but be patient. Community trust-building takes time and consistent effort.

As you and your community partners work toward community goals, we encourage you to celebrate each progressive step in the work, no matter how small it may seem (celebrated accomplishments). Community building and partnership development require hard work, and observable outcomes seldom happen quickly. Well-designed goals and objectives (see chapter 7) should measure incremental progress, and can therefore serve as milestones of success. And nothing contributes to the momentum of capacity building quite like the celebration of success.

Cultural Competence and Humility

We would be remiss if we did not caution you about the potential challenges of partnership development and capacity building. Imagine attempting to establish a partnership with a community that you know nothing about, and having to rely on what you *think* you know about that community based upon what you *think* you know about its history, culture, and perspectives.

Consider, for example, the case of a health professional who mistakenly assumed that all Latina women in a community adhered to traditional Catholic views about using birth control, and shaped recommendations for community health promotion accordingly. Or the health professional who suspected an eating disorder when an adolescent female consistently refused to eat when others were eating, only to discover the young female was observing Ramadan, the Islamic month for prayer and spiritual cleansing, and could only eat after sundown and before sunrise (F. Youssefi, personal communication, April 4, 2000). As in these cases, you may discover a tendency to act on stereotypes (oversimplified and distorted images or descriptions of a group) or faulty assumptions that can cause you to inadvertently misinterpret, misadvise, and impede trust in the community you wish to serve.

Many health professionals are aware that understanding and adapting to varying levels of cultural influence on individuals and groups is essential for effective capacity building. However, some become frustrated with the wide variety of terms and concepts, and disagreements about what those terms mean, that can confuse and hinder their efforts to develop culturally relevant skills. We have chosen to introduce and discuss a few of those concepts here as a starting point.

Cultural competence in community health education and promotion, has been defined as "the ability of an individual to understand and respect values, attitudes, beliefs, and mores that differ across cultures, and to consider and respond appropriately to these differences in planning, implementing, and evaluating health education and promotion programs and interventions" (Gold & Miner, 2002, p. 4). We believe this definition of cultural competence is a good place to begin because it implies that we need to invest time and effort in learning about the individuals and populations with whom we work in order to effectively partner with them for capacity building. This definition integrates **cultural awareness** (gaining descriptive knowledge about cultural norms and practices) with **cultural sensitivity** (understanding and respecting the values and beliefs that shape those norms and practices). Cultural awareness and sensitivity, coupled with basic guidelines for effective cross-cultural communication, can enhance our levels of cultural competence or ability to work with a specific individual, group, or community.

However, there is some risk in using the term *cultural competence* because many view competence as a state of being, of having arrived at a high skill level that renders one fully capable in all situations. From this "perfection-laden" viewpoint, it is virtually impossible for any of us to ever become fully culturally competent in any community because of individual differences, historical variations, the emergence of blended cultures, and evolving societies.

This realization has led to a shift from the end-product perspective of competence to a more process-oriented approach called *cultural humility.* Cultural humility has been defined as the "ability to maintain an interpersonal stance that is other-oriented (or open to the other) in relation to aspects of cultural identity that are most important to the [person]" (Hook, Davis, Owen, Worthington, & Utsey, 2013, p. 2). This process has been characterized as a life-long commitment to self-evaluation and self-critique, a desire to fix power imbalances in communities, and an aspiration to develop partnerships with people and groups who advocate for others (Tervalon & Murray-Garcia, 1998; Waters & Asbill, 2013).

Cultural humility begins with an awareness of differences between one's personal cultural perspectives and those of community members, and progresses to a respectful insight into the reasons behind those differences. As adults, these differences can sometimes be shaped by our **cultural luggage.** The influence of culture has been described as mental programs or ways of assigning meaning that a person learns during childhood from caregivers/families, schools, and communities (Hofstede, 2001). These mental programs are the cultural "luggage that each of us carries around for our lifetime" (Spector, 2013, p. 9). This cultural influence can shape the way an individual interacts and connects with others. For example, if you were taught as a child that direct eye contact with a person of authority is disrespectful, you may automatically misinterpret the behavior of a person who was taught that direct eye contact is a way of showing respect. A culturally competent response to eye contact, or the lack of it, can then be based on an understanding of and appreciation for the culture-based reasons behind that behavior.

When we use the word *luggage,* we do not mean to imply that these ways of thinking are negative. Most cultural luggage contains both positive and negative elements. The utility of this term is that it serves as a reminder that most individuals, including health professionals, are influenced by the cultural luggage they still carry as adults, even if they are not aware that it exists. When you are in the early stages of learning how to appropriately interact in a culture that is different from your own, you will likely make some mistakes along the way. A teachable attitude and a willingness to apologize when those mistakes happen (cultural humility) will positively impact your trust-building efforts in the community.

Be patient and realistic in your expectations when working toward cultural competence in a community of interest. Because true cultural competence in all contexts is virtually impossible to achieve, it is more accurately described as a developmental process rather than an arrival point. It often takes months to begin to gain some basic understandings of a particular culture group and years to develop a significant level of competence in effectively working with that group. True cultural competence is a life-long developmental process. You will know that you are moving in a positive direction toward cultural competence if you:

- Engage in ongoing self-analysis to identify and address your personal perspectives and any existing cross-cultural biases.

- Actively seek to view life through the eyes of others and, through that, develop a greater level of sensitivity for the values and life challenges of other groups.

- Participate in hands-on training opportunities for practice and feedback that can help you master new skills and refine existing techniques that enhance cultural competence.

- Seek opportunities to engage in cross-cultural interactions in all aspects of life. (Doyle, 2008, p. 165)

In general, your ability to identify and appreciate a community's collective heritage (culture, ethnicity, religion) as a source of social capital will enable you to interact from a culturally competent standpoint. Self-identified ethnic communities or subgroups often have a strong sense of pride and community identity that can be a valuable capacity-building asset.

≡ Community Health Partnerships and Settings

In chapter 1, we talked about the importance of interprofessional collaboration to effectively address complex health issues. But, collaborative health professionals are not the only partner groups of value when working to promote the health of a community. Engaging community members and other organizations in a community is also essential (USDDHS, 2011, *Principles*). We refer to this community-engaged collaboration, one in which interprofessional groups collaborate with community entities, as *community health partnerships*.

The *Healthy People* initiative (USDHHS, 2014a) is a good place to begin learning about community health partnerships. For three decades, leaders of this initiative have been working to:

- Encourage collaborations across communities and sectors.

- Empower individuals toward making informed health decisions.

- Measure the impact of prevention activities. (USDHHS, 2014a, para. 1)

The vision, mission, and overarching goals of *Healthy People 2020* serve as a road map for partnership efforts to promote population health. The *Healthy People 2020* mission includes efforts to "engage multiple sectors to take actions to strengthen policies and improve practices that are driven by the best available evidence and knowledge" (para. 4). This and other parts of the mission have driven a focus on the social determinants in Figure 2.2.

When you visit the *Healthy People 2020* website, you'll find a list of topic areas. Each topic area contains a primary goal, measurable objectives, data relevant to outcomes measured to date, and related evidence-based resources. One of those topic areas is called *Educational and Community-Based Programs*. The primary goal of work related to this topic is to "increase the quality, availability, and effectiveness of educational and community-based programs designed to prevent disease and injury, improve health, and enhance quality of life" (USDHHS, 2014c, *Goal*, para. 1). These programs and strategies are often designed to reach people through the existing social structures one of four commonly-identified settings: schools, worksites, health care settings, and communities. We invite you to visit the *Healthy People in Action* section of the www.healthypeople.gov website to read stories about how communities are working together to promote health.

Another source of information about partnered efforts to promote healthy communities is the Division of Community Health within the National Center for Chronic Disease Prevention and Health Promotion (NCCDPHP), which is part of the Centers for Disease Control and Prevention. This division promotes partnered approaches to community action through such programs as the *Partnerships to Improve Community Health* and the *Racial and Ethnic Approaches to Community Health (REACH)* (CDC, 2016a).

We offer below a brief introduction to some common settings in which community health partnerships often occur and some organizations engaged in health promotion within each setting. We invite you to also visit the websites of organizations and programs mentioned in this chapter to learn more about current community health partnerships and settings.

School Setting

Schools can play a critical role in promoting health over the 13-year span (kindergarten through 12th grade) of a young person's life. Though the extent to which health is part of the K–12 curriculum in the United States differs from state to state, most states include health in the public school curriculum at some learning level.

But, school health includes more than what happens in the classroom. In 1987, the CDC adopted an eight component model called *Coordinated School Health Model* to guide curriculum development for health education and physical education as well as to coordinate efforts related to other aspects of the school environment, such as student services and safety, health promotion among school employees, and family/community partnerships. The CDC then partnered with the Association for Supervision and Curriculum Development (ASCD) to launch in 2014 a new, expanded model called the *Whole School, Whole Community, Whole Child (WSCC) Model* (ASCD, 2017; CDC, 2015c).

The WSCC Model (Figure 2.5) contains the original components of the Coordinated School Health Model integrated with tenets of the whole child approach to education developed by the ASCD (ASCD, 2017; CDC, 2015c). It provides a strong framework through which school administrators, educators, nurses, nutrition specialists, counselors, worksite wellness experts (for school staff), parents, leaders of community organizations and public health agencies, and other community members can work together to promote wellness among school children. Measures of success can be monitored through the Youth Risk Behavior Surveillance System (YRBSS), a national database of priority health-risk behaviors; the School Health Index, a self-assessment and planning tool that schools use to enhance health-related policies and programs; and capacity-building support for nongovernmental organizations

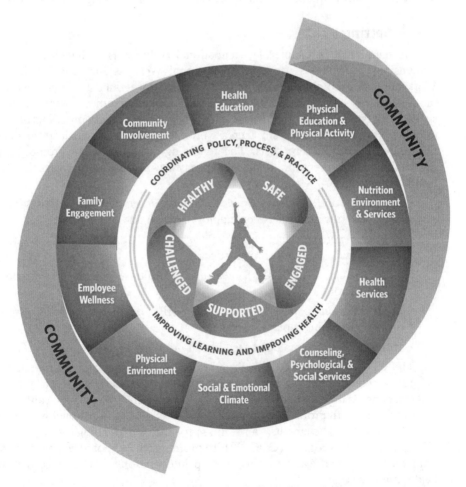

Figure 2.5   Whole School, Whole Community, Whole Child (WSCC) Model.

From *Whole School, Whole Community, Whole Child,* Centers for Disease Control and Prevention/Association for Supervision and Curriculum Development, 2018, March 1. Retrieved from http://www.cdc.gov/healthyyouth/wscc/index.htm

(NGOs) to help prevent HIV infection and other priority health problems in schools and high-risk youth populations.

Though college and university campuses are not always viewed as part of the concept of school health, we have included here some information about this academic setting. The American College Health Association (ACHA) led in the development of *Healthy Campus 2020*, a framework for promoting healthy campus communities that is linked to *Healthy People 2020* efforts (ACHA, 2016). The Healthy Campus framework includes national health objectives for students and faculty/staff, an action model, and a toolkit for use in promoting wellness on college campuses. We also encourage you to read a report from the Institute of Medicine and National Research Council (IOM & NRC, 2014) called *Investing in the Health and Well-Being of Young Adults*, a report about the health, development, and social needs of young adults aged 18 to 26.

Work Setting

As mentioned in chapter 1, occupational wellness is included as one of Six Dimensions of Wellness used by the National Wellness Institute (Hettler, 1976). Worksite health promotion and employee wellness programs are important for promoting healthy communities because of the amount of time so many Americans spend in workplace settings. Business leaders who support these programs often do so to reduce employee absenteeism, increase productivity and job satisfaction, and lower insurance and health care costs. The following worksite health promotion terms (Partnership for Prevention, 2009, p. 65) may be of use if you engage in worksite health promotion:

- *presenteeism* and *health and productivity management:* terms used to describe, promote, and track links between employee health and productivity
- *demand management* and *medical self-care:* terms that relate to appropriate use of health services and self-care practices
- *health risk appraisals* (HRAs): measures of health risk based on behaviors and genetic history
- *population health management:* the use of HRA databases as health assessment and programming tools
- *virtual wellness:* technology-based health promotion

The CDC Workplace Health Program (CDC, 2017b) "is a coordinated set of programs, policies, benefits, and environmental supports designed to meet the health and safety needs of all employees" (para. 3). Recommended worksite health interventions include health promotion programs supported by organizational policies, benefits, environmental elements, and links to the surrounding community. The Workplace Health Program (CDC, 2017b) promotes the use of assessment, planning, implementation, and evaluation to develop interventions that produce measurable health outcomes.

The *CDC Worksite Health ScoreCard* (2017b) is designed for assessing health promotion programs in worksite settings, identifying gaps or needs, and developing evidenced-based approaches to preventing heart disease, stroke, and related conditions. These strategies include health promoting counseling services, environmental supports, policies, health plan benefits, and other worksite programs shown to be effective in preventing heart disease, stroke, and related health conditions.

Worksite health promotion programs vary greatly. Some companies initiate their own programs, while others contract out for part or all of their health promotion efforts. Virtual programs (e.g., webinars) and/or face-to-face seminars and workshops may address a variety of health topics such as stress management, fitness, smoking cessation, nutrition, weight management, parenting, drug abuse prevention, and chronic disease awareness and prevention. Health fairs, screenings, and HRAs are regular components of most programs. Some programs consist of after-work and weekend recreation activities that involve employees and their families in friendly sports competitions. Company picnics, marathons, ropes courses for professional development, and other one-time events may also fall under the worksite health promotion umbrella in some settings. Management of facilities, equipment, and personnel is part of the job in larger programs.

Health Care Setting

Health care providers are in a unique position to improve the health of individuals in several ways. The most obvious avenue of influence is through diagnosis and treatment that can help an individual move away from illness on the illness-wellness continuum (chapter 1). However, as we explained, healing and recovery to the point of the absence of illness is not the full definition of health. Professionals working in health care settings can and do contribute to high levels of wellness, holistic health, and quality of life. Teachable moments arise when patients interact with health care providers about specific health conditions. The influence of health care providers on health behavior can be powerful.

Collaboration between health care and public health professionals in the United States has resulted in a number of significant improvements in American health. These include increased life spans, reductions in infant mortality and childhood illnesses, improved management of cardiovascular disease and stroke, and effective treatment of pneumonia (Fielding & Teutsch, 2009). Though "public health professionals generally think about how to improve health at a population level, whereas clinicians generally address the needs of individuals" (Fielding & Teutsch, 2009, p. 317), integrating health promotion into health care settings and linking those efforts to community partnerships is promoted by national and international health leaders (Agency for Healthcare Research and Quality, 2015; McManus, 2013; USDHHS, 2014f; WHO, 2017b).

For example, the Agency for Healthcare Research and Quality (AHRQ, 2014b) developed a *Guide to Clinical Preventive Services*. This guide contains an extensive array of recommendations about screening, counseling, and preventive medication for adults and adolescents/children. The screening recommendations include such diverse topics as suicide risk, hepatitis infections, testicular cancer, and illicit drug use screening. Counseling recommendations include those related to breastfeeding, falls in older adults, healthful diet and physical activity, skin cancer, and motor vehicle occupant restraints. Aspirin and folic acid are among recommended preventive medications. Recommendations related to behavioral counseling for alcohol misuse and interventions to prevent child maltreatment are also available.

The effective application of these AHRQ recommendations calls for partnered approaches that include health care professionals, health education specialists, and a number of other professional partners. In many instances, these approaches would also benefit from a strong clinic-community partnership link where teams of health professionals work with community leaders and volunteers to provide a more holistic approach to health promotion and prevention (AHRQ, 2015b; CDC, 2016g; Fielding & Teutsch, 2009; USDHHS, 2014f). For example, the American Medical Association (AMA, 2014) partnered with the YMCA of the Greater Twin Cities in Minnesota to encourage physicians to refer individuals with prediabetes to the YMCA's Diabetes Prevention Program. These effective partnerships are often supported by a physician champion, a volunteer physician leader who promotes the cause and advises/encourages others in the practice to engage (AHRQ, 2014a).

Community Setting

It may seem a bit confusing to talk about community settings as *one* of four distinct areas in which community-based programs occur, especially when the other three settings (schools, worksites, and health facilities) are also considered channels to the broader community. Our earlier statement about how communities are defined by what people have in common may be helpful in understanding the rationale. Health promotion programs implemented in the other three settings impact three loosely defined groups in America: working adults, school- and college-aged young people, and medical patients who are eligible for and need health care services. However, those three channels of access do not reach all members of the broader American community. That is why a community setting, one that allows for a wide variety of approaches to community-based programming, is needed.

The community setting can include "public facilities; local government and agencies; and social service, faith, and civic organizations that provide channels to reach people where they live, work, and play" (USDHHS, 2000, sect. 7). A major contributor to these community-based efforts is the **public health system**. Though both public and private organizations are considered part of this system, governmental health agencies are the backbone of public health (IOM, 2002, 2003; National Association of County and City Health Officials [NACCHO], 2016). The 10 **essential public health services** listed in FYI 2.2 serve as a guide for U.S. public health agencies at the national/federal, state, and local levels (CDC, 2014e). We will begin our description of community-based public health efforts with a description of local health departments; that is, the units most likely to actively engage as partners in your community-based health promotion efforts.

LOCAL HEALTH DEPARTMENTS

According to NACCHO (2016), **local health departments** (LHDs) are the "foundation of the local public health system that comprises public- and private-sector health care providers, academia, business, the media, and other local and state governmental entities" (para. 1). LHDs are primarily responsible for public health promotion in local communities. Their jurisdictions or service areas can encompass a single county or city, a combined city-county jurisdiction, or a district or region of multiple counties or cities. Most of their funds come from a mixture of local county/city governments and

2.2   10 Essential Public Health Services

1. **Monitor health status** to identify and solve community health problems.

2. **Diagnose and investigate** health problems and health hazards in the community.

3. **Inform, educate, and empower people** about health issues.

4. **Mobilize community partnerships** and action to identify and solve health problems.

5. **Develop policies and plans** that support individual and community health efforts.

6. **Enforce laws and regulations** that protect health and ensure safety.

7. **Link people** to needed personal health services and assure the provision of health care when otherwise unavailable.

8. **Assure competent** public and personal health care workforce.

9. **Evaluate effectiveness, accessibility, and quality** of personal and population-based health services.

10. **Research for new insights** and innovative solutions to health problems.

Source: *The Public Health System and the 10 Essential Public Health Services*, Centers for Disease Control and Prevention, 2014, May 29. Retrieved from http://www.cdc.gov/nphpsp/essentialServices.html

state and federal sources, but some portion can come from private foundations and fees charged to local residents. We mention this to point out that LHDs aren't solely government funded; local community partnerships are important.

An essential component of LHD services includes the ability to respond to disease outbreaks, environmental hazards, natural disasters, terrorist attacks, and bioterrorism (NACCHO, 2016). Though specific services and activities vary, many LHDs provide (or partner with other organizations to provide) adult and child immunizations, communicable/infectious disease surveillance and screenings (for example, tuberculosis and sexually transmitted diseases/infections), chronic disease surveillance and prevention (high blood pressure and cancer screenings, tobacco use prevention, physical activity and healthy eating promotion, etc.), food service inspections and food safety education, and environmental health surveillance and protection. Maternal and child health services are offered by a large number of LHDs, while a smaller number also offer behavioral/mental health services, substance abuse services, oral health care, home health care, and primary health care and treatment services (NACCHO, 2006).

Whether you work in a nongovernmental organization or a government agency, the LHD that serves your community of interest will be a critical ally in your community health education and promotion efforts. This is true not only because of LHD connections with local community groups but also because LHDs are often linked to available information and resources from state and federal health agencies.

STATE HEALTH AGENCIES

The Association of State and Territorial Health Officials (ASTHO, 2014) is the national nonprofit organization that represents U.S. state public health agencies (also U.S. territories and the District of Columbia). The structure of state health agencies can differ in structure (freestanding or part of a larger agency), authority over local health agencies, rules for the appointment of state health officials, and how the agencies partner with other agencies and nongovernmental organizations. But, despite these variances, most state health agencies promote access to health care with specific attention to rural health and populations at risk to health disparities. Primary prevention, screening, and treatment services are also common; the most commonly offered services focus on tobacco use, HIV, and sexually transmitted diseases. Surveillance, epidemiology, data collection, and laboratory functions (for example, testing for bioterror agents, food-borne illness, and influenza type) are common activities. Maternal and child health services, as well as environmental health activities, are often included.

Though the nature of the relationships between state health agencies and local/regional public health departments differ, most report being highly collaborative with local departments. They report providing technical assistance, exchanging information, and partnering on projects with local departments, in addition to hospitals, community health centers, health providers, schools, faith communities, the media, and law enforcement.

State health agencies may also be responsible for federal initiatives. The most common of those are the CDC's Public Health Emergency Preparedness cooperative agreement; Title V Maternal and Child Health funding; vital statistics for the National Center for Health Statistics; CDC's Preventive Health and Health Services Block Grant; the ASPR Hospital Preparedness Program; CDC's National Cancer Prevention and Control

Program Grant; immunization funding; the Special Supplemental Nutrition Program for Women, Infants, and Children (WIC); *Healthy People*; and CDC's Injury Center effort.

FEDERAL HEALTH AGENCIES

In addition to local and state efforts, the federal government promotes community-based programs through the **U.S. Department of Health and Human Services** (USDHHS). The USDHHS is the U.S. government's principal health agency. Agency personnel work "to enhance and protect the health and well-being of all Americans. We fulfill that mission by providing for effective health and human services and fostering advances in medicine, public health, and social services" (USDHHS, n.d., *About HHS*, para. 1).

The USDHHS oversees 10 operating divisions, many of which you are likely familiar. The previously mentioned AHRQ and the National Institutes of Health (NIH) support research that addresses health care quality/cost-effectiveness (the AHRQ) and biomedical/behavioral research (the NIH). The Food and Drug Administration and the Agency for Toxic Substances and Disease Registry protect the public from exposure to environmental hazards, harmful foods, and other harmful factors. The Health Resources and Services Administration, Centers for Medicare & Medicaid Services, Administration for Community Living, and Administration for Children and Families focus on providing quality health services to medically underserved and vulnerable populations. The Substance Abuse and Mental Health Services Administration promotes prevention and treatment of addictive and mental disorders. The Indian Health Service provides health services for American Indians and Alaska Natives.

The CDC, a USDHHS operating division, is one of the primary *public health service agencies* within the USDHHS. The CDC is charged with protecting America "from health, safety and security threats, both foreign and in the U.S. Whether diseases start at home or abroad, are chronic or acute, curable or preventable, human error or deliberate attack, CDC fights disease and supports communities and citizens to do the same" (CDC, 2017f). Our nation often turns to the CDC for accurate health information and help in promoting and protecting our health.

The CDC promotes the empowerment of communities through a number of initiatives. The CDC's Division of Community Health (CDC, 2016b), focuses on outreach at the community level by supporting community efforts to achieve health equity, address the built environment, and build community awareness about important health issues. National organizations receive guidance and funding support for use in more localized community capacity-building efforts. Online resources and funding programs that directly support specific community projects are also among the array of efforts invested in supporting communities.

A number of other guides exist that communities and health professionals can use to promote health in their communities. Among those is *MAP-IT: A Guide to Using Healthy People 2020 in Your Community* (USDHHS, 2014f), a community-based program planning guide provided as part of the *Healthy People 2020* initiative. Another, *The Community Guide* (CDC, 2016g), includes information about program and policy interventions that have been proven effective in other communities. We encourage you to visit the websites of the national health agencies and develop a general familiarity with their contribution to community health promotion.

OTHER HEALTH ORGANIZATIONS

NGOs are also part of the community setting targeted by *Healthy People* objectives. These largely nonprofit organizations often serve as essential partners in community-based programs because of the health-related expertise, cultural competence, community connections, and funding support they can provide. For example, **voluntary health agencies** (VHAs) such as the American Heart Association and the American Cancer Society contribute to community health through public education, patient services, research, and advocacy related to a specific health issue or special population.

Faith-based organizations and other **nonprofit community organizations** with established roots in, or connections to, a local community can open doors for you, both literally and figuratively, to establish community partnerships. Local community residents who work or volunteer in these organizations, and the professionals who work with them, can help shape the program in ways that meet community interests and needs in a culturally appropriate format.

Private and grant-making **foundations** not only provide needed funds for NGOs and public health agencies, but also can provide expertise and support to community-based partnership groups. The Robert Wood Johnson Foundation (RWJF) and the W. K. Kellogg Foundation (WKKF) are examples of grant-making foundations that actively support community-based health promotion programs and other community empowerment initiatives. The RWJF (2017) funds a variety of health-related initiatives including child and family well-being, vulnerable populations, and various aspects of public health and health care. The WKKF (n.d.) has promoted capacity-building efforts that improved the lives of vulnerable children (and their families and communities) in the United States, southern Africa, South America, and the Caribbean.

A commitment to global health is evident in the activities of several U.S. organizations and agencies. For example, the USDHHS **Office of Global Affairs** maintains a website called *globalhealth.gov* and collaborates with other agencies and governments to address global health issues. The CDC (2017a) maintains a *Global Health* Web page and partners with WHO on a variety of global health initiatives.

The **World Health Organization** (WHO), part of the United Nations system, leads the world in global health promotion. WHO's (2017a) six leadership priorities are achieving universal health coverage; supporting the International Health Regulations; increasing access to medical products; addressing social, economic, and environmental determinants; responding to noncommunicable diseases; and working toward the health-related Millennium Development Goals. WHO is headquartered in Geneva, Switzerland, with six regional offices strategically placed around the world. The Pan American Health Organization (PAHO), headquartered in Washington, DC, serves as the WHO regional office to the Americas. We encourage you to become familiar with WHO and other global health organizations. As we discuss in chapter 14, you will likely discover a global health connection to your work, even if you never work outside of the United States.

≡ In Conclusion

Health professionals from a wide variety of disciplines are working in community-based partnerships to build capacities, empower communities, and promote the concept of *healthy communities*. Your ability to develop cultural competence and form strong partnerships will impact your level of success in the community you serve. A number of public health organizations (both government and nongovernment) are working toward solutions to community health needs. A community's ability to assume leadership and provide health-enhancing opportunities for its members is the true key to becoming a healthy community. We invite you to consider the perspectives and processes described in subsequent chapters in light of the community and cultural concepts presented here.

REVIEW QUESTIONS

1. Define healthy communities and describe what they do for their community members.

2. Describe Maslow's hierarchy of needs and the model of heritage consistency and explain how they contribute to social connectedness.

3. List some social determinants of health and explain how they impact the health of individuals and whole communities.

4. Define community capacity and describe its elements.

5. Justify why community empowerment, community building, and community organizing are important in community health promotion.

6. Describe the model for community capacity building and recommended approaches to community partnership development.

7. Explain what it means to exhibit cultural humility and how it relates to community partnership development and capacity building.

8. Describe settings in which the *Healthy People* initiative and other public health efforts are implemented to establish educational and community-based programs.

9. Analyze the role of public health agencies at the local, state, and national levels. What role do nongovernmental organizations play in community health partnerships?

FOR YOUR APPLICATION

Neighborhood Windshield Tour

Conduct a windshield tour or a walk-through in a local low-income neighborhood. (Be sure to find out about neighborhood safety before you go and take needed precautions.) Go with a friend who can help you note the condition of store fronts, housing, and automobiles; existing and missing resources (food stores, gas stations, banks, health clinics) and access to private (cars) and public transportation (buses, taxis, subways); the nature and content of prominent signs and/or graffiti; and the types of activities and interactions of people who live and work there. Visit the neighborhood at different times of the day and on different days of the week to note the ebb and flow of community life. If possible, sit in a local eatery or public place and observe patterns of activity. Then, drive through a more economically developed neighborhood and note similarities and contrasts. Create a list of your impressions for both types of neighborhoods. Identify factors that contribute to these neighborhood differences and any health-related implications.

3

Epidemiological Considerations

You have just started a new job at the local public health department. The director notifies you that a local physician has reported a case of E. coli (a foodborne organism that produces a toxin). He says that he and other health officials are concerned about the potential for an epidemic. You are not absolutely sure what he means or how they will know an epidemic has started. In fact, even though almost everyone has heard about E. coli, you can't remember many specifics of its causes, transmission, or symptoms. You wonder what role you will play if there is an epidemic.

Chapter Objectives

1. Describe the epidemiological approach to understanding patterns of disease and disease-related behaviors among humans.
2. List the purposes of epidemiology.
3. Compare current and historical life expectancies in the United States.
4. Identify measures of mortality and morbidity.
5. Classify causes of disease.
6. Describe the factors that influence morbidity.
7. List sources of epidemiologic data.
8. Describe concepts related to infectious disease, such as agent, host, environment, mode of transmission, and spectrum of disease.
9. Identify concepts related to noninfectious disease, such as acute illness, chronic illness, and web of causation.

≡ The Epidemiological Approach in the Community

The word *epidemiology* originally comes from Greek. If you have studied medical terminology, you know that the suffix *ology* means "study of" and the prefix *epi* means "among or upon." The root word *deme* means "commune or group of people." Therefore, the literal definition would be "the study of groups of people." We think a good working definition of **epidemiology** is the study of disease, the determinants of health, and the behaviors that prevent or cause disease or injury among groups of people. This definition implies that epidemiology serves many purposes. Some of these purposes are to

- study past or current trends in health status or level of disease
- identify causes of death
- establish **etiology** (cause) of disease
- define risk factors and determinants of disease
- determine need for health services
- identify feasible disease-prevention and health promotion strategies

- suggest need for future research in health and disease
- predict future disease outbreaks

An **epidemiologist** is a specialist in **epidemics**, or outbreaks of disease. In a sense, epidemiologists are detectives. They seek answers. In general, epidemiologists consider the population as a whole, or the community, in their investigations. They ask questions of individuals so that they can understand the disease or prevention strategy in the group. You may not be preparing to be an epidemiologist; however, you will need to understand their work. You may be part of a team that studies specific issues related to health or you may use an epidemiologist's report to support your work in prevention. In any case, basic knowledge of the field is imperative to your success.

If you were responsible for gathering information about diseases, and there was an outbreak of a disease in your community, how would you start your investigation? Some obvious questions might be "How many people are sick now and what do they have in common?" and "How quickly is it spreading?" With our hypothetical case of E. coli, you would first find out as much as possible about the organism and the illness it causes. Even if you already knew a lot about the disease, you would find out if new information had been discovered. Next, you would interview the girl who had E. coli, her physician, and family. Other people with similar symptoms would be interviewed to determine if more cases of E. coli were present in the community. The long-term purpose of your investigation would be to protect the community from an epidemic.

Even if you weren't yet sure of the name of the disease or its cause, you would still start with questions like "How many cases?" and "How fast is it spreading?" to determine the incidence and prevalence. You may have heard the words before, but they are sometimes used incorrectly even in professional literature. **Incidence** is the number of new cases of a specific disease among a specific group of people at a specific period of time. For example, in 2013 there were 522 new cases of E. coli in the United States (CDC, 2014). **Prevalence** is the total number of cases (not just the new ones) of a specific disease among a specific group of people at a specific period of time. For example, "An estimated 1.1 million people in the United States were living with HIV at the end of 2015" (CDC, 2016e, para. 4).

As the investigating health professional, you should determine incidence and prevalence in order to make decisions about whether an outbreak, or epidemic, of a disease is present. That's important because an epidemic is an increase in the normal incidence of a disease. You might plot an epidemic curve to assist in the decision-making process. The epidemic curve would illustrate the first infection (**index case**) and the number of new cases at selected intervals in time until there are no further new cases. In our E. coli example, the case reported to the health department would be the index case. Any others that were found during interviews would be plotted. Historical incidence rates for E. coli in the community would be compared to the current rate. If the current rates are higher, an outbreak is occurring. If people die as a result of a disease outbreak, you might also determine disease-specific death rates early in the investigation.

Mortality

Of course, you would want to move as quickly as possible in collecting epidemiological information to minimize risk of mortality. **Mortality** means death. Epidemiologists compute crude mortality, or death, rates in order to get an overall picture of the level of death in a community. Mortality rates are computed by dividing the number of deaths in a specific place by the number of people in the population at a given period of time. FYI 3.1 lists formulas commonly used in epidemiology. A **crude mortality rate** cannot be used to estimate the degree of risk an individual has of dying in a community because many factors have powerful influences on death rates. The most powerful is age. If the community you are investigating has a large number of older individuals, it will have a higher mortality rate than a community with many young individuals—not because it is a riskier place to live, but because older people are more likely to die.

What if you suspect that a disease outbreak is specific to a particular age group? To test your assumption, you can compute rates. Sometimes epidemiologists will compute **age-specific mortality** rates in order to study the frequency of death among people of a selected age group. This mortality rate is computed by dividing the num-

FYI

3.1   Formulas for Selected Rates and Ratios Used in Epidemiology

Rates and ratios play important roles in epidemiology. They are not difficult to use when you know the formulas. Some of the most common are listed here.

Morbidity

$$\text{Incidence} = \frac{\text{Number of new cases of a disease}}{\text{Total number of people at risk}} \text{ over a period of time} \times 100{,}000$$

$$\text{Attack Rate} = \frac{\text{Number of people sick}}{\text{Number of people both sick and well}} \text{ during a period of time} \times 100$$

$$\text{Prevalence} = \frac{\text{Total number of people with a disease}}{\text{Average number of people}} \text{ during a period of time} \times 100{,}000$$

Mortality

$$\text{Crude mortality} = \frac{\text{Number of deaths in a selected year}}{\text{Number of people in the population}} \times 100{,}000$$

$$\text{Infant mortality*} = \frac{\text{Number of infant deaths during a year}}{\text{Number of live births during a year}} \times 1{,}000$$

$$\text{Disease-specific mortality} = \frac{\text{Number of deaths due to a specific disease}}{\text{Number in population}} \times 100{,}000$$

$$\text{Age-specific mortality} = \frac{\text{Number of deaths in a specific age group}}{\text{Number of people in the same age group}} \times 100{,}000$$

*Infant deaths are defined as deaths among babies from 0 to 365 days old.

ber of deaths among people in a specific age group (for example, 13–18 year olds) by the number of people in the age category at a specific period of time. You can also compute the mortality for other age groups to compare across groups. Performing calculations to remove age influences on crude mortality rates makes it more feasible to compare risk of death between communities because you have removed the effect of the factor that influences rates the most.

Morbidity

Morbidity means illness. We've already stated that incidence and prevalence are morbidity rates commonly used by epidemiologists and other health professionals to determine the level of illness in a community. The morbidity rates of different types of diseases that affect communities vary over time, according to the place, and with the characteristics of the people. If you review Figure 3.1 (on the next page) you will note shifts in the types of disease that caused death in the 20th century. As you can see, the types of disease that were the leading causes of death early in the 20th century are completely different than the leading causes of death early in the 21st century.

Major causes of disease-related morbidity come from two categories of disease, infectious and noninfectious. Infectious diseases such as tuberculosis (TB), pneumonia, and gastroenteritis were more common causes of death in the early 1900s than were noninfectious diseases (Friis & Sellers, 1999). Today, noninfectious diseases are leading causes of death, although we may see another shift if infectious diseases like avian flu become prevalent in the United States. In 2013, 611,105 people died of heart disease, 584,881 of cancer, 149,205 of chronic lower respiratory diseases, and 128,978 of stroke. However, 56,979 people died of influenza and pneumonia (CDC, 2015). Morbidity and mortality influence both life expectancy and quality of life, which are two issues that make the understanding of epidemiology imperative for health educators.

Life Expectancy

Fluctuations in morbidity and mortality rates in a community will, of course, affect the life expectancy of its residents. **Life expectancy** refers to the average number of years groups of people are expected to live. Life expectancy rates have changed over time. Advances in available treatments, prevention methods, and healthier lifestyles have contributed to the change. In 1900 the life expectancy in the United States was 47.3 years, whereas in 2016 the U.S. life expectancy was 77.8 (Xu, Kochanek, Murphy, & Arias, 2011). Figure 3.2 (on p. 59) graphs life expectancies for men and women and Blacks, Hispanics, and Caucasians in the United States. The reasons behind the differences in genders, ethnicities, and racial groups are not easy to understand; however, it is imperative to both seek the causes of the differences and actively address them.

According to Marmot and Wilkinson (2006), differences in life expectancy are directly related to poverty. Low socioeconomic status influences insurance coverage, which in turn, influences access to medical care. Even if medical care is accessible, poor people may not be able to afford nutritious food or even enough food. Their housing may be inadequate and safety may be a major issue. Education may not be attainable; and this problem alone influences all of the aforementioned. Poverty and its influence on health will be discussed in more detail in later chapters.

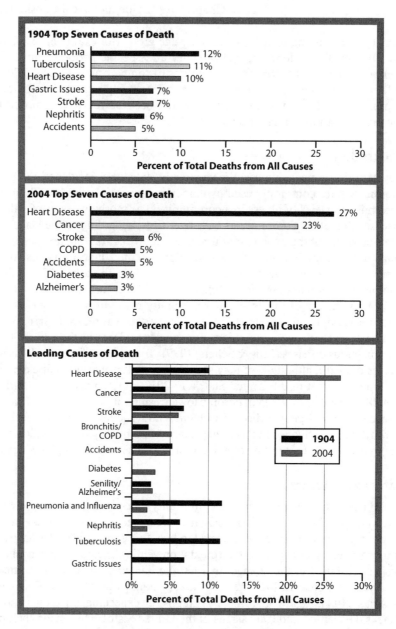

Figure 3.1 Shifts in causes of death from 1904 to 2004.
As you can see from these graphs, the types of diseases that caused death shifted over the 100 year period illustrated. In 2004, even though we saw some infectious diseases, such as influenza, pneumonia, and chronic lower respiratory diseases, becoming more prevalent, the major causes of death were related to lifestyle choices.

Sources: "Deaths, Percent of Total Deaths, and Death Rates for the 15 Leading Causes of Death: United States and Each State, 1999–2004," Centers for Disease Control and Prevention, 2007. Retrieved from http://www.cdc.gov/nchs/data/dvs/LCWK9_2004.pdf; "Deaths and Death Rates for Leading Causes of Death: Death Registration States, 1900–1940." Retrieved from http://www.cdc.gov/nchs/data/dvs/lead1900_98. pdf.

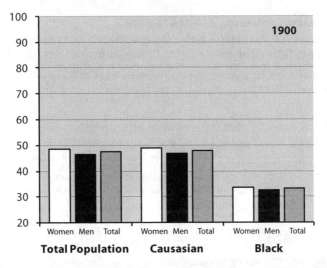

Figure 3.2   Life expectancy charts, United States, 1900 and 2016.
Life expectancy has increased dramatically over time for all people in the United States; however, disparities still exist between people of different ethnicities. These charts illustrate both the increase in life expectancy and some of the disparities.

Source: *Chartbook on Long-Term Trends in Health*, National Center for Health Statistics, 2017, Hyattsville, MD. Retrieved from https://www.cdc.gov/nchs/data/hus/hus16.pdf#015

Figure 3.3 illustrates the life expectancies of people in selected regions of the world. Note the differences in life expectancies and try to identify some of the reasons they exist. Life expectancy rates sometimes differ as a result of the level of development of a country or region. Some regions just don't have the technology to address medical problems that is available to developed countries. Other regions have environmental

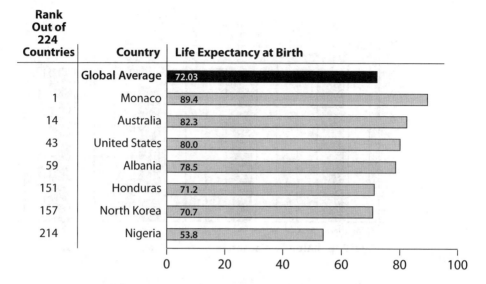

Figure 3.3   Life expectancies for selected regions.
Life expectancies have not increased for all regions of the world. As you can see from this chart, some countries fall well below the United States and other developed countries.

Source: "Country Comparison—Life Expectancy at Birth," World Factbook, 2017. Retrieved from https://www.cia.gov/library/publications/the-world-factbook/rankorder/2102rank.html

problems or cultural practices that influence life expectancies. For example, a nuclear power plant accident could cause dramatic increases in several types of cancer. Health professionals have an opportunity to broaden the scope of their work in communities by seeking answers to root causes of death and disease. In order to do so, they must understand where to get information about how disease impacts the population.

Sources of Data

Prevention efforts should begin with the collection of health-related data or epidemiological research. Plans for health education programs of all types should be based on assessment of relevant information. There are two major places from which information can be gathered for the epidemiological investigation. These include primary and secondary sources.

Primary Sources

Using primary sources of data involves the active process of collecting specific information through research. In our example, you would need to collect data on how many individuals have E. coli; their ages; the disease status of their families, friends, associates; and commonalities between those infected, especially in food intake. This strategy helps you accomplish two things. The most obvious is that it can provide accurate, community-specific data about the problem and potential solutions. If conducted appropriately, the process can also help you establish important relationships with community members.

In primary data collection efforts, epidemiologists use four major types of studies to discover patterns, compare numbers, and establish causation. These study types include cross-sectional, cohort, case-control, and experimental designs. We will learn more about the research process itself in chapter 9, but for now let's examine these four study designs.

CROSS-SECTIONAL STUDIES

These studies involve a "snapshot" of a group of people. A **cross-sectional study** is a one-time data-collection effort (by survey or some other means) that often uses a self-report format. **Self-report** simply means that no clinical or official measurement is made; rather, people report information about themselves. This type of study is also called a *prevalence study* if the researcher is studying the presence of a disease. Why would a cross-sectional study determine prevalence? If you review the definition of prevalence given earlier in the chapter, you will remember prevalence has to do with the total number of cases at a given time; therefore, if the correct questions are asked, a cross-sectional study collects that information. The title of the study (cross-sectional) describes the sample; a cross section of the population is selected to participate in the study. Many types of information can be gathered during the data-collection process, from health behaviors to attitudes and beliefs.

Cross-sectional studies can identify relationships; for example, if you conducted a survey in an urban community, you might find that many people report a concern about pollution and many people also recycle trash. You can compute a type of statistic called a **correlation** to see if there is a mathematical relationship between the number of people who have concern about pollution and the number who recycle. Unfortunately, if there is a mathematical relationship, it does not prove that having a concern about pollution causes a person to recycle or vice versa. It just means there is a relationship of some sort. Let's look at another example that will make this easier to understand. If you went to a very small town, a medium size town, and a large city and counted both the number of churches and the number of crimes, what do you think you would find? If you computed a correlation, you would find that there is a mathematical relationship (high correlation) between the number of churches and the number of crimes; where there are more churches, there are more crimes. So, should you hold a news conference and declare that churches cause crime? Absolutely not! All you found from your study is that there is a relationship in the numbers—when one number goes up, so does the other. Why do you think we would find more crime in places where there are more churches? Hopefully you realized immediately that when there are more people, there will be both more churches and more crimes. We could just have easily counted the number of grocery stores and crimes and discovered the same correlation. Although cross-sectional studies can provide you with a lot of information about relationships, you must be careful not to make unwarranted assumptions about cause and effect.

COHORT STUDIES

These studies are sometimes called *incidence studies*. As you know, the frequency of new cases of a disease is used to compute an incidence rate. In a **cohort study**, a cohort of healthy people is followed through time to see if they develop a specific disease of interest. Other information is also collected, such as health behaviors, beliefs, and exposures. As a result, the incidence rate for the disease of interest can be computed. Cohort studies allow comparisons of incidence rates between people who report a specific behavior (such as physical activity) and those who report they do not engage in the specific behavior (no physical activity).

A **cohort** is any group whose members have something in common. The commonality might be age, place or location, gender, occupation, or virtually any other characteristic. Cohort studies cost more than other types of studies because they are carried out over a long period of time. These studies are also referred to as *longitudinal studies* because of the length of time they take, or *prospective studies* because they are generally future-oriented. One of the classic cohort studies was the Framingham Heart Study, in which more than 5,000 people in one community were assessed and followed over many years. The study provided some outstanding information about risk factors for heart disease. Recent information from this ongoing study included the discovery of hundreds of new genes that are related to heart disease (Hajar, 2016).

The U.S. Department of Defense began a large cohort study in 2001 because of concerns regarding the long-term health effects of serving in the military. The project currently has 150,000 participants who were randomly selected for the sample. The study will address issues such as posttraumatic stress disorder (PTSD), depression, alcohol misuse, respiratory illnesses, and brain injuries (Naval Health Research Center, n.d.). Data will be collected every three years until 2022. Some important information has already been identified; for example, "service members who had experienced prior violent or sexual assault in their lives were more vulnerable to posttraumatic stress disorder after deployment. It was also found that exposure to actual combat rather than deployment itself was a factor in the onset of PTSD symptoms" (Force Health, 2008 p. 4). There have been very few differences in levels of depression or diagnosis of PTSD between National Guard Reservists and active duty military members (Schaller, et al., 2014).

CASE-CONTROL STUDIES

In **case-control** studies, a specific disease is generally the focus of the research. In the most common use of this type of study, a number of people with the disease are selected to be *cases* in the study. A second group of people, without the disease but otherwise very similar to the first in regard to characteristics like age, gender, ethnicity, and socioeconomic status, are selected to be *controls*. Researchers ask people in both groups to recall behaviors or health determinants from the past, or they use retrospective (past) medical records to study how the two groups differ. The objective is to discover how and/or why the disease occurs.

D'Souza and associates (2007) conducted a case-control study with 100 oropharyngeal cancer patients and 200 controls. They sought evidence that the human papillomavirus (HPV) played a role in oropharyngeal cancer. They determined that even when cancer patients did not smoke or use alcohol, there was a strong association between infection with HPV and the presence of oropharyngeal cancer.

In 2014, Chen, Malone, and Li responded to media concern that there might be a connection between the type of bras women wore and breast cancer. They conducted a population-based case-control study in which 454 ductal carcinoma patients, 490 lobular carcinoma patients, and 469 controls were compared. No associations between bra type and breast cancer was found.

EXPERIMENTAL STUDIES

A true scientific experiment is the only type of study from which researchers can determine the cause of a disease or the effectiveness of treatments. In an **experimental study**, participants are randomly selected from the population of interest. A computerized process, much like throwing every person's name into a hat and drawing out the number needed, is used to randomly choose those who will be in the study. This **random selection** process gives each person the same chance of being in the study. In other words, one type of person won't be intentionally over- or underrepresented in the study. Participants are also randomly assigned to either the intervention or control group. Participants in the control group will not receive the treatment or intervention but will be treated the same in every other way. Differences in the groups will be analyzed in order to determine the efficacy of the intervention.

The U.S. Food and Drug Administration (USFDA, 2007) conducted an experimental study to determine if the type of health message on food products impacted participants' perceptions and intent to purchase the food. This study was conducted via the Internet, which is an increasingly popular method for communicating with study participants. The participants were not randomly selected from the total U.S. population, but the study was still experimental in nature because a legitimate sampling technique was used and an intervention occurred. An experimental study must have an intervention. In the USFDA study the findings showed that if a food product had a label giving both the name of a nutrient and the positive health effect to be expected, participants were more likely to consider buying it. Participants were least likely to consider buying a food product that had a label with only a nutrient content message.

Secondary Sources

Secondary data consists of information that has already been collected by national, state, or local sources. Going back to our E. coli example, it would be wise to identify data that has been collected by other cities regarding E. coli cases. Secondary data helps you determine how your outbreak compares to those of other communities who face similar issues. You can learn about effective and ineffective approaches attempted in other places and may gain some insight otherwise missed. You can then consider the specific characteristics and needs of your community and adapt what you learned from those secondary sources.

The World Health Organization (WHO) is a good source of secondary data because it assesses the global burden of disease (GBD). The first assessment, sponsored by the World Bank with the help of the Harvard School of Public Health, was conducted in 1990. At that time the project goals, still in use today, were detailed (Murray, Lopez, Mathers, & Stein, 2001). The study introduced a way of looking at the burden of disease called *DALY* (disability-adjusted life year). The DALY is a mathematical formula that takes the years of life lost from premature death into account. This complex data-collection process is a great example of the use of numerous sources of data. The WHO sources include epidemiologic research (primary data collection) and disease registries, population surveys, and health facility data (secondary data sources). If you are interested in learning more about the GBD, check out the World Health Organization data resources at http://ghdx.healthdata.org/gbd-2015.

DISEASE REGISTRIES

Disease registries involve databases that list numbers of new cases of diseases. Certain diseases that occur in the United States are considered notifiable. Physicians or other health care providers who diagnose these illnesses are required to record and report the diseases to the state in which they practice (CDC, 2008d). The state officials then compile and report the numbers to the CDC. As you can see in FYI 3.2, E. coli is on the notifiable list for 2015. Changes in the specific diseases that require notification occur as new infections emerge or as the incidence declines dramatically over a long period of time.

FYI

3.2   National Notifiable Infectious Diseases, United States 2015

- *Anaplasma phagocytophilum* Infection
- Anthrax (http://wwwn.cdc.gov/nndss/conditions/anthrax/)
- Arboviral diseases, neuroinvasive and non-neuroinvasive California Serogroup Virus Diseases
- Babesiosis
- Botulism / *c. botulinum*
- Botulism, Foodborne
- Botulism, Infant
- Botulism, Other
- Botulism, Wound
- Brucellosis
- Campylobacteriosis
- Chancroid
- Chikungunya Virus Disease* (not OMB PRA approved)
- *Chlamydia trachomatis* infection
- Cholera
- Coccidioidomycosis / Valley Fever
- Congenital Syphilis
- Crimean-Congo Hemorrhagic Fever virus
- Cryptosporidiosis
- Cyclosporiasis
- Dengue
- Dengue Fever (DF)
- Dengue Hemorrhagic Fever (DHF)

- Dengue-like illness* (not OMB PRA approved)
- Dengue, Severe
- Dengue Shock Syndrome (DSS)
- Dengue virus infections
- Diphtheria
- Eastern Equine Encephalitis Virus Disease
- Ebola virus
- Ehrlichiosis and Anaplasmosis
- *Ehrlichia chaffeensis* Infection
- *Ehrlichia ewingii* Infection
- Giardiasis (http://wwwn.cdc.gov/nndss/conditions/giardiasis/)
- Gonorrhea (http://wwwn.cdc.gov/nndss/conditions/gonorrhea/)
- *Haemophilus influenzae*, invasive disease
- Hansen's disease / Leprosy
- Hantavirus infection, non-Hantavirus pulmonary syndrome* (not OMB PRA approved)
- Hantavirus pulmonary syndrome (HPS)
- Hemolytic uremic syndrome, post-diarrheal (HUS)
- Hepatitis A, acute
- Hepatitis B, acute
- Hepatitis B, chronic
- Hepatitis B, perinatal infection
- Hepatitis C, acute
- Hepatitis C, past or present

- HIV Infection (AIDS has been reclassified as HIV Stage III) (AIDS/HIV)
- Influenza-associated pediatric mortality
- Invasive Pneumococcal Disease (IPD) / *Streptococcus pneumoniae*, Invasive Disease
- Lassa virus
- Legionellosis / Legionnaire's Disease or Pontiac fever
- Leptospirosis
- Listeriosis
- Lujo virus
- Lyme disease
- Malaria
- Marburg virus
- Measles / Rubeola
- Meningococcal disease
- Mumps
- New World Arenavirus – Guanarito virus
- New World Arenavirus – Junin virus
- New World Arenavirus – Machupo virus
- New World Arenavirus – Sabia virus
- Novel influenza A virus infections
- Pertussis / Whooping Cough
- Plague
- Poliomyelitis, paralytic
- Poliovirus infection, nonparalytic
- Powassan Virus Disease
- Q fever, acute
- Q fever, chronic
- Rabies, animal
- Rubella, congenital syndrome (CRS)
- Salmonellosis
- Severe Acute Respiratory Syndrome-Associated Coronavirus Disease (SARS)
- Shiga toxin-producing *Escherichia coli* (STEC)
- Shigellosis
- Smallpox / Variola
- Spotted Fever Rickettsiosis
- St. Louis Encephalitis Virus Disease
- Streptococcal toxic-shock syndrome (STSS)
- Syphilis
- Syphilis, Congenital
- Syphilis, Early Latent
- Syphilis, Late Latent
- Syphilis, late with clinical manifestations (including late benign syphilis and cardiovascular syphilis)
- Syphilis, Primary
- Syphilis, Secondary
- Syphilitic Stillbirth
- Tetanus / *c. tetani*
- Toxic shock syndrome (other than Streptococcal) (TSS)
- Trichinellosis / Trichinosis
- Tuberculosis (TB)
- Tularemia
- Typhoid fever
- Undetermined Human Ehrlichiosis/Anaplasmosis
- Vancomycin-intermediate *Staphylococcus aureus* and Vancomycin-resistant *Staphylococcus aureus* (VISA/VRSA)
- Varicella / Chickenpox
- Varicella deaths
- Vibriosis
- Viral Hemorrhagic Fever (VHF)
- West Nile Virus Disease
- Western Equine Encephalitis Virus Disease
- Yellow fever

From "National Notifiable Diseases Surveillance System," Centers for Disease Control and Prevention, 2015. Retrieved from https://wwwn.cdc.gov/nndss/

POPULATION SURVEYS

Health-related data are collected systematically in the United States through **population surveys**. One example of such a survey is the Behavioral Risk Factor Surveillance System (BRFSS). This survey tracks access to health care, presence of diseases and other conditions, and behaviors (preventive and risk) through a self-report telephone survey. Data collection is continuous in all of the states and approximately 350,000 U.S. adults are interviewed each year (CDC, 2008b).

The National Health Care Surveys are a set of surveys conducted among a representative sample of health care providers and health care settings. They provide data about resources for health care, types of procedures and disease management, and characteristics of patients and providers. The information collected can be invaluable for researchers, public health personnel, and policy makers (CDC, 2008c).

CENSUSES

Censuses originated in combination with the process of taxation in ancient Egypt and Rome. In the United States, the census occurs every 10 years in order to determine seats in the U.S. House of Representatives. Federal funding of some health and social services programs also depends on the number and distribution of people as measured by the U.S. census. As in all self-report surveys, caution is needed when using census data. For example, the ethnic and racial categories listed on the census survey have stirred controversy. There is such diversity in this country that many experts wonder if it is necessary or even possible to categorize ethnicity and race. Other data collected in censuses include gender, age, marital status, type of housing, ancestry, language spoken in the home, year the residence was built, place of birth, education level, employment status, plumbing and kitchen facilities, telephone and vehicle availability, and type of heating and cooling. Combining census data with data about disease helps health professionals gain a clearer picture of a community's health status.

VITAL STATISTICS

In the United States vital life events are recorded and then counted. For example, each newborn receives a birth certificate, and death certificates are generated for each person who dies. The numbers of marriages and divorces also become vital statistics.

With censuses and other kinds of record keeping, there are inaccuracies. Sometimes diseases aren't diagnosed properly or the cause of death is inaccurately listed. As time progresses, diagnostic criteria may change, making comparisons of vital statistics between years less meaningful. Nevertheless, vital statistics provide a great deal of information that helps health professionals. Of course, the reason for collecting data, whether from primary or secondary sources, is to improve the health of individuals and communities. Although health is a great deal more than the prevention of disease, prevention remains one of the primary roles of the health educator.

≡ Prevention

Helping people get the information they need to make healthy choices is one important aspect of prevention. You may even think that your involvement in prevention occurs only before an individual becomes ill. But two of the three categories of prevention take place after the onset of disease.

Primary Prevention

Efforts that occur before individuals become sick are called **primary prevention**. Programs that help people stop smoking before they develop heart disease or cancer reflect primary prevention tactics. Another example of primary prevention is vaccination of children against infectious diseases. Vaccinations trigger the production of antibodies, which in turn prevents future cases of the disease. These types of primary prevention impact the host. It is also possible to change the environment to bring about primary prevention. For example, mosquito control and water fluoridation programs are primary prevention efforts.

Secondary Prevention

Once a disease occurs in an individual, efforts to prevent its progression are called **secondary prevention**. Screening tools like mammography (breast x-rays that screen for cancer) are secondary in nature. They may identify a cancerous lesion at an early stage when it can be treated successfully, thereby preventing progression. Many women believe that if they have yearly mammograms they will not get breast cancer. In fact, mammograms do not prevent breast cancer. Regardless of the disease, any program that screens for disease is a secondary prevention program.

Tertiary Prevention

Tertiary prevention is concerned with the quality of life of individuals with disease. Regardless of a disease's effect on a person, tertiary prevention is practiced when efforts are made to improve the quality of life as much as possible. This may not seem like prevention at all, but the idea is to prevent situations from becoming worse. In other words, to help people with serious diseases live their best lives. Home health care and hospice care are two examples of tertiary prevention programs.

Think of some actions that you could take to improve the quality of life for someone who has suffered major mobility issues due to the West Nile virus. Then work backward and consider how you would help prevent the individual from getting the virus in the first place. To do this, you will need information about the virus and how it spreads. It's wise to have some general information about disease transmission.

☰ Infectious Disease

Infectious diseases spread from individual to individual or from insects, animals, or other carriers to humans. They are often caused by an easily identified single organism. Important aspects of infectious disease include causative organisms, modes of transmission, reservoirs, spectrum of disease, epidemic curve, immunity, and prevention.

Although many models have been used to illustrate the basic concepts of the epidemiology of infectious disease, the triangle is still relevant and easy to understand (Figure 3.4). The three apexes of the triangle represent the agent, host, and environment. The **agent** is the cause of the disease or causative organism. Another term used for agent in infectious diseases is **pathogen** (disease-causing microorganism). The **host** is the recipient of the disease. Anything internal within the host that influences the disease process should be considered part of the host. The **environment** consists of the external surroundings that influence the host.

Figure 3.4   The epidemiological triangle.
There are three major factors that influence whether an individual gets an infectious disease. They are the agent, external environments, and host (individual or internal environment).

Agent

The most common agents in infectious disease are viruses, bacteria, fungi, and worms. Viruses are the smallest agents and most difficult to treat. **Antibiotics**, which are substances that arrest the growth of or destroy pathogens, do not kill viruses. They do kill bacteria, which are also microscopic and come in shapes that range from rectangular to spiral. Although some bacteria are becoming antibiotic-resistant due to misuse among populations, most are still controllable with standard treatments. Some of the antibiotic-resistant strains can be controlled through the use of a combination of antibiotics called a *cocktail*. Fungi, yeast, and molds cause many common conditions, such as vaginal yeast infections and athlete's foot. Worms such as tapeworms, which can be many feet long, cause a variety of illnesses. See Figure 3.5 for common biological agents and examples of the diseases they cause.

The effects of agents on a host depend on many characteristics, such as their virulence, infectivity, pathogenicity, resistance, and the number of microorganisms that enter the host. For example, rabies is a very severe illness that almost always causes death in humans. The virus that causes it is **virulent**. An agent that can easily enter a body and multiply is **infective**. A highly infective agent causes measles. Measles is also a disease of high **pathogenicity**; once in the body, the measles agent almost always causes full-blown disease, not just a light case. HIV has low **resistance**, which means that outside of the body it is easy to kill.

You need to know the common biological agents because as a health educator you may be asked to teach people about the causes of their infectious diseases. Understanding terms like *virulence, infectivity, pathogenicity,* and *resistance* will allow you to help others communicate with their health care providers.

Host

The host is the individual who has the disease; *host* can be thought of as a person's internal environment. Think about the internal things that influence you. Did you come up with things like what you eat, how much you sleep, the presence of other diseases or disorders, genetics, and the ability to develop immunity? If so, you are absolutely right. Anything that influences the body internally has the potential to influence the outcome of a disease. Even factors like stress, physical activity, and body temperature influence disease processes in the body. These factors don't cause the disease but rather determine, to some extent, how an individual will react to or fight a disease.

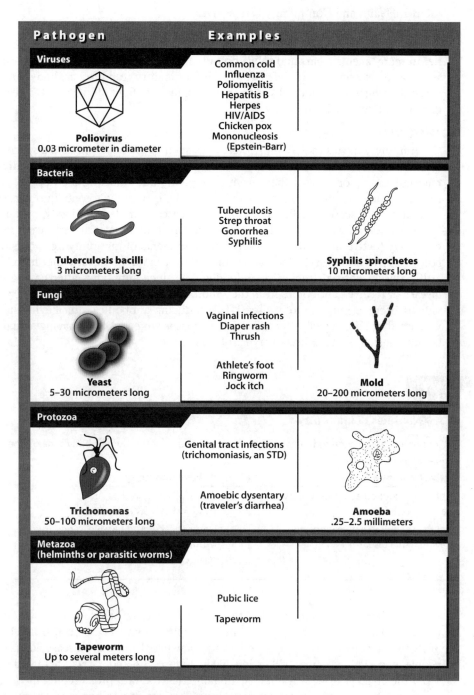

Pathogen	Examples	
Viruses		
Poliovirus 0.03 micrometer in diameter	Common cold Influenza Poliomyelitis Hepatitis B Herpes HIV/AIDS Chicken pox Mononucleosis (Epstein-Barr)	
Bacteria		
Tuberculosis bacilli 3 micrometers long	Tuberculosis Strep throat Gonorrhea Syphilis	**Syphilis spirochetes** 10 micrometers long
Fungi		
Yeast 5–30 micrometers long	Vaginal infections Diaper rash Thrush Athlete's foot Ringworm Jock itch	**Mold** 20–200 micrometers long
Protozoa		
Trichomonas 50–100 micrometers long	Genital tract infections (trichomoniasis, an STD) Amoebic dysentary (traveler's diarrhea)	**Amoeba** .25–2.5 millimeters
Metazoa (helminths or parasitic worms)		
Tapeworm Up to several meters long	Pubic lice Tapeworm	

Figure 3.5 Common biological agents.
Infectious diseases are caused by a number of organisms. Some of the most common are shown in this illustration along with the types of diseases they cause.

Adapted from *Environmental Health*, 2nd ed., by M.T. Morgan. © 1997 Brooks/Cole, a part of Cengage Learning, Inc. Used with permission.

The host's first line of defense is skin. What an amazing organ! It serves as a barrier to many agents. Tears and saliva do the same. The body's inflammatory response serves as the second line of defense. In an inflammatory response, the body sends fluids containing white blood cells and other substances to fight off the agent. The body's third line of defense is immunity.

IMMUNITY

Immunity means that an individual is resistant or not susceptible to a specific disease. Immunity occurs when antibodies are produced in the body. **Antibodies** kill microorganisms or prevent them from multiplying and infecting the host. A person isn't immune to all diseases just because he or she is immune to one. In other words, immunity is disease-specific, and not all diseases stimulate antibody production. There are several ways in which immunity occurs. Individuals can produce it in their own body (**active immunity**) or receive the ingredients of immunity from outside the body (**passive immunity**). Both active and passive immunity occur either naturally or artificially. In **natural immunity**, individuals produce antibodies after having had a disease or received antibodies from their mother in utero. In **artificial immunity**, individuals become immune to a disease by producing antibodies after having had the weakened or killed agent responsible for the disease injected or by having actual antibodies injected. FYI 3.3 lists the types of immunity.

FYI

3.3   Examples of Immunity

Immunity can be acquired in two ways. Immunity is one of the human body's major lines of defense against disease.

Active Immunity	Passive Immunity
Artificially acquired active immunity (Vaccination)	Artificially acquired passive immunity (Antibodies injected)
Naturally acquired active immunity (Having had a disease)	Naturally acquired passive immunity (Antibodies passing from mother to baby)

Herd immunity occurs when a significant number of people in a population are immune to a disease. If many people in a community have a disease, it is much more likely that the disease-free people will get it; if few people have the disease, its spread to people who aren't immune will be less likely. Figures 3.6 and 3.7 will help you understand the concept of herd immunity. Imagine that the rain drops represent a disease agent and the umbrellas represent immunity. The first figure illustrates that most people in a group of 12 people will get wet (become infected with the agent) if there are only two umbrellas. The second figure illustrates an increase in the number of people in the group who stay dry (uninfected) if there are more umbrellas. If a large number of people become immune—by vaccine, for example—a protective barrier is created for those who are susceptible. People who don't have the disease, due to immunity or no contact, won't spread it. Almost the entire population or "herd" is protected.

As a health educator, you may help people gain the knowledge necessary to make good decisions about health. The range of information people might need concerning the internal environment of the host may vary from healthy food choices to reducing stress to the side effects of vaccines as well as their benefits. As we have mentioned before, it is important for you to be able to access information; in this case, you would need to research host issues.

Environment

The external environment influences both the outcomes of disease and the very presence of the disease. The external environment has physical aspects (such as terrain, precipitation, and temperature) as well as social aspects (such as cultural characteristics). The numbers of people, plants, and animals influence the external environment. Insects or animals spread some diseases. If an insect carrier (vector) of a

Figure 3.6   Herd immunity—low.
Low immunization levels fall short of protecting individuals within a group.

Figure 3.7   Herd immunity—high.
A high level of immunization within the group affords a good level of protection to most of the individuals within the group.

specific disease doesn't live in an environment, the disease is less likely to be present in the environment. If a disease is spread via tiny droplets in the air, a place crowded with people is going to have disease spread at a higher rate than will a location with very few people. Certain organisms live and spread best in places that are very hot and humid. The cultural environment influences everything from food choices to types of housing and stress-coping strategies. Although all cultural characteristics do not influence the external environment, all influence an individual's likelihood of contracting certain diseases. As a community health professional you will need to be prepared to answer questions about the environment and how it affects disease. If, for example, you live in a place where deer ticks, which carry Lyme disease, are common, your job may be to teach people that tick bites can be prevented by wearing long sleeves and tucking in loose clothing.

The interactions among agent, host, and environment produce the overall parameters of infectious disease. One example of the interaction occurs in the mode of transmission of disease. Characteristics of hosts, agents, and environments affect how the agent is transmitted from one person to another.

Mode of Transmission

The way in which an agent travels from one host to another is its **mode of transmission**. Some agents travel through the air, whereas others have to be picked up from a hard surface. As noted earlier, insects and animals also carry some agents from one host to another. Modes of transmission are direct or indirect. A *direct* mode of transmission means that an agent is passed directly from one person to another (person to person). *Indirect* modes involve a third element—an animal, insect, hard surface, or food. All modes of transmission fall within these two broad categories. Airborne transmission occurs when the agent is carried on small droplets of moisture or dust. Small droplets, forcefully expelled from someone's mouth or nose via a cough or a sneeze, can travel great distances if they aren't blocked. Vectorborne transmission occurs when an animal or insect serves as the agent's transportation. **Vectors** are living but nonhuman. **Fomites** are inanimate objects, such as cups, tables, doorknobs, and toys that can also serve as a means of transportation for some agents. Sometimes an agent remains in a **reservoir** and multiplies until it is transmitted to a host. Anything living or nonliving might serve as a reservoir, including the human body. Some humans or animals carry an agent and transmit it to others but do not get sick themselves. These *carriers* make prevention a challenge because their carrier status often goes undetected until many people around them get the disease. Typhoid Mary is the most famous example of the carrier phenomenon.

Mode of transmission involves the way agents get from person to person but do not determine how an agent enters the body (*portal of entry*) or exits the body (*portal of exit*). Portals of entry and exit and modes of transmission play important roles in the prevention as well as transmission of diseases.

Under the right conditions, once an agent enters a body the disease will progress through a fairly consistent set of stages. These phases are illustrated in Figure 3.8. The *incubation period* is the time from the agent's entry in the body (*point of infection*) to the occurrence of signs or symptoms of disease. Signs and symptoms are actually different things. *Signs* are measurable changes in the body such as body temperature or number of white blood cells. *Symptoms* are subjective changes in the body such as pain or dizziness. Signs and symptoms begin to appear during the *prodromal period*. A disease is at its peak during the *fastigium period*, and signs and symptoms decline during the *defervescence period*. The individual recovers during *convalescence*.

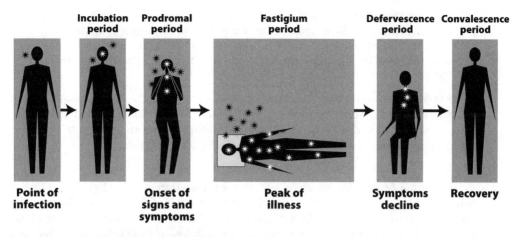

Figure 3.8   Progression of an infectious disease.
In this case, the disease affects the respiratory tract.

Noteworthy Infectious Diseases

Some infectious diseases are short term, or **acute**, and others are long term, or **chronic.** Although there are many acute and chronic diseases that we might discuss, we will discuss three that have been in the news in the recent past. Other significant infectious diseases and their modes of transmission are listed in Table 3.1.

ESCHERICHIA COLI

Some forms of the bacterium *Escherichia coli* (E. coli) are virulent pathogens and many are carried by food products. You may have heard about recent outbreaks from contaminated foods. One such announcement was made on November 1, 2007. It stated,

Table 3.1   Critical Biological Agents

Easy to Spread Agents	Moderately Easy to Spread Agents	Emerging Agents to Watch in Future
Anthrax Bacterium spread by contact with infected animals	E. coli Bacteria spread by eating undercooked food products that contain the E. coli toxin	Hantavirus Spread through exposure to infected rodent droppings
Botulism Spread by eating food containing botulism toxin	Cryptosporidium Parasite spread through contaminated water	
Smallpox Virus spread through air, person to person	Mycobacterium Tuberculosis Bacterium spread through air, person to person	

Source: "CDC's List of Critical Biological Agents." *NSF Live Safer.* Retrieved from www.nsf.org/consumer/bioterrorism/bioterrorism_agents.asp#anthrax=

General Mills Operations, a Wellston, Ohio, establishment, is voluntarily recalling approximately 3.3 million pounds of frozen meat pizza products because they may be contaminated with E. coli O157:H7 and may be linked to an outbreak of E. coli O157:H7 illnesses, the U.S. Department of Agriculture's Food Safety and Inspection Service announced today. (USDA, 2007, para. 1)

Individuals who contract the illness caused by the O157:H7 strain frequently have bloody diarrhea for short periods of time. Unfortunately, some individuals—especially very young children—die as a result. This illness is severe and acute in nature but can be prevented by adequate heating of the food reservoirs.

EBOLA

The name *Ebola* came about because the first recognized cases (1976) were by the Ebola River in the Democratic Republic of the Congo (CDC, 2014c). Most cases today are still found in Africa; however, on September 30, 2014, the first case of Ebola was diagnosed in the United States. This case was diagnosed in Dallas, Texas, but was related to travel from Africa. The individual with Ebola died from the disease because his diagnosis came too late and his health was poor prior to contracting the disease. On October 12, 2014, a health care worker in Dallas also tested positive for Ebola. This individual was treated successfully (CDC, 2014c).

Transmission of Ebola occurs through direct contact with the blood or body fluids of sick individuals when symptoms occur. Transmission can also occur through contact with infected wildlife and contaminated objects (CDC, 2014c). Symptoms generally occur around eight days after exposure but can occur between 2 and 21 days. Symptoms include fever, headache, muscle pain, weakness, diarrhea, vomiting, stomach pain, and most worrisome—hemorrhage (CDC, 2014c). While there are ways to diagnose the illness, no vaccine has been approved at this time. Primary prevention is key, which means that although this disease is rare in the U.S., all health care professionals and facilities must be prepared with the knowledge and skills to prevent transmission.

ZIKA VIRUS

There's no doubt that most of us have heard about the *Zika Virus* due to media coverage before and during the 2016 Olympics in Rio De Janeiro. Like West Nile Virus, Zika spreads most often through mosquito bites. The types of mosquitoes that carry the virus live in many parts of the U.S. and around the world (CDC, 2018a). One difference between West Nile and Zika is that Zika can also be spread through sexual contact. If a woman with the virus becomes pregnant, her fetus can become infected. Zika can cause birth defects in the fetus, the most serious of which is microcephaly, or poor brain development (CDC, 2018a).

Since there is no vaccine available, mosquito control—such as eliminating all standing water; controlling tall grass and shrubbery where mosquitoes like to live; using mosquito-repelling plants; fogging key parts of communities; and putting out mosquito killers, zappers, and magnets—will be important. Using mosquito repellent and mosquito repelling shirts are also good ways to prevent infection. Many people who are infected with the Zika Virus experience few or no symptoms, but that doesn't mean the threat to public health should be ignored. In fact, during the summer of 2016, several areas in Florida were found to have mosquitoes carrying the Zika Virus (CDC, 2016). In order to prevent serious health issues caused by this virus, communities and individuals must act responsibly.

Noninfectious Disease

The definition of noninfectious disease seems simple enough: diseases that are not transmitted from one person to another. However, there is nothing simple about most noninfectious diseases. These diseases are caused by chemical, metallic, electrical, psychosocial, genetic, or any number of other agents. The agent is not generally a pathogen, although it can be. In fact, noninfectious diseases are commonly caused by a combination of agents. A visual schematic of how agents work together to cause disease is found in Figure 3.9 on the next page. The schematic, called a *web of causation*, demonstrates the relationship between agents. Finding the agents that cause a noninfectious disease or discovering how several agents work together to cause the disease is not simple. In the United States and most other developed countries, the burden of noninfectious chronic diseases is very heavy. The four leading causes of death in 2013 were chronic diseases and were responsible for about 57% of all deaths in the United States that year (CDC, 2014). The statistics were nearly the same for 2006, with diseases of the heart (26%), malignant neoplasms (23.1%), cerebrovascular diseases (5.7%), and chronic lower respiratory diseases (5.1%) accounting for 60% of all deaths (Heron et al., 2009). Diabetes, although not a leading cause of death, burdens many millions of people with serious consequences and in some cases death.

Heart Disease

In 2016, 28.1 million adults had diagnosed heart disease (CDC, 2017d). The category "heart disease" encompasses over 20 different conditions that make it difficult for the heart to function (CDC, 2017d). These disorders range from myocardial infarction, a heart attack, to congenital heart disease, something that occurred in the heart's development before birth. However, coronary artery disease is by far the most frequently occurring disorder.

Coronary artery disease is a condition in which the blood vessels on the heart get too narrow for blood to flow normally. You have probably heard of atherosclerosis, which is the collection of fatty plaque on the walls of arteries. The collection of plaque is what narrows the arteries, sometimes to the extent that no blood flows through them. When this happens in arteries on the heart, the result will be a heart attack.

The cause of diseases of the heart is multifaceted. Review the web of causation seen in Figure 3.9. You will see that food choices, body fat, use of tobacco, blood pressure, physical activity, personality characteristics, other illnesses, and genetics can all play a role. While not all of these are under a person's control, many are. As a health professional, you may be asked to help individuals or groups understand their illness or change their negative health behaviors.

Cancer

All cancers combined account for the second leading cause of death in the United States. Lung and bronchus cancers are the most common cancers among Americans; 221,200 new cases were diagnosed in 2015 (American Cancer Society [ACS], 2015). While not always easy to treat, lung cancer is the most preventable. Tobacco use, whether through cigarette, cigar, or pipe smoking, has the largest impact on the number

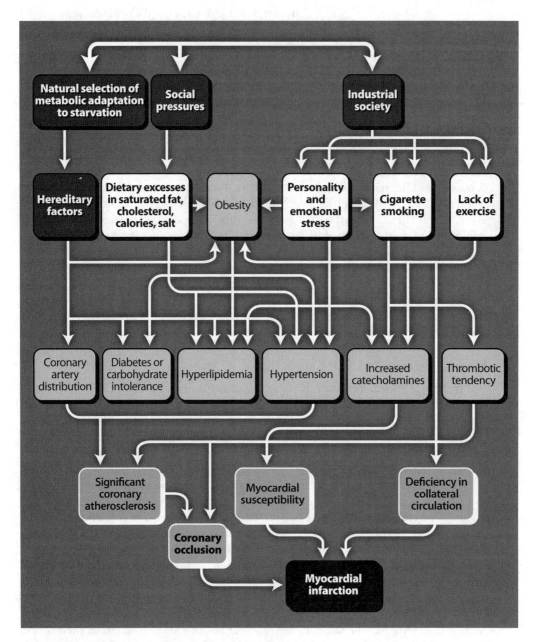

Figure 3.9 Web of causation for heart disease.
The cause of a myocardial infarction, or heart attack, is not simple to track. As you can see from this illustration, many things influence the onset of heart disease. In this illustration, the dark gray boxes are the factors outside the control of individuals, while the white boxes are behaviors or characteristics that people can change. The pale gray boxes are the first level of consequences, leading to the second level of consequences in the white-bordered boxes. The black box is the ultimate result.

Adapted from *Primer of Epidemiology*, 4th ed., p. 4, by G. D. Friedman, 1994, New York: McGraw-Hill.

of lung cancer cases. Eight out of 10 lung cancers result from the use of tobacco. Don't forget that secondhand and thirdhand smoke play important roles in cancer deaths.

> The number of new cases of cancer (cancer incidence) is 439.2 per 100,000 men and women per year (based on cases from 2011 to 2015). The number of cancer deaths (cancer mortality) is 163.5 per 100,000 men and women per year (based on deaths from 2011 to 2015). (National Cancer Institute, 2018, para. 4)

The five most common cancers by rank from 2010 to 2014 were female breast, prostate, lung and bronchus, and colon and rectum (U.S. Cancer Statistics Working Group, 2017). The leading cancer sites among men include prostrate, lung and bronchus, and colon and rectum; the leading cancer sites among women include breast, lung and bronchus, and colon and rectum (U.S. Cancer Statistics Working Group, 2017).

The diminished quality of life and death caused by cancer are tragic. However, those aren't the only issues that receive attention. The cost of cancer in 2009 exceeded $216 billion in the United States (NIH, 2012). The burden of cancer does not have to be so high! Many cancers can be prevented. As a health professional, you will want to have basic information about the leading cancers and how they can be prevented.

Diabetes

"The dramatic increase in the prevalence of childhood overweight and its resultant comorbidities are associated with significant health and financial burdens, warranting strong and comprehensive prevention efforts" (American Academy of Pediatrics, 2003). Childhood obesity leads to obesity in adults, and around 44 million Americans are considered obese as measured by body mass index. From 1991 to 2001 the number of obese adults increased by 74% (CDC, 2008h). In 2016, around 37.8% of adults were considered obese and 70.4% of adults were considered overweight (CDC, 2017). Unfortunately, there is a strong correlation between obesity and diabetes.

Diabetes is actually a group of diseases in which insulin is not produced correctly or the action of insulin is not adequate. Consequences of uncontrolled diabetes include blindness, kidney damage, cardiovascular disease, and even death. Type I diabetes, which usually begins in childhood or young adulthood, occurs when an individual's immune system destroys the cells in the pancreas that regulate insulin. Insulin, in turn, controls blood sugar (CDC, 2007b). Most individuals with Type I diabetes require injections of insulin. Type II diabetes, which generally occurs in older individuals, is highly associated with obesity. The body does not use insulin well in this type of diabetes. Over 90% of diabetes cases are Type II.

As a health professional, you may have the task of helping an individual who is predisposed to Type II diabetes. You will need to let him or her know that the disease is influenced by many factors, including genetics, metabolism, behavior, environment, culture, and socioeconomic status. Because behavior and environment play such an important role, prevention may be possible. What an outstanding opportunity to implement the skills you will gain from this book and your other courses.

☰ In Conclusion

Epidemiological studies provide much valuable information to health educators. Morbidity (incidence and prevalence) and mortality rates alone can assist health educators in helping individuals and communities obtain information about prevalent infectious or noninfectious diseases and plan appropriate education and prevention programs.

The epidemiological triangle is a guide to understanding how agent, host, and environment interact in the spread of disease. Understanding agents that are commonly found in a community will help determine the types of information that might be presented in an educational program. If highly infectious diseases are present, ill people may need to learn the importance of remaining at home or away from the uninfected population. On the other hand, if a disease that is highly resistant to normal treatments is present, people may need very specific information on what preventive measures to take.

Health educators play an important role in keeping the external environment healthy. You may be asked to help plan a recycling program or determine ways to solve overcrowding. Your largest role, however, may well be in helping people change their internal environments. You may have an opportunity to plan programs about food choices, physical activity, or other lifestyle matters that affect the host.

You may be involved in determining what epidemiological information is needed to plan effective health programs. As a health educator you will need to know how to use the vast amount of epidemiological data available for the benefit of your community. Epidemiology is likely to be an important aspect of your job.

REVIEW QUESTIONS

1. Define incidence and prevalence.

2. Consider the question, "Can the incidence rate of any disease be higher than the prevalence rate for the same disease, at the same time and place, and with the same people?" Explain your answer.

3. Define morbidity and mortality.

4. Consider the question, "Can the mortality rates of two very different cities be compared to determine in which city there is more risk of death?" Explain your answer.

5. Define life expectancy.

6. Give possible reasons for disparities in life expectancies between ethnic groups in the United States.

7. Give examples of agents, host issues, and environmental issues that influence the spread of disease.

8. Briefly describe how the agent, host, and environment interact with one another in infectious diseases.

9. Give examples (other than those listed in the text) of each of the three types of prevention.

10. Describe the four types of epidemiological studies described in the chapter.

11. Identify and analyze a health issue that is currently in the news and the response of health officials.

FOR YOUR APPLICATION

You may have already selected or been assigned a partner community for a project. If not, just select a community. It's time to get to know the community by searching data sources for epidemiologic information about its members. You will want to find information such as life expectancy, leading causes of death, and leading causes of illness. Your search shouldn't stop with morbidity and mortality statistics but should also include health behavior information. As you know, behaviors such as tobacco use, drug and alcohol use, dietary intake, physical activity, and other choices seriously impact health, so collect as much data as possible. If you will remember our discussion about the relationship between poverty and health, you'll realize that you also need information about average socioeconomic status, education levels, and common types of employment for your community members. (The entire needs assessment process is covered in chapter 6.) You should write a summary of the information you collected to add to your project report. Don't forget to use appropriate citations in the text of your summary and begin a reference list for the final report.

4

Health Equity

You've decided to work on gaining some community experience and building your résumé as you work through your degree program. Bravo! You volunteer at a local community center whose clientele is primarily in a low-income bracket. The director asks you to develop a one-day workshop that teaches local residents about healthy eating. You enthusiastically agree, but you discover that this group lives in a food desert with no easy access to fresh vegetables and fruits. Local grocers say they can't keep these food items in stock because people don't buy it "before it goes bad," and they have to increase prices to off-set their costs and potential losses. Local residents say they can't afford these items and have no transportation to other locations where these items may be more available and affordable. It's not as simple as just providing information about what to eat and why. Where do you begin?

Chapter Objectives

1. Define *health equity* and *health disparity*, and explain their significance in addressing health issues in the United States.

2. Explain how social determinants, socio-ecological factors, and structural inequities impact the prevalence and nature of health issues across the life span.

3. Describe specific health issues within selected population groups within the context of socio-ecological influences and health equity.

4. Describe and apply essential elements for promoting health equity.

≡ Faces of America

America continues to grow older and more diverse. Life expectancy in the United States increased from 47.3 years in 1900 to 78.8 in 2014 (National Center for Health Statistics, 2016a; USDHHS, 2015a). According to the U.S. Census Bureau (Colby & Ortman, 2015, March), one in five Americans is projected to be at least 65 years of age by 2030, more than half of Americans will belong to a minority group by 2044, and one in five of the nation's total population will be foreign born by 2060.

At least historically, the overall picture of health in America has improved in comparison to previous decades. According to a NCHS data brief (Hoyert, 2012), the age-adjusted risk of dying declined by 60% from 1935 to 2010 for all Americans (see Figure 4.1). Though declines in dying risk were detected for heart disease, cancer, and stroke, they all remained among the top five leading causes of death across that 75-year span; heart disease and cancer ranked as numbers one and two respectively. The risk of dying for children ages one through four years across that same time span decreased by 94% while the decline for adults aged 85 or more years was 38%. The risk of dying for all race subgroups tracked across that time span also decreased though differences between groups (the disparity gap) persists (with the widest gaps most evident between 1988 and 1996).

These general trends in lower death rates for the total population are encouraging. But, do these numbers tell the whole story about the health status of Americans? Despite

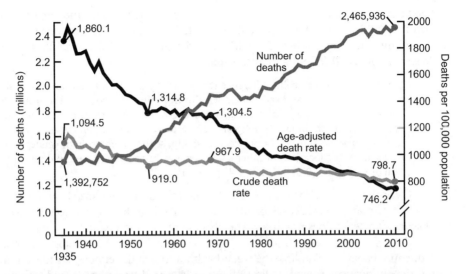

Figure 4.1   Trends in age-adjusted risk of dying in the U.S. 1935–2010.

Notes: 2010 data are preliminary. Crude death rates on an annual basis are per 100,000 population; age-adjusted rates are per 100,000 U.S. standard population. Rates for 2001–2009 are revised and may differ from rates previously published.

From *75 Years of Mortality in the United States, 1935–2010*, by D. L. Hoyert, 2012, March, NCHS data brief, no 88. Hyattsville, MD: National Center for Health Statistics. Retrieved from http://www.cdc.gov/nchs/data/databriefs/db88.htm#male

increasing longevity, on average, Americans have reported that they suffered poor mental health on at least 3.7 of the last 30 days and suffered from poor physical health on at least 3.9 of the last 30 days (United Health Foundation, 2017). Though these numbers may seem small, they actually serve as a significant indicator of some important health issues. Experiencing poor physical health days is an indicator of pervading illnesses (chronic and acute) and health issues that continue to plague many Americans. Poor mental health days can be used to predict health-related quality of life, mental distress and illness, the number of office visits and hospitalizations, and, in extreme cases, suicide, which is the 10th leading cause of death for all ages and the 2nd leading cause of death among adults aged 25 through 34 (United Health Foundation, 2017). Both of these indicators, poor physical and mental health days, are directly related to quality of life.

Another important consideration when examining the health status of America is the existence of health disparities across groups that we briefly mentioned in previous chapters. Leaders of *Healthy People 2020* (2016, June 6, Disparities) pointed out that reducing and, then, eliminating health disparities has been an overarching goal for decades. Though some strides have been made toward achieving that goal, disparities still exist. For that reason, the goals of achieving health equity and improving the health of all groups were added to the goal of eliminating disparities as one of the four overarching goals. These leaders addressed the terms health equity and health disparity and explained the importance of these goals as follows. *Healthy People 2020* defines health equity as the "attainment of the highest level of health for all people. Achieving health equity requires valuing everyone equally with focused and ongoing societal efforts to address avoidable inequalities, historical and contemporary injustices, and the elimination of health and health care disparities" (USDHHS, 2014b, para. 5). *Healthy People 2020* defines a **health disparity** as

> a particular type of health difference that is closely linked with social, economic, and/or environmental disadvantage. Health disparities adversely affect groups of people who have systematically experienced greater obstacles to health based on their racial or ethnic group; religion; socioeconomic status; gender; age; mental health; cognitive, sensory, or physical disability; sexual orientation or gender identity; geographic location; or other characteristics historically linked to discrimination or exclusion. (USDHHS, 2014b, para. 6)

Over the years, efforts to eliminate disparities and achieve health equity have focused primarily on diseases or illnesses and on health care services. However, the absence of disease does not automatically equate to good health.

Powerful, complex relationships exist between health and biology, genetics, and individual behavior. The links between health and health services, socioeconomic status, the physical environment, discrimination, racism, literacy levels, and legislative policies are also complicated. These factors, which influence an individual's or population's health, are known as determinants of health. (USDHHS, 2016, June 6, *Disparities*).

Though the overall trends in the health status of Americans are encouraging, some subgroups in the U.S. population (women, older adults, and some ethnic communities) are more vulnerable to the effects of poverty and face unique health challenges. Table 4.1 and Figure 4.2 illustrate differences in income by ethnic groups in the United States, a factor that significantly impacts health equity across these populations. Measures of health and mortality for the total U.S. population can cloud the true picture of health and quality of life among Americans in different stages of the life span and from different walks of life.

In this chapter, we will examine health issues that impact communities within communities and analyze how social determinants and socio-ecological factors influence the etiology and severity of disease. As a future health professional, it is vital that you understand how social determinants play a role in the development of disease and contribute to health inequities. In describing select populations, we will approach this with a wide net, moving beyond categorizations based on skin color, to discuss communities within communities tied together by a common characteristic (or characteristics); examples include occupation, age group, culture, ethnic background, gender, and/or an environmental setting in which residents share exposure to a unique health risk. The role of social determinants and socio-ecological factors are explained through a number of examples.

Table 4.1   Living in Poverty: 2014

Group	% of group
White, Non-Hispanic	10.1%
Hispanic or Latino (any race)	23.6%
Black or African American	26.2%
Asian	12.0%
Total U.S. Population	**14.8%**

Source: *Income and Poverty in the United States: 2014,* Current Population Reports, P60-252, by C. DeNavas-Walt and B. D. Proctor, 2015, U.S. Census Bureau. Washington, DC: U.S. Government Printing Office. Retrieved from https://www.census.gov/content/dam/Census/library/publications/2015/demo/p60-252.pdf

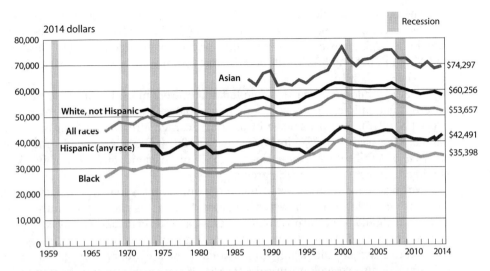

Figure 4.2   Real median household income by race and Hispanic origin: 1967–2014.

Note: The 2013 data reflect the implementation of the redesigned income questions. Median household income data are not available prior to 1967. For more information on confidentiality protection, sampling error, nonsampling error, and definitions, see <ftp://ftp2.census.gov/programs-surveys/cps/techdocs/cpsmar15.pdf>.

From *Income and Poverty in the United States: 2014,* Current Population Reports, P60-252, by C. DeNavas-Walt and B. D. Proctor, 2015, U.S. Census Bureau. Washington, DC: U.S. Government Printing Office. Retrieved from https://www.census.gov/content/dam/Census/library/publications/2015/demo/p60-252.pdf

≡ Health Through the Life Span

One of the four overarching goals of *Healthy People 2020* is to "promote quality life, healthy development, and health behaviors across all life stages" (USDHHS, n.d., p. 1). This goal is based on evidence that health status, along with the risk factors and determinants related to health, vary across the life span.

America's Children

The Federal Interagency Forum on Child and Family Statistics (FIFCFS, 2016) was founded to facilitate a collaborative approach to collecting and reporting federal data about U.S. children and families. The FIFCFS reports, which can be obtained from their website at www.childstats.gov, contain information about population growth trends among children living in the U.S. and information about key indicators within seven domains: family and social environment, economic circumstances, health care, physical environment and safety, behavior, education, and health. Focusing on these domains to better understand child health within context is in harmony with the attention to social determinants of health used to frame the *Healthy People 2020* mission (see chapter 2).

The number of children living in America was expected to grow to 76.3 million by 2030 in comparison to 72.4 million in 2000 (FIFCFS, 2016). By 2050, 39% of children in the U.S. are expected to be White, non-Hispanics (compared to 74% in 1980 and 52% in 2015) and 32% will be Hispanic (compared to 9% in 1980 and 25% in 2015) (FIFCFS, 2016).

In 2014, children in married-couple families were much less likely to be living in poverty than children living in female-householder families with no spouse present (FIFCFS, 2016). The percentage of all American children living with two married parents decreased from 77% in 1980 to 64% in 2014. When grouped by race/ethnicity, 74% of White-alone (non-Hispanic), 58% of Hispanic, and 34% of Black-alone children lived with two married parents.

We must be careful to avoid making assumptions about the impact of family structure on child health, however, some evidence is in place that family structure matters. It should be no surprise that, in some cases, a single parent may struggle with health care costs, challenges inherent to juggling work and family care, and other factors that can impact child health. Grandparents who are primary care givers for young children can also struggle to remain abreast of current health information, care for their young charges, and care for their own health and other needs.

Though birth rates in the overall U.S. population have recently decreased, increases in births to unmarried women are impacting child health. Low birth weight, infant mortality, and poverty are more prevalent among children of unmarried women (FIFCFS, 2015). Low birth weight (LBW) is of particular importance because of its association with serious infant health conditions such as respiratory distress syndrome and problems related to brain, heart, and intestinal development; and its relationship with long-term health problems such as obesity, diabetes, and heart disease (March of Dimes, 2017).

Because these risks are more likely among women of younger ages, it is important to note that the birth rate among women ages 15 to 19 has been on a relatively steady decline from its last peak in 1991 at 62 per 1,000 to 24 per 1,000 in 2014 (Child Trends Data Bank, 2016). This is highly significant in light of reports from the Child Trends Data Bank (2016) that children born to mothers in this age group are more likely to be born prematurely, at low birth weight, and at higher risk to infant death than infants born to mothers ages 20 and older. Infants of teen moms are also more likely to exhibit poorer academic skills, such as math and reading scores, language and communication skills, social skills, and behavioral skills. They are also more likely to struggle with physical and emotional well-being than children of older mothers.

If the child has working parents or grandparents, another contributing factor to his or her health and well-being is the time spent in childcare and the quality of the childcare received. Involvement in extracurricular activities (e.g., the arts, sports, religious activities, and community service) can be important to child development and safety. The extent to which children are left to care for themselves is a critical factor (FIFCFS, 2015). In 2012, 61% of America's children not yet in kindergarten were in center-based care (an increase from 55% in 2007). Though the nature of the impact of center-based care on child health is debatable, these trends serve as an indication that attention to the type of care and its impact are important.

In 2014, about 22% of all school-aged children spoke a language other than English at home, and 5% of school-aged children spoke another language at home and had difficulty speaking English (FIFCFS, 2016). These language barriers can impact child health and well-being as children struggle to succeed in schools and, later, in job markets where English is the primary language used. Language can also be a barrier for the parents and immediate caregivers of some of these children—those who may also struggle to navigate the English-dominated health system in the U.S.

You have probably noted that economics have permeated this discussion about child health. Low income can be a direct causal factor when, for example, parents cannot afford adequate health care nor provide a health-enhancing living environment for their children. It can also be part of a life-long cycle when impoverished children, including those who face language barriers, struggle in school and therefore miss employment opportunities, contributing to low income and poor health in their adulthood. The following quotation provides further explanation of this complex web of impact.

> Children living in poverty are vulnerable to environmental, educational, health, and safety risks. Compared with their peers, children living in poverty, especially young children, are more likely to have cognitive, behavioral, and socioemotional difficulties. Additionally, throughout their lifetimes, they are more likely to complete fewer years of school and experience more years of unemployment. (FIFCFS, 2016, p. 12)

Even in cases where poverty is not a factor, America's children are at risk to conditions that are critical for health and well-being. Leaders of *Healthy People 2020* (USDHHS, 2017b) have identified the following as some critical risks for America's children: developmental and behavioral disorders, child maltreatment, asthma and other chronic conditions, obesity, dental caries, and unintentional injuries. You can learn more about these and other child health issues by visiting the *Early and Middle Childhood* topic section of the *Healthy People 2020* website (USDHHS, 2017b).

When the health of a nation suffers, its children are among those who suffer most. Conversely, when community partners work together to improve the lives of community members, children are among those most likely to gain. We encourage you to consider how you can become part of the support system for America's children.

America's Adolescents

The future of a nation is in many ways dependent on the health of its youth. Leaders of *Healthy People 2020* (USDHHS, 2017a) have included the health of adolescents (ages 10 to 19) as an important focal area for promoting America's health. These leaders indicated that "adolescence is a critical transitional period that includes the biological changes of puberty and the need to negotiate key developmental tasks, such as increasing independence and normative experimentation" (USDHHS, 2017a, para. 5). Their list of highlighted examples of important adolescent health issues include homicide, suicide, motor vehicle crashes (including those caused by drinking and driving), substance use and abuse, smoking, sexually transmitted infections (including human immunodeficiency virus), teen and unplanned pregnancies, and homelessness.

The primary health issues of adolescents are strongly influenced by social environments, mediated by behavioral choices, and largely preventable (USDHHS,

2017a). FYI 4.1 contains some research-based highlights of environmental factors that influence adolescent health. Social influences from family, school, neighborhoods, and the media influence health-impacting behaviors among adolescents.

According to *Healthy People 2020* leaders (USDHHS, 2017a), the ethnic diversity of American adolescents is rapidly increasing with high growth rates occurring among Hispanic and Asian Americans in particular. Thus, strong attention to culturally-sound health promotion efforts will be important in the coming decades. Because of the prevalence of poverty and other social barriers in some ethnic groups, a focus on interventions that include a strong development perspective has been recommended.

Leaders of the Office of Adolescent Health (2016), established by the U.S. Department of Health and Human Services, provided more detailed information about adolescents that may be of particular use when developing adolescent health interventions. Developmental, physical, and behavioral differences exist between

4.1   Environmental Influences on Adolescent Health: Research Highlights

Family
- Adolescents who perceive that they have good communication and are bonded with an adult are less likely to engage in risky behaviors.
- Parents who provide supervision and are involved with their adolescents' activities are promoting a safe environment in which to explore opportunities.
- The children of families living in poverty are more likely to have health conditions and poorer health status, as well as less access to and utilization of health care.

School
- Academic success and achievement are strong predictors of overall adult health outcomes. Proficient academic skills are associated with lower rates of risky behaviors and higher rates of healthy behaviors.
- High school graduation leads to lower rates of health problems and risk for incarceration, as well as enhanced financial stability during adulthood.
- The school social environment affects students' attendance, academic achievement, and behavior. A safe and healthy school environment promotes student engagement and protects against risky behaviors and dropping out.

Neighborhoods
- Adolescents growing up in distressed neighborhoods characterized by concentrated poverty are at risk for a variety of negative outcomes, including poor physical and mental health, delinquency, and risky sexual behavior.

Media Exposure
- Adolescents who are exposed to media portrayals of violence, sexual content, smoking, and drinking are at risk for adopting these behaviors.

Source: "Adolescent Health," *Healthy People 2020*, United Stated Department of Health and Human Services, 2016, June 1. Retrieved from https://www.healthypeople.gov/2020/topics-objectives/topic/Adolescent-Health

younger (ages 10 to 14) and older (ages 15 to 19) adolescents, and between genders within each group. For example, older adolescents are more likely to engage in risky behaviors—such as drug use and sexual activity—than younger adolescents. Male adolescents are more likely than female adolescents to use and abuse tobacco, alcohol, and other drugs and are less likely than their female counterparts to seek health care as they get older. Female adolescents are more likely than male adolescents to be physically inactive and engage in eating-related behaviors (skipping meals, intentional vomiting) that can lead to weight management issues and eating disorders.

The percentage of adolescents in the total U.S. population is expected to decrease from 13.2% in 2014 to 11.2% in 2050 (Office of Adolescent Health, 2016). However, this projected proportion shift will occur because more Americans are living longer, so older adults now represent a growing proportion of the American population. Despite this shift, the actual number of American adolescents is expected to grow from an approximate 42 million in 2016 to almost 45 million by 2050. This growth in adolescent numbers, coupled with the potential impact of adolescent decisions on long-term health, renders this period of the life span a critical moment for health promotion.

The challenge of working with adolescents is sometimes tough, and the stakes can be very high. Yet fostering family and school connectedness and instilling in adolescents an optimistic sense of purpose about their future have been proven to positively affect risk-taking behavior. The more equipped you are with adolescent-specific knowledge and skills, the more likely you are to make a difference. You can impact the viability of the nation and influence tomorrow's health leaders through your efforts to promote health among today's adolescents.

America's Adults

The term *adult* can be misleading because it is commonly used to describe a wide range of ages and experience. You can obtain adult mortality data from the NCHS's Health Data Interactive website. The data tables include, among other things, mortality rates for all adults 18 years old and over (the total U.S. adult population) and for subgroups clustered by age ranges: 18–34, 35–44, 45–64, 65–84, and 85+ years. These age ranges pose some challenges in interpreting the data. For example, the youngest adult age range (18–34) could include a single 18-year-old college student living in a dorm *and* a 34-year-old homeowner with a spouse, two children, and a mortgage. Differences in socioeconomic status, age, geographic location, education, ethnicity, and a wide variety of other factors exist among adults in these groups. However, despite these limitations, these data sets provide valuable information about the general health of U.S. adults in each age range and as a whole. This information can be used to compare the status of U.S. citizens to that of other countries, and it can be used by you to compare the status of local populations with which you work to national norms for specific age groups. We have reported information in the following sections to highlight a few important health issues and social determinants that impact well-being in some selected age groups.

COLLEGE STUDENTS

In 2015, roughly one in three American adults (33%) had completed a bachelor's degree or higher (Ryan & Bauman, 2016). Though this proportion of the adult population may seem relatively small, growth trends over time indicate a steady increase since 1940, when only 5% of American adults had completed a college degree. Though online degrees and non-traditional study opportunities are impacting the typical college student profile, health issues and contributing factors unique to the traditional college student (ages 18 to 24) have gained the attention of leaders of the Centers for Disease Control and Prevention (CDC, 2015a; 2016f), the American College Health Association, and other health-focused organizations (The Nemours Foundation, 2016; United States National Library of Medicine, 2017).

For the typical first-year college student who moves to a campus, the transition to living in a campus-oriented environment can be highly stressful as this student develops new relationships, learns to navigate academic systems, and adjusts to new routines (The Nemours Foundation, 2016). According to the CDC (2015a; 2016f), traditional college students can be at risk to weight gain (the freshman 15), physical inactivity, sleep deprivation, binge drinking, substance abuse and smoking, sexually transmitted infections, sexual assault, exposure to illnesses from other students, and inadequate health care.

Members of the Healthy Campus Coalition, sponsored by the American College Health Association (2016), developed a Healthy Campus 2020 program that is linked to the *Healthy People 2020* initiative. Coalition members are interested in helping professionals in higher education promote the health and well-being of their campus communities. You can learn more about health issues and ongoing initiatives through the websites of organizations mentioned in this section.

WORKING ADULTS

Adults aged 25 to 64 are usually included in discussions about the health and well-being of "working adults." However, marked differences across this age range exist. Figure 4.3 contains a snap shot of the leading causes of death by age group in 2016 (CDC, 2017a). As can be noted there, the order and makeup of the five leading causes of death shift by decade with unintentional injury, suicide, and homicide dominating among adults aged 25 to 34 and gradually giving way to malignant neoplasm (cancer) and heart disease as age increases. It is notable that unintentional injuries are among the top three causes of death for adults in each decade of the 25 to 64-year-old life span, and suicide ranks among the top five causes on the list for adults in three age groups (25 to 54 years).

These trends in causes of death across the working adult life span are associated with some common lifestyle patterns. **Controllable risk factors** that contribute significantly to heart disease and cancer are chronic physical inactivity, unhealthy dietary patterns, obesity, and tobacco use. These lifestyle habits are often formed early in life with the resulting chronic conditions emerging at an older age.

Unintentional injuries and suicide are of high concern for all subgroups of this age group (25 to 64 years). The majority of deaths from unintentional injuries result from motor-vehicular accidents (NCHS, 2016a). Though suicide ranked higher as a cause of death among younger adults in 2014, the rates of suicide deaths were higher among males aged 45 to 64 and 65 and older, and among females aged 45 to 64, than they were among younger adults in that year (NCHS, 2016a).

Most adults know that regular physical activity, proper diet, and abstinence from tobacco use are good for them. They also know that risky behaviors such as drinking and driving can result in life-impacting physical harm. So, why don't they do "the right thing" when it comes to these behaviors? To understand this, other influencing factors must be considered. Working adults aged 25 to 64 years old are a diverse group with a variety of needs and interests. Some common health-influencing factors for this age group include financial pressures at all levels of the socioeconomic scale, relationship and responsibility stressors at home and work, and low motivation to attend to personal health in light of these other pressures. The suicide rates previously discussed

Rank	25–34	35–44	45–54	55–64	65+	Total
1			Malignant Neoplasms 41,291	Malignant Neoplasms 116,364	Heart Disease 507,118	Heart Disease 635,260
2		Malignant Neoplasms 10,903	Heart Disease 34,027	Heart Disease 78,610	Malignant Neoplasms 422,927	Malignant Neoplasms 598,038
3		Heart Disease 10,477			Chronic Low-Respiratory Disease 131,002	
4	Malignant Neoplasms 3,791			Chronic Low Respiratory Disease 17,810	Cerebro-vascular 121,630	Chronic Low-Respiratory Disease 154,596
5	Heart Disease 3,445		Liver Disease 8,364	Diabetes Mellitus 14,251	Alzheimer's Disease 114,883	Cerebro-vascular 142,142
6	Liver Disease 925	Liver Disease 2,851	Diabetes Mellitus 6,267	Liver Disease 13,448	Diabetes Mellitus 56,452	Alzheimer's Disease 116,103
7	Diabetes Mellitus 792	Diabetes Mellitus 2,049	Cerebro-vascular 5,353	Cerebro-vascular 12,310	Unintentional Injury 53,141	Diabetes Mellitus 80,058
8	Cerebro-vascular 575	Cerebro-vascular 1,851	Chronic Low. Respiratory Disease 4,307		Influenza & Pneumonia 42,479	Influenza & Pneumonia 51,537
9	HIV 546	HIV 971	Septicemia 2,472	Septicemia 5,941	Nephritis 41,095	Nephritis 50,046
10	Complicated Pregnancy 472	Septicemia 897		Nephritis 5,650	Septicemia 30,405	

Figure 4.3   Ten leading causes of death: 2016.

From *10 Leading Causes of Death and Injury: 2016*, Centers for Disease Control and Prevention, 2017, May 2. Retrieved from https://www.cdc.gov/injury/wisqars/LeadingCauses.html

should serve as a strong indicator that mental and emotional pressures for adults in this age group should be an important consideration. The health professional who understands these needs will be better equipped to work in adult-based health promotion settings.

OLDER ADULTS

As longevity increases in the United States, health and quality of life among older Americans (aged 65 and older) has become a critical topic in discussions about national health. As the baby boomer generation has moved into this span of life, some have redefined what it means to be *older* as some continue to work or pursue totally different interests long after the traditionally expected retirement age.

Yet, as these Americans live to older ages than were the norm for previous generations, common chronic health conditions and quality of life in this age group are an important focus. The leading causes of death for adults aged 65 and older are heart disease, cancer, and lower respiratory diseases (see Figure 4.3). Cerebrovascular disease, Alzheimer's disease, and diabetes rank fourth, fifth, and sixth respectively. According to the NCHS (2016b), a significant number of older adults struggle with complications related to obesity.

Because health-risk behaviors and conditions impact multiple body systems, it is common for some adults to develop more than one chronic health condition. The U.S. Department of Health and Human Services (2015, October 18) launched an initiative to address **multiple chronic conditions (MCC)**. The following information from their MCC website provides a clear explanation of MCC.

> Chronic conditions are conditions that last a year or more and require ongoing medical attention and/or limit activities of daily living. They include both physical conditions such as arthritis, cancer, and HIV infection. Also included are mental and cognitive disorders, such as ongoing depression, substance addiction, and dementia.
>
> MCC are concurrent chronic conditions. In other words, multiple chronic conditions are two or more chronic conditions that affect a person at the same time. For example, either a person with arthritis and hypertension or a person with heart disease and depression, both have multiple chronic conditions. (USDHHS, 2015b, *About the chronic conditions initiative*, para. 3)

According to the USDHHS (2015, October 18), three out of four older Americans (aged 65 or older) have MCC. MCC is associated with poor day-to-day functioning and high mortality risk, and accounts for 66% of America's health care spending. Based on age-adjusted life expectancy rates (NCHS, 2016b), a 65-year-old man can expect to live another 17.9 years, and a woman of that age can expect to live another 20.5 years. Your contributions as a health professional to the well-being of older Americans have the potential to impact your own quality of life as an older adult.

≣ Root Causes of Health Inequity

As you read about health issues through the life span, you probably noted that poverty, social environments, low family connectedness, language barriers, parenting pressures, and other life stressors were highlighted as factors that influence the health status of individuals and specific groups. We highlighted those because, as indicated by leaders of the Office of Minority Health (OMH), "the conditions in the places where people are born, grow, live, work, play, learn, and age have significant impact on the health outcomes of individuals, families, and their communities" (OMH, 2017, *Welcome*, para. 2).

The Impact of Social Determinants on Health Inequity

As we explained in chapter 2, understanding the impact of social determinants on health is critical to your effectiveness as a health professional. It is particularly important in shaping your perspectives regarding the health inequities that exist in the United States for many ethnic groups and other subpopulations. That is because these health disparities are largely attributable to differences in resources, opportunities, and risk. Leaders of the Office of Minority Health described this phenomenon and its importance as follows:

> Health disparities—the differences in health and well-being—have a significant impact on our nation and among racial and ethnic populations in particular. Minorities are less likely to get the preventive care needed to stay healthy, less likely to receive quality care, and more likely to face poorer health outcomes. . . . Healthier communities mean lower health care costs, which translate into a stronger economy and a more productive, competitive America.
>
> Our work and the work of our partners creates bridges that help make high quality education, safe neighborhoods, quality housing, reliable transportation, clean surroundings, nutritious food, and stable employment available to all Americans. It is work that touches the everyday lives of American communities: transportation that makes it possible to get to a well visit; neighborhoods where it is possible to exercise or play outdoors; and accessible grocery stores that make it possible to eat a well-balanced diet. (OMH, 2017, *Learn More*, para. 1–2, 4).

In 2017, the National Academies of Sciences, Engineering, and Medicine (NASEM) released a report called *Communities in Action: Pathways to Health Equity* (NASEM, 2017), in which the authors described the underlying root causes of health inequity and recommended community-based solutions to promote health equity. These leaders stated that health inequity "arises from social, economic, environmental, and structural disparities that contribute to intergroup differences in health outcomes both within and between societies" (p. 124). They used the term *structural inequities* to refer to "the systematic disadvantage of one social group compared to other groups with whom they coexist that are deeply embedded in the fabric of society" (p. 127). This structure is shaped by policies, law, governance, and culture that contribute to an unequal distribution of power and resources across groups. These structural inequities and the resulting health inequities have been evidenced for groups that differ from the mainstream in terms of race and ethnicity, gender, sexual orientation, disability status, and religious identity.

Examples of Health Inequity

We created Figure 4.4 to further illustrate our point that the influence of social determinants and socio-ecological factors on an individual's health goes beyond his or her lifestyle and individual behaviors; social determinants include various levels, including social/cultural and community support, workplace/occupational hazards, and public policies. We invite you to refer to this figure as you read the following examples about how some aspects of social determinants and socio-ecological factors are impacting the health status of specific groups. These examples are not intended to serve as an exhaustive list of all health disparity issues. We recommend that you visit the website of the Office of Minority Health at www.omh.gov as a starting point for gaining an in-depth understanding of health disparities.

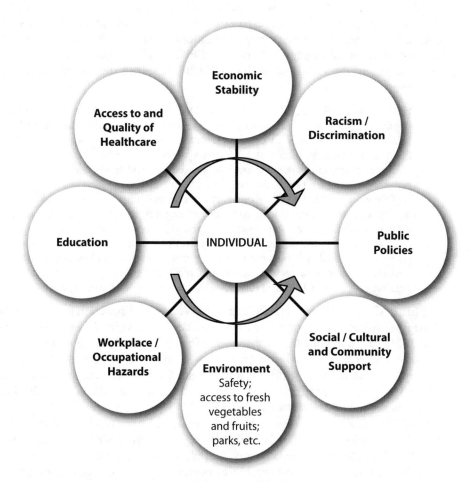

Figure 4.4. Examples of social determinants that affect individual health.
Factors that impact the individual include external/environmental socio-ecological influences. For example: culture, environment, education, working conditions, access to medical care, and community infrastructure all have a positive or negative impact on one's health and well-being. Therefore, external determinants such as social support and elements of the community should be considered when planning health education and public health programs, activities, and campaigns (Clark & Utz, 2014).

TYPE 2 DIABETES IN LATINX POPULATIONS

Type 2 diabetes is the sixth leading cause of death in the United States and one of the leading chronic killers among adults (CDC, 2018b). The rates of diabetes among those who are Latinx, a gender neutral term that has replaced the term *Hispanics* in some settings, are almost double the rates of non-Latinx Whites (see "Hispanic" in Figure 4.5) and even higher among African Americans and American Indian/Alaska Natives (CDC, 2018b). However, the reason behind these higher rates has more to do with social determinants and socio-ecological factors than ethnicity.

Most research and resulting clinical strategies for various populations with diabetes have focused on individuals with short-term health improvements that have not been maintained over time. More recently, researchers have recognized the need to consider the social determinants of diabetes and health along with individual factors. For example, Clark and Utz (2014) explored the link between social determinants of health and diabetes. In their review of peer-reviewed literature, they found that several social determinants such as physical environment, education, and social/community support were commonly associated with diagnosis of diabetes. Moreover, Vega, Rodriguez, and Gruski (2009) published findings about the role of social determinants on Latinx morbidity and mortality in relation to type 2 diabetes. Strengthening the argument that factors external to the individual have more influence on overall health status than genetics, the results of their epidemiological study emphasized that "there is no viable evidence to support an explanation of genetic determinants of differential morbidity and mortality outcomes by nativity in this population" (p. 2). Second, Vega and colleagues illustrated how socioeconomics and acculturation play a role in the

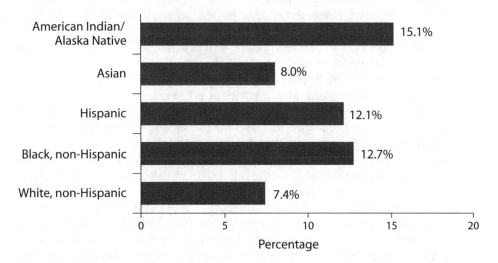

Figure 4.5   Percentage of U.S. adults aged 18 or older with diagnosed diabetes, by racial and ethnic group, 2013–2015.

From *Diabetes Report Card 2017*, Centers for Disease Control and Prevention, 2018, Atlanta, GA: Author, U.S. Department of Health and Human Services. Retrieved from https://www.cdc.gov/diabetes/pdfs/library/diabetesreportcard2017-508.pdf

development of diabetes: "Latinx immigrants have lower income and educational status and experience superior mortality outcomes compared to wealthier and better-educated US-born Latinx" (p. 7).

Research has also demonstrated a direct relationship between socioeconomic status and health outcomes. According to Patton (2016) and the Pew Research Center, women and men of color earn significantly less than White men and women, although this varies by ethnic population. According to this report, Latinx males earn less than Asian and African American males and only 69% of what White males earn hourly. Latinx women also earned less than Asian and African American women and only 58% of the median hourly wage for White men (Patton, 2016). Socioeconomics is also strongly associated with other social determinants, such as education, stress, depression, and unhealthy eating and obesity, which can compound to increase rates of diabetes (WHO, n.d.).

Access to health care and quality of care also influences the development of diabetes. Immigrant Latinx adults are least likely to receive preventative care, to have a usual source of health care, to have health insurance coverage, or to receive guideline-based health information compared to non-immigrant Latinx or White adults (CDC, 2014; Clark & Utz, 2014). Components of the physical environment also play a role in the development of diabetes among Latinx populations. Transportation, neighborhood safety, and healthy food are examples of components of the physical environment. Inadequate access to resources among marginalized populations means fewer resources are available to overcome barriers, thus effects are magnified. For example, limited transportation for Latinx adults in rural areas may require traveling far distances to gain access to health care providers or grocery stores with fresh food options. Due to higher crime rates, lack of sidewalks, and lack of places for recreation, residents of urban communities may be less physically active and/or obese, both attributing to diabetes risk.

Education level is commonly linked with health outcomes (WHO, n.d.). The incidence and prevalence of type 2 diabetes increases as education levels decrease (Hill, Nielson, & Fox, 2013). Research has also shown that individuals with higher levels of education are more likely to participate in preventive health care including eating healthier foods, being more physically active, and avoiding obesity. This is largely because the level of education increases the likelihood of socioeconomic stability and access to resources and care (Clark & Utz, 2014). Education level can also refer to a lack of information. For example, if culturally tailored health information about the disease is not made available, that may also impact risk as well as self-management of type 2 diabetes in Latinx populations (Melancon, Oomen-Early, & del Rincon, 2009).

Culture/social and community support includes individuals' "formal and informal relationships that give rise to a belief that one is cared for or supported emotionally in a defined situation such as working toward improving health outcomes" (Clark & Utz, 2014, p. 298). The degree of social support may vary between individuals and among ethnic groups; for example, research revealed that Latinx individuals diagnosed with diabetes prefer group and family medical visits for self-management support, whereas individuals from non-Latinx groups are more likely to indicate that they have no preference (Clark & Utz, 2014). Just as greater social support correlates with improved self-management outcomes, the perception of negative or low levels of social support has been shown to increase the risk of fewer self-management behaviors among Latinx adults (Melancon, Oomen-Early, & del Rincon, 2009). Diabetes is perceived as a "family disease" for many Latinx adults living with the disease, and this can be both a positive and negative factor. A participant in a study by Melancon, Oomen-Early, and del Rincon (2009) explained it this way:

> It (type 2 diabetes) takes a lot of patience and support from everyone in your life. I'm terrified and don't want this for my family. They can see I am different now and blame the changes on diabetes. At times I have trouble seeing, and I get confused. But love from my family keeps me trying to fight it. (p. 6)

Workplace conditions including exposures to toxic chemicals (such as pesticides); unstable employment; confronting work-related trauma; assault; and/or persistent social stressors, such as discrimination, are determinants which also impact rates of disease and injury. Unfortunately, marked employment disparities have been noted among racial and ethnic groups in the U.S., with Latinx and other non-White populations overrepresented in service occupations and manual labor segments such as construction, agriculture, hospitality, and factory positions (Mora, 2015). These positions usually provide lower wages and increased risk for physical injury and chronic conditions. Exposure to hazardous materials or chemicals, physically taxing labor, or jobs that require more sedentary behaviors can also produce a confounding effect on biological factors that increase risk to diabetes, such as increased cortisol levels, development of metabolic syndrome, sleep irregularities, and obesity.

INFECTIOUS DISEASE AMONG REFUGEES

Refugees are "men, women and children fleeing war, persecution and political upheaval who have crossed borders to seek safety in another country" (Rescue Organization, 2017, *Overview*, para. 1). Many refugee communities currently exist in the United States and they are expected to grow. In fact, since the 1980 Refugee Act, around three million refugees have resettled in the United States (Krogstad & Radford, 2017). When the Soviet Union broke up, many refugees came to the United States from those areas; recently, refugees have arrived from Syria and the Democratic Republic of Congo due to political turmoil (Igielnik & Krogstad, 2017). Unfortunately, because we often hear about refugees in only a political context (good or bad; cost-effective or cost-draining), we rarely talk or hear about refugees as members of a community.

Refugees often come from countries that struggle with infectious diseases due to lack of resources as a result of the conflicts occurring. One of the most prevalent communicable diseases among refugees is tuberculosis. Other less serious conditions, such as skin infections, can also cause distress. The social determinants we have discussed thus far also impact the health of refugees. In 2015, the health of children in a large Somali community in Minnesota (Guo, 2015) was impacted by the same misinformation that has occurred among many Americans. While the vast majority of Americans get their children vaccinated today, in the past, many parents chose not to due to an unfounded belief that vaccines were related to autism. The misinformation spread quickly through journalists, movie stars, athletes, and parents. Today, a small population still chooses not to have their children vaccinated.

In 2017, a measles outbreak occurred among the Somali children in the community mentioned above; at one point, 76 children in the community had measles. The outbreak was related to fear and misinformation. The following is an excerpt from a KAALTV article, which offered comments regarding the cause of the outbreak and its solution as viewed by Sahra Noor, the CEO of a community health clinic in the area. Noor said,

> If you ask any Somali, whether they are doctors or the person that just arrived from the refugee camp, they know that the Department of Health has said there's no link (between measles and autism). They don't believe it. They are not buying it. (Fazal, 2017, para. 12)

Noor explained that Somali parents are worried that instances of autism are higher in their community and they feel that most parents in their community are vaccinating their children. They don't see any research studying the reason for the high rates of autism and have determined it is due to the vaccinations because of this correlation. She said the answer to the measles crisis is inside the Somali community.

> We need Somali providers to speak up, we need Somali parents to speak up, we need religious leaders to speak up and policy makers who look like us to speak up. Once we own the issue, it's easier to solve. (Fazal, 2017, para. 16)

It's important to remember that depending on the prevalent health issues in the place from which refugees come, the resources they had before fleeing, and the trials of the journey to safety, health issues and therefore health disparities may already exist prior to arrival in the U.S. People seek refuge due to "persecution based on race, gender, political and religious beliefs, and nationality" (Lopez, 2014), but the unfortunate truth is that these same factors may further negatively impact the health of refugees once in the United States and deepen health disparities among them.

EMOTIONAL DISTRESS, DEPRESSION, AND SUICIDE AMONG LGBTQ YOUTH

Accumulating evidence indicates that adolescents who identify as lesbian, gay, bisexual, transgender, and queer (LGBTQ) experience greater feelings of isolation and discrimination than heterosexual youth (Almeida, Johnson, Corliss, Molnar, & Azrael, 2009). LGBTQ youth are also more likely to exhibit symptoms of emotional distress, including depressive symptoms, suicidal ideation, and suicide attempts (Almeida et al., 2009; Ueno, 2005). For instance, data from the 2015 Youth Risk Behavior Surveillance (YRBS) system showed that 30% of youth who identified as lesbian, gay, or bisexual had seriously attempted suicide, while roughly 46% had considered it. This is significantly higher than heterosexual youth who considered taking their lives (26%). The report also revealed that lesbian, gay, and bisexual students are as much as *three times more likely* to experience physical and sexual dating violence than their heterosexual peers.

The social stigma associated with homosexuality, and deviation from socially-prescribed gender roles in general, remains pervasive, particularly for young people. LGBTQ adolescents live in social environments in which they may be exposed to negative experiences, including social rejection and isolation, diminished social support, discrimination, and verbal and physical violence. When combined with other risk factors and a lack of support, such violence can put young people at high risk for suicide. Despite growing evidence of the emotional toll negative experiences related to LGBTQ stigma has on youths, gaps in knowledge remain. The good news is that expanding supportive policies and services in schools for LGBTQ adolescents may help to counter the detrimental effects of discrimination. Studies have reported the positive impact of LGBTQ support groups (e.g., Pride and Gay-Straight Alliances) and other efforts to improve the climate for LGBTQ high school students (Almeida et al., 2009).

As Almeida et al. (2009) reported:

> Lesbian, gay, and queer high school students who attended schools with support groups *had half the risk of reporting victimization* and were *less than one third as likely to report multiple suicide attempts.* In addition, lesbian, gay, and bisexual students who perceived that there was a school staff member who they could turn to for help had a lower likelihood of reporting multiple suicide attempts. (p. 1105)

High levels of victimization appear to be more detrimental to the mental health of gay, queer, and transgender youth as compared to heterosexual youth. This fact still remains largely unexamined. It is possible that those youth have less social support or fewer resources to cope with victimization experiences, or that their victimization experiences are more severe (Dunbar, 2006). Taking into account the entire body of literature on health among adolescents who report being LGBTQ, it is important to better understand the experiences of these youths and support initiatives that address creating safe and supportive environments to ensure their emotional well-being. As the Trevor Project website admonishes, "We have been reminded countless times that a threat against any one community is a threat against all of us, and that we must take notice and action . . . moving forward with love and acceptance for all" (The Trevor Project, 2017, para. 4).

MUSLIM AMERICANS AND DEPRESSION

According to the Pew Research Center, approximately 3.3 million American citizens identify themselves as Muslim (Mohamed, 2016). Although there are areas in which larger numbers of American Muslims live, such as New York, they have homes across the entire United States (American Arab Institute, 2015). While the ancestral history and cultural roots of American Muslims come from a number of geographical locations, including all Arab and various other countries, there are consistent beliefs stemming from Islam. Muslims value knowledge; in fact, more Muslim Americans hold higher education degrees than the general American population (Yan, 2015). Islamic foundations do not discourage innovation nor prevent followers from benefiting from innovation. Yan (2015) reported that around 90% of female Muslim Americans agree that women should be allowed to work outside the home and that many work in professional settings.

We know that beliefs, including religious beliefs, influence people's behaviors and, thereby, their health. Unfortunately, there is very limited research regarding connections between Islamic-related beliefs and health outcomes (Padela, 2015). However, there is evidence that fear and misunderstandings among those who know little about the Islamic faith may be impacting the mental health of Muslim Americans, a phenomenon significantly exacerbated by a historical event commonly referred to as *9/11.*

On September 11, 2001, the perceptions of safety in America and the world changed. After the horrific 9/11 attacks, Americans and all people of the world were told to be wary, report anything out of the norm, and expect travel rules to change as needed. The attacks in 2001 constituted the worst terrorist attacks on American soil.

Unfortunately, the by-product was that people who looked and dressed in ways that were associated with Muslim culture were viewed with fear since the attacks were perpetuated by Muslims (Clay, 2011).

A rise in anti-Muslim sentiments and actions since 9/11 has created a stressful environment for many Muslim Americans (Clay, 2011; Jost, 2006; Kishi, 2017). Jost (2006) described the environment that has emerged as follows.

> Within the United States, meanwhile, Muslims bore the brunt of a crackdown aimed at ferreting out terrorists, potential terrorists or terrorist sympathizers. Government investigators asked hundreds of foreign Muslims legally in the United States to submit to voluntary questioning about terrorists in or outside the United States. Later, immigration officials moved to track down Muslim immigrants who had failed to comply with deportation orders issued before the attacks. The Council of American-Islamic Relations accused the government of "sacrificing the civil rights of Arabs and Muslims in the name of fighting terrorism." At the same time, the group blamed "anti-Muslim agitation on television and radio" for what it described as "the worst" wave of anti-Muslim hate crimes in U.S. history. (Jost, 2006, *War on Terror*, para. 3)

According to findings in a Gallup (2016) poll, *Islamaphobia*—which is defined as "an exaggerated fear, hatred, and hostility toward Islam and Muslims that is perpetuated by negative stereotypes resulting in bias, discrimination, and the marginalization and exclusion of Muslims from social, political, and civic life" (Gallup, para. 3)—persists. Researchers have indicated that Islamaphobia contributes to depression, anxiety, and fear among Muslim Americans (Amer & Hovey, 2012; Clay, 2011; Hodge, Zidan, & Husain, 2016; Kishi, 2017).

A number of experts on Islam and the common beliefs and practices of traditional Muslim Americans maintain that Islamaphobia is steeped in misinformation. Jost (2006) explained that because piety, virtue, and tolerance are strong tenets of Islam; Muslims are not as likely to become terrorists as some may believe. Starting after the terrorist attack in 2011 through 2014, the number of Americans killed (50) by terrorists who were Muslim Americans was less than half the number killed (136) in terrorist mass shootings perpetrated by non-Muslim Americans (Yan, 2015).

Also contrary to the perceptions of many U.S. citizens, many American Muslims condemn terrorism, especially when perpetuated by Muslims (Yan, 2015). Researchers at Duke University found that more terrorism suspects and perpetrators were brought to the attention of law enforcement by members of the Muslim-American community than were discovered through U.S. government investigations (Yan, 2015). Though Muslim Americans are resilient (Clay, 2015), depression, anxiety, and other mental health issues related to discrimination continue to be disparate among them.

WOMEN AND SEXUAL VIOLENCE

Sexual violence is a major public health problem with long-term consequences. It is a complex issue because it can occur in many forms that can be difficult to describe and detect. Sexual violence experts (Black et al., 2011) of the Centers for Disease Control and Prevention used a nationwide survey called the *National Intimate Partner and Sexual Violence Survey* (NISVS) to measure five types of sexual violence: rape (forced penetration), being made to penetrate someone else, sexual coercion (unwanted penetration due to nonphysical pressure), unwanted sexual contact (e.g., being fondled or grabbed), and non-contact unwanted sexual experiences (e.g., exposing sexual body parts, flashing, or masturbating in front of victim; making victim show his/her body parts or participate in sexual photos or movies).

Survey results (Black et al., 2011) indicated that more than one in three women (35.6%; more than one in four men, 28.5%) had experienced rape, physical violence, and/or stalking by an intimate partner. Over 79% of female rape victims were raped before the age of 25, and 42% were raped before the age of 18. Onc in six women (16.2%; 1 in 19 men, 5.2%) had experienced stalking victimization in which they feared for their or another's safety. The majority of female sexual violence victims had one perpetrator in their lifetime—usually a current or former intimate partner—who exerted multiple forms of violence (e.g., rape, physical violence, and stalking) on the victim (Black et al., 2011).

Sexual violence survivors experience physical injury, mental health consequences (e.g., depression, anxiety, low self-esteem, suicide attempts, post-traumatic stress disorder), and other health consequences (e.g., gastrointestinal disorders, asthma, diabetes, substance abuse, sexually transmitted infections, gynecological or pregnancy complications) at higher rates than those who never experienced sexual violence (Black et al., 2011). They are also more likely to report frequent headaches, chronic pain, difficulty with sleeping, and activity limitations (Black et al., 2011).

Racial and ethnic minority women (and men) are more likely to be victims of sexual violence, stalking, and intimate partner violence than White women (and men). The CDC (Black et al., 2011) has maintained that this disparity is likely due to stressors linked to social determinants in some ethnic communities (e.g., low income, education, resources, and services). They recommend that communities and organizational partners work together to change societal norms so that respectful, nonviolent relationships are valued and sexual violence is not perpetuated as an acceptable element of masculinity. New and existing laws and policies are needed so that victims and potential victims receive protection and services related to legal, housing, and mental health needs in a timely and effective manner. Health professionals must be trained and encouraged to detect signs and symptoms of sexual violence and ensure that appropriate treatment, counseling, protection referrals, and follow-up care are provided when sexual violence has occurred. Insurance coverage for detection, prevention, and treatment is also needed.

≡ Promoting Health Equity

The concepts of building community capacity and community-engaged partnerships that we introduced in chapter 2 are important elements of any approach to promoting health equity and social justice. However, as indicated earlier in this chapter, social determinants and structural inequities may negatively impact your community partners' access to the power and resources that are needed for significant change.

Community Perspectives

The introductory scenario described in this chapter can serve as a useful example of how social determinants and structural inequities impact health. One of our textbook authors recently engaged with community partners in her community to assess factors impacting healthy eating and physical activity in a low-income area. The partners were already aware that neighborhood residents lived in a food desert where fresh fruits and vegetables were neither readily available nor affordable when offered in the neighborhood stores. Local vendors revealed a catch-22 situation in which they reported that they lost money when they attempted to consistently pay for a steady supply of fresh produce that local residents didn't consistently purchase. The residents explained that they did not try to buy produce locally because of high prices and poor quality. Additionally, public transportation to better produce sources was lacking.

In focus groups conducted among ethnic-specific groups, participants talked about culturally-linked eating habits and preferences. They indicated that most "healthy food options" offered to their children in school cafeterias and vegetables often touted as "good for you" in the news and through advertising were not a part of eating norms in their cultural heritage. Some indicated they believed that "outside professionals" who recommended healthy eating solutions to their community were out of touch with their needs and preferences.

The assessment participants also identified a number of barriers to physical activity in their neighborhood. Several neighborhood streets lacked walkable sidewalks, and the walking tracks on school properties were often closed after school hours. Existing parks were in need of bathroom facilities and more safety patrols. Though a local YMCA was frequently named as a commonly used site for physical activity, some indicated the membership fees were beyond their means. Some participants strongly lamented that local city swimming pools once used by neighborhood families had been closed years ago, and biking lanes were requested but had not been paved; both of these barriers contributed to perceptions that decision-makers in city government had abandoned the neighborhood. According to key informants, the fact that most residents in this low-income area were African American perpetuated a neighborhood belief that racism contributed to structural inequities.

This real-world example illustrates some of the concepts we have discussed regarding social determinants and health inequities. Addressing healthy eating and physical activity in this local community has called for the engagement of a wide number of professional, volunteer, and community resident groups. The good news is that partnership building in this community is well underway, but needed changes for a complex problem of this magnitude often occur more slowly than most would prefer. Ongoing collaboration and community engagement, combined with careful and deliberate approaches to addressing those structural inequity factors, are vital elements for success.

Communities in Action

We now return to the NASEM (2017) report called *Communities in Action: Pathways to Health Equity* for ideas about how to promote health equity and address the factors that impact it. The NASEM leaders and their partners developed a conceptual model for a successful community based on their review of community-based solutions. The model contains three essential elements, which we have named and briefly summarized below. We encourage you to read the report for more details.

Multi-sector collaboration: Multi- or cross-sectional partnerships that include community groups and individual community members, government agencies, universities, nonprofit organizations, and private and for-profit entities are often much more effective in fostering broad-based policies, resources, and other support needed to address social determinants and structural inequities than are individual organizations or partnership groups that only include health professionals.

Health equity as a shared vision and value: When health equity is a shared vision among partners and is clearly articulated as a motivating theme, collaborators are more likely to be able to work together despite differences. This shared vision can drive the establishment of policies and practices that result in positive outcomes.

Community capacity to shape outcomes: A sense of belonging and trust among neighbors can foster community ownership. Developing this social capital contributes to a community's capacity for community-led action to promote health equity.

The NASEM leaders also provided some specific steps that we should all consider when working to promote community-engaged and multi-partnered approaches to promoting health equity in any community. They are listed below.

- Leverage existing efforts whenever possible.
- Adopt explicit strategies for authentic community engagement, ownership, involvement, and input throughout all stages of such efforts.
- Nurture the next generation of leadership.
- Foster flexibility, creativity, and resilience where possible.
- Seriously consider potential community partners, including nontraditional ones.
- Commit to results, systematic learning, cross-boundary collaboration, capacity building, and sustainability.
- Partner with public health agencies whenever possible, no matter the focus of the effort. (NASEM, 2017, p. 25)

You have probably already begun to imagine the depth of careful thought, time, and effort needed to implement these recommendations. Many of the health inequities and influencing socio-ecological factors we have discussed in this chapter are deeply entrenched. However, we encourage you to not lose heart as you explore ways to apply the concepts and strategies we have described here and in other chapters. A good place to begin is to use the "For Your Application" activity provided in this chapter to identify ways in which those essential elements for promoting health equity are being used in various communities.

≡ In Conclusion

A strong understanding of health equity and socio-ecological influences is essential if you plan to help promote health across a broad socioeconomic spectrum of individuals, populations, and communities. We encourage you to use this chapter as a frame of reference as you discuss the theoretical frameworks addressed in chapter 5 and consider specific steps (e.g., assessment, planning, implementation) in the process of promoting health that we address in later chapters.

REVIEW QUESTIONS

1. Define *health equity* and *health disparity*, and explain their significance in addressing health issues in the United States.

2. Explain how social determinants, socio-ecological factors, and structural inequities impact the prevalence and nature of health issues across the life span.

3. Describe specific health issues within selected population groups within the context of socio-ecological influences and health equity.

4. Describe and apply essential elements for promoting health equity.

FOR YOUR APPLICATION

Applying the Essential Elements to Promoting Health Equity

Select a health issue and a specific population (for example, diabetes in Latinx communities). Search the Internet and/or talk to community leaders and other experts to gather evidence of the three essential elements for promoting health equity related to your selected health issue and population: *multi-sector collaboration, health equity as a shared vision and value, community capacity to shape outcomes* (see details and examples under *Communities in Action* in this chapter). The following questions may be useful as a starting point of your exploration and discussion: What barriers or challenges to promoting health equity are evident or assumed for this health issue in this population? What organizations/agencies are collaborating to promote health equity for this health issue in this population? What are those collaborative groups doing and/or trying to accomplish? Do their stated mission/vision statements focus on promoting health equity? Do they provide data and other information that could be used to better understand health equity factors? Is it clear that community members are involved in these partnership efforts? What specific community-led organizations or groups are or should be involved in these efforts?

5

Theory-Based Approaches

You realize that understanding health behavioral theories is important to your work. You've been told that we apply theory to our lives every day—but how so? Every time you've seen an illustration of a theory, it seemed like a jumbled collection of boxes, circles, and lines. When you tried to review more than one, it became just plain overwhelming. How can we break down theories and models so they are more understandable and can be applied in our professional practice? How do we know which theories or models to select?

Chapter Objectives

1. Describe the primary components of individual behavioral theories such as the health belief model, theory of planned behavior, transtheoretical model, and the precaution adoption process theory.

2. Explain how the interpersonal behavioral theory—social cognitive theory—differs from individual behavioral theories.

3. Discuss how the PEN-3 model can be used to distinguish between positive, existential, and negative cultural influences on health.

4. Explore the ways in which social network analysis can increase understanding of the many complex relationships that impact health.

5. Detail how PRECEDE/PROCEED would be a useful model for identifying factors that influence community health problems.

6. Analyze how behavioral theory relates to public health.

≡ Importance of Theory to Health Education

Having to memorize theories and models for a college course can be a nuisance. You may suspect that some professors include them in required materials just to keep you busy or to satisfy some egotistical "ivory tower" personality quirk. We don't deny that in some cases you could be correct. However, theories and models are meaningful in the real world when they serve as a framework for accuracy and efficiency in health program planning. Used appropriately, they enable you to competently evaluate large, complex issues. To illustrate the value of using a model in needs assessment, program planning, or evaluation, we invite you to consider a fictitious story we lovingly refer to as "The Elephant Story."

Our story is derived from a well-known poem called "The Blind Men and the Elephant" written by John Godfrey Saxe in the 1800s (Bornstein, 1996). The poem was fashioned after a portion of the Udana, canonical Hindu scripture (Ireland, 1999). Both are about blind men who believed they understood all there was to know about an elephant but, in reality, understood only certain parts. Our elephant story helps make the point about needing to see the whole picture. We hope it will help you in your quest to unscramble the meaning behind behavioral theories and their use.

The Story

Once upon a time, there were a number of different research groups who were all attempting to assess a certain health phenomenon called "The Elephant." Part of the problem inherent in seeing the full picture of this elephant phenomenon was that the research groups were not cooperating with each other. Members of each group feared that sharing information with others would threaten their access to limited resources. The result was that each group had only a partial picture of the whole elephant issue. This, of course, distorted the truth about the elephant phenomenon and crippled any effective attempts to address the issue as a whole.

One day, a student who had recently joined one of the research teams voiced the unspeakable. She suggested that all of the teams be invited to a conference to share what they'd learned about the elephant phenomenon. She even launched an awareness campaign to help each team realize the advantages of being able to see the whole elephant picture. She then booked the conference in the Bahamas to add to the appeal. Miraculously, it worked. The teams came.

On the first day of the conference, all of the big names in elephant phenomenon research entered the conference hall, and the excitement (not to mention the competitive tension) was high. The first research team representative walked to the podium and the crowd expectantly hushed. He started speaking: "Ladies and gentlemen, I am honored to be the first to speak on this momentous occasion about the phenomenon we all know to be the elephant. As you know, our research team has been tirelessly working for a number of years to carefully assess the elephant and we have clearly identified some interesting physical characteristics and movement patterns. We now know that the elephant is shaped much like a tree trunk, is flat on the bottom, and often appears in clusters of four" (Figure 5.1). With a self-satisfied look on his face, the researcher returned to his seat.

A representative of another research group then came to the podium with a slight frown on her face. She leaned into the microphone and stated, "Ladies and gentlemen, I respectfully submit that the previous speaker may think he's been researching the elephant. However, I can only surmise that he must be mistaken." The first speaker gasped from his seat, and his face turned red. But she continued, "My team

Figure 5.1
The elephant story.
The "elephant story" illustrates how a model can be used to create a more complete picture of a community health issue from previously isolated pieces of information.

has been researching the elephant phenomenon for over a decade and we've found our data to accurately reflect its characteristics." She paused for effect. "The elephant is not at all shaped like a tree trunk, nor does it move in clusters of four." The first speaker angrily grasped the arms of his chair. "To the contrary, elephants almost always move in pairs. (We believe they mate for life.) They are shaped much like a huge, flat fan and, under certain conditions, may move in wavelike motions." She shot a pointed look at the first speaker and returned to her seat.

The tension mounted as a representative of yet a third research group approached the microphone. He solemnly eyed his audience and, with a thoughtful expression, said: "Distinguished colleagues, I am perplexed by what we have heard today. There is nothing in my 20-year experience of elephant phenomenon research to validate the previous two speakers' descriptions. In our assessments, we have never encountered elephants in close proximity to each other. Each elephant is shaped like a garden hose and often behaves like one with an occasional spray of water coming out the end." He sat down amidst the hubbub of agitated whispers and angry looks between research teams.

Just as total crowd chaos was about to break forth, a tall, white-haired, distinguished-looking gentleman suddenly stood from the back of the room and shouted above the noise "Enough!" Heads turned toward his voice and in the ensuing hush you could have heard a pin drop. This man was recognized by all as a long-time researcher and scholar in the field. Though he, too, had selfishly guarded his findings over the years, he remained a recognized authority in elephant research, predominantly because he'd been researching the longest. All eyes were on him as he purposefully made his way to the front of the room. He turned his intense gaze onto the hushed audience and said, "I've heard enough! I am appalled at your lack of understanding and true knowledge about a phenomenon that affects the lives of so many people. This elephant phenomenon is no joking matter!" Fixing his fiery gaze on each of the three speakers, he virtually shouted, "You have embarrassed our profession with your misguided attempts to describe the elephant! The elephant is like . . . it's small . . ."

The crowd leaned toward him, sensing that what he was about to say would change forever how they saw the elephant. But the intensity of the moment became too much and, before he could finish his sentence, the gentleman fell to the floor in a dead faint. The crowd rushed to his aid, almost smothering him in the process. Some were shouting instructions to unbutton his collar, get him some water, call 911. Others shouted for the crowd to back up and give him some breathing space. In a moment, the gentleman came to and instantly grabbed the collar of the researcher who kneeled beside him. Pulling him close, the gentleman urgently whispered in a hoarse, strained voice, "The elephant is like a very large, stiff worm with no eyes." Those close enough to hear him looked at each other in surprise. "A worm?" someone asked incredulously. "Yes," he hissed. "A worm that grows out of the rump of a hill." He paused to catch his breath and then moaned, "But, to this day, I can't for the life of me determine the source of that awful smell."

The Meaning

Okay, so it's a silly story. It's difficult to imagine any thinking human having difficulty seeing the full picture of an elephant. After all, we all know what an elephant looks like, right? But what if we were talking about a real community health issue that was a little more difficult to define and assess? What if it were something that affects the well-being of a large number of community members, such as violence in schools? Think about the many instances in our country in which a person walked into a school and opened fire on students and teachers with an automatic weapon or other gun. The aftermath was devastating in every situation, and people across the country participated in trying to assess what happened and why.

The discussions sounded a lot like the comments of those researchers who saw only parts of the elephant. Some blamed the school systems for loose security and called for metal detectors at all doors or specialized training for school personnel. Others pointed to violent media sources and demanded that they be banned. The parents were certainly scrutinized, and some argued for more counseling programs for troubled families or for stricter laws holding parents accountable. Still others called for broader and tougher gun control laws, including banning certain types of guns and increasing age limits for gun purchases. Most assuredly, a large array of resources and potential solutions have been suggested, some of which might actually work within the context of the whole picture. However, without a general understanding of all potential influences and solutions, some parts of the "elephant" might be overlooked.

That's how theories and models help. They provide a framework through which we can accurately assess large, complex health issues and their potential solutions. They remind us to look for common relationships between factors and help us ask the right questions. A number of theories and models are used in the health education field. We will address only a portion of them in this textbook. Most are useful in a number of ways, including needs assessment; program planning, implementation, and evaluation; and program marketing. The theories you use will depend on your unique work situation, the participants, and the target behaviors. For that reason, we encourage you to learn enough about the commonly used theories and models to gain some idea of where to start when selecting a theoretical foundation for your work.

Commonly Used Theories in Health Education

Words abound when discussing theories and models so let's start by considering a few definitions. Some individuals use the word *theory* to mean simply an idea about how something works. However, most fields that are grounded in science use the word *theory* only when that idea has been studied through research and determined to be true in at least one circumstance. When we talk about behavioral theory, especially behaviors related to health, we are talking about the scientific use of the word *theory*. A theory, then, can be used to understand and organize the processes in health decision making as well as envision the resulting consequences. Because human behavior is complex, behavioral theories are generally multifaceted; that is, they contain several concepts and/or constructs that work together to explain a behavior. **Construct** is a term for a theoretical concept that was created for a specific theory (Glanz, Rimer, & Viswanath, 2008). As a theory is studied, relationships between concepts are clarified and put together to explain why a behavior occurs.

According to Glanz, Rimer, and Lewis (2002), a model uses concepts or constructs from several theories to explain a phenomenon or behavior. In a sense, it's like melding several theories into a new theory. When a theory is studied through research, concepts and constructs are called **variables**. Of course, it would be easier if the same words were used, but research and evaluation carries a set of specific terms that have meaning to researchers, so it is important for you to understand how those terms relate to your work. You will learn more about research and evaluation in an upcoming chapter.

One of the reasons that studying behavioral theories becomes frustrating is the sheer number of them. There are theories that work best with individuals, while others were created for use with entire communities. Some theories focus on attitudes and beliefs, while others regard consequences of actions as most important. An appropriate first step is to become familiar with some of the commonly used behavioral theories in health education. The following sections will assist you in this endeavor.

Health Belief Model

The **health belief model** (Hochbaum, 1958) was initially created to explore people's willingness to participate in screening x-rays for tuberculosis and to evaluate that willingness in relationship to their perceptions of susceptibility to the disease and perceptions of disease severity. It is a model that helps explain the behaviors of individuals. Although the theory originated out of a study of individuals in a screening program, it can be applied to other behaviors.

Did you ever watch a film or video in school that was designed to deter you from drinking and driving? If so, you may still remember some of the more graphic scenes of automobiles ripped in half and human blood everywhere. Did the scare tactics work? If so, for how long did the message influence your behavior?

What if you had been the person hired to make that video? Would you have done it any differently? You might have, if you understood the average adolescent mind-set. Adolescents who take risks rarely believe that behavioral consequences affect them. They may fully accept statistical evidence that shows a high correlation between fatal accidents and drinking while driving. But they may not fully believe themselves to be at risk, even though they drink and drive. Their attitude may be, "I know it can happen to the other guy—that doesn't mean it's going to happen to me." In some cases, showing a dozen graphic videos about the severity of the consequences may do little to change that perception.

As illustrated in Figure 5.2, an individual's perception of the severity of a behavioral consequence plus the perception of their personal susceptibility to the consequence will determine their perception of threat from the behavior. In other words, risk-taking adolescents are more likely to refrain from drinking when they drive if they

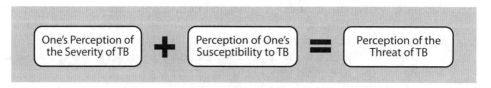

Figure 5.2   Perceived threat in the health belief model.

truly feel threatened or at risk of experiencing the potentially awful consequences. So, how would you convince them they are at risk? How would you increase their levels of perceived threat? The graphic video might not work if it addresses only one of the two types of individual perceptions that often influence perceived threat. An adolescent can truly believe bad stuff can happen when a person drinks and drives (high perceived severity) but still think, "It won't happen to me!"

According to the health belief model, adequate levels of both perceived severity and perceived susceptibility must be present for perceived threat to be a behavioral motivating factor. Even with both those elements in place, other modifying factors sometimes come into play (Strecher & Rosenstock, 1997), as illustrated in Figure 5.3. Of course, we already know that differences in age, personality, culture, experience, and so forth can influence perceptions about threat. For example, an adolescent who has been in a car hit by an intoxicated driver will certainly have different perceptions of threat than other adolescents.

Perceived benefits and barriers (pros and cons) to engaging in healthy behavior also increase the likelihood of behavior change if the benefits outweigh the barriers (Nardi & Petr, 2003). Adolescents may believe that their friends want them to drink, which may serve as a powerful momentary barrier that may outweigh the benefit of keeping their moms and dads happy. So, the key is that perceptions of barriers must be decreased while the perceptions of benefits increased.

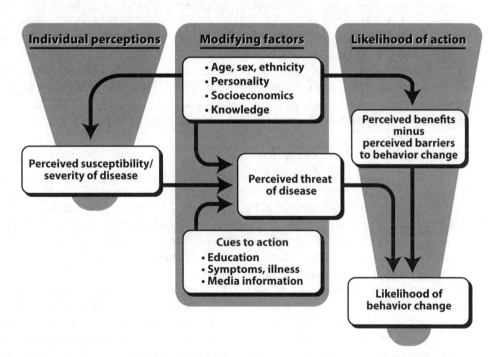

Figure 5.3   Health belief model.
According to the health belief model, adequate levels of perceived severity and perceived susceptibility must both be present for perceived threat to be a behavior-motivating factor

Even with all those health-enhancing components in place, individuals may still need a little nudge to help them get started on changing behavior for the better. In the health belief model, that little nudge is referred to as a cue to action, usually a single event that serves to jump start behavior change. In our example, a cue to action among adolescents might be the death of an admired celebrity in an alcohol-related accident. Any event that brings the threat closer to home can serve as a cue to action.

The construct of self-efficacy was added to the health belief model (Rosenstock, Strecher, & Becker, 1988) when the model started being used for more complex behaviors. Self-efficacy is a perception about how well one can perform a specific task. If adolescents don't believe they can say no to alcohol being offered by peers, they have low self-efficacy regarding this behavior. We will learn more about self-efficacy in the discussion about social cognitive theory, the theory for which it was created.

The state of Idaho provides a real-life example of the role of the health belief model in drinking and driving. State health officials conducted a needs assessment related to substance abuse prevention that compiled information from several sources, such as the CDC Youth Risk Behavior Surveillance Survey, the Idaho Department of Education Safe and Drug-Free School Survey, and the Substance Abuse and Mental Health Services Administration National Survey on Drug Use and Health (Idaho State Epidemiological Outcomes Work Group, 2015). Factors related to substance abuse were determined in the final analysis. Among other things, the analysis documented that students' perceptions of the level of risk in alcohol use correlated with less drinking, and that the number of fatal car crashes related to substance abuse was also correlated with less drinking (2013). I hope you will note that these findings match components of the health belief model (perceived susceptibility and perceived severity).

Now that you've learned about the health belief model, what tactics would you use to increase the likelihood that adolescents would choose to refrain from drinking and driving? Even with your new knowledge, it won't be an easy task and other theories and/or models might better fit the adolescents in your community.

Theory of Planned Behavior

Have you ever done something you knew was risky? Though you may have had a number of reasons, none may have been related to your perceptions about the severity of the consequences or your susceptibility to them. That's why the health belief model doesn't work in every situation. There are times when people know all about severity and susceptibility and still forge ahead. So we encourage you to consider some of the influencing factors in Figure 5.4, which illustrates another individual behavior change theory, the **theory of planned behavior** (Ajzen, 1991).

Like the health belief model, the theory of planned behavior includes an attitude component that reminds us to think about behavior-related perceptions, beliefs, and expected outcomes. An individual's belief about a behavior (what will happen if a behavior is performed) plus his/her judgment about that outcome (positive or negative) make up the attitude toward the behavior which, in turn, impacts the intention to perform a behavior. The behavioral intention, then, influences the actual behavior. For example, a woman who believes that quitting smoking will improve health but does not value her health or believes that quitting will be physically and emotionally difficult will have a negative attitude toward the quitting behavior. That negative attitude will lessen the intention to quit.

The theory also prompts us to think about another common influencing factor we've not yet discussed. It's called **subjective norm** (see Figure 5.4). A person's subjective norm is made up of his or her perceptions about whether others approve or disapprove of the behavior (normative belief) plus the degree to which he or she values their opinions (motivation to comply). In our smoking example, the woman may believe that her doctor wants her to quit, but there would also have to be a motivation to comply with the doctor for the behavioral intention to be increased. A more likely scenario is that friends of the smoker, who also smoke, don't want her to quit. There may be stronger motivation to comply with friends, which would lessen the behavioral intention.

Perceptions of behavioral control, made up of control beliefs and perceived power, will influence both the behavioral intention and the actual behavior. The perception that there are factors that facilitate or prevent a behavior are *control* beliefs, while the weight that an individual gives each of those factors determines whether there is a negative or

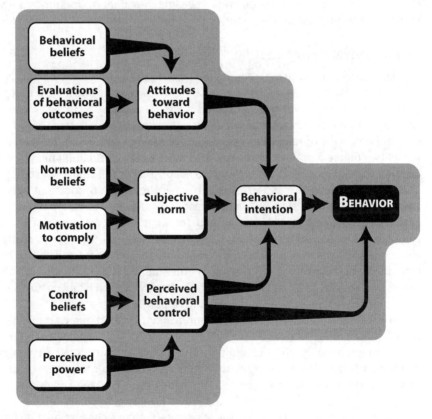

Figure 5.4   Theory of planned behavior.
In the theory of planned behavior, subjective norm is measured as a person's perceptions about and motivation to comply with the opinions of others.

positive perception of behavioral control. Our smoker will have a positive perception of behavioral control if she believes there are useful factors that will help her quit.

Hukkelbers, Hagtvet, and Icovac (2014) found that intentions to quit smoking increase if components of the theory of planned behavior interact with one another. They discovered that when attitudes toward a behavior and subjective norms work together, the intent to quit smoking is higher. They also discovered that when attitudes toward a behavior and perceived behavioral control work together, the intention to quit smoking increases. Therefore, smoking cessation programs may be more successful if they helped smokers link their attitudes, beliefs about how others feel, and control beliefs.

If all of the people in your community of interest acted like clones, if they all had the same perceptions and moved at the same pace in their decision-making processes, we could end our discussion of theory here. After all, we've already discussed different types of behavior-related attitudes and beliefs (health belief model) and the powerful influence of peers (theory of planned behavior). What we haven't covered, however, is how the behavior-change process can evolve over time. We think that's important because we don't want you to become impatient or discouraged if you don't witness immediate results with your health education efforts.

Transtheoretical Model

The process of educating a community about health and observing positive changes is sometimes like planting a seed and watching it slowly grow into a flowering plant. You have to be patient and willing to "feed and water" the behavior-change process along the way. You also have to understand what that process needs at each stage of growth. That's one of the benefits of referring to the **stages of change** portion of the **transtheoretical model** (see Figure 5.5). It will help you determine where community members are in the decision-making process as well as ways to adapt your health education strategies.

In our previous discussions about behavior-related attitudes and beliefs, we've assumed that our participants had already formulated some opinions about the health-related behaviors of drinking and smoking. However, some of those participants, even the ones who drink and drive or smoke, may have never really thought about it at all. They may have been too busy with the ups and downs of life to contemplate the risks of drinking and driving or smoking. According to the transtheoretical model (Prochaska, Redding, & Evers, 1997), those who haven't given any thought to a particular behavior would be in the **precontemplation** stage.

What if most of the adolescents in our drinking and driving example had already thought about it a great deal due to some recent alcohol-related deaths in their school? In that case, spending all your limited time and money on an awareness campaign might be a waste. The majority would be in the **contemplation** stage, meaning that they have been thinking about the need to change their drinking and driving habits but are, perhaps, hesitating because of what they'd have to give up.

As you have probably guessed, each stage of change has its own characteristics and information needs. Individuals in the **preparation** stage have already decided to make a change and are planning to do something about it in the very near future. They are the ones who need more information about how to avoid drunk driving situ-

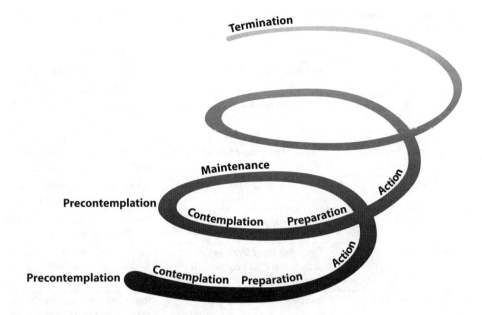

Figure 5.5 Transtheoretical model.
The transtheoretical model (stages of change) illustrates how a person can progress through a series of stages, from not even considering a behavior change to actually infusing the behavior change into one's lifestyle. Loops and repeated stages depict potential relapse and repeated change cycles.

From "The Transtheoretical Model of Change and HIV Prevention: A Review," by J. O. Prochaska, C. A. Redding, L. L. Harlow, J. S. Rossi, and W. F. Velicer, *Health Education and Health Behavior* 21(4): 471–486. © 1994 by Sage Publications. Used with permission.

ations in the face of peer pressure. On the other hand, it would be a waste to start with this "how to" information if individuals are in the precontemplation stage and haven't even decided yet that they need such information.

Those in the **action** and **maintenance** stages have already been practicing the desired behavior at different levels of success. Different health education strategies are required to promote consistency in practicing the newly acquired behavior change and prevent relapse. Strong support groups can help individuals who have reached these last stages to continue making good choices.

Other aspects of the transtheoretical model demonstrate, once again, how important beliefs, perceptions, and attitudes are in making behavior changes. Decisional balance and self-efficacy are core constructs of the transtheoretical model. Decisional balance describes concepts we discussed earlier; simply, the pros and cons of making a behavioral change. And as you know already, self-efficacy is one's belief that he/she can perform a task.

The transtheoretical model goes beyond theoretical concepts and offers actual strategies for helping individuals move through the stages of change. These strategies are termed **processes of change** and include the actions listed in Table 5.1.

Table 5.1   Processes of Change

Process	Goal	Interventions
Consciousness Raising	Increase awareness	Feedback, education, confrontation, and media campaigns
Dramatic Relief	Increase emotional experience	Psychodrama, role-playing, grieving, personal testimonies, and media campaigns
Environmental Reevaluation	Assess thoughts and feelings	Empathy training, documentaries, and family interventions
Social Liberation	Increase social opportunities	Advocacy, empowerment procedures, and appropriate policies
Self-reevaluation	Assess one's self image	Value clarification, healthy role models, and imagery
Stimulus Control	Decrease negative cues to action and add positive cues to action	Avoidance, environmental re-engineering, and self-help groups
Helping Relationships	Increase social support	Rapport building, a therapeutic alliance, counselor calls, and buddy systems
Counter Conditioning	Learn healthy behavior	Examples—relaxation can counter stress; assertion can counter peer pressure; nicotine replacement can substitute for cigarettes; and fat-free foods can be safer substitutes
Reinforcement Management	Add consequences and rewards for specific behaviors	Examples—a day off after 6 days of physical activity; a special low-calorie food treat after several days of very low-calorie meals
Self-liberation	Increase belief that one can change and stick with it	New Year's resolutions, public testimonies, and multiple rather than single choices can enhance self-liberation

Source: "How Do We Do It: Health Behaviors," Center for Health Communication Research, 2008. Retrieved from http://chcr.umich.edu/how_we_do_it/health_theories/healththeories5/chcr_document_view

Precaution Adoption Process Model

We want to give you a very brief introduction to the **precaution adoption process model (PAPM)**. This model has seven stages that document an assumption that behavior change is dynamic and occurs over time (Elliott, Seals, & Jacobson, 2007). The stages include the following: unaware, unengaged, deciding about action, deciding not to act, deciding to act, acting, and maintenance. Do you see the similarities to the stages of change in the transtheoretical model? The stages are much the same in both processes but we include PAPM because it addresses individuals who choose not to act.

In the stages of change, people who have no knowledge of a new healthy behavior and those who know about the healthy behavior but choose not to act are placed together in the precontemplation stage. In reality, a different strategy may be needed to motivate people who have decided not to act compared to those who just don't know about the healthy behavior. We believe this issue is important because you will be working with many people who choose not to act. For example, how many people do you know who smoke and have no idea that the behavior is unhealthy?

Weinstein and Sandman (1992), who developed the model for the precaution adoption process, believe that concepts and constructs from other theories such as perceptions of susceptibility and severity (health belief model), self-efficacy (social cognitive theory), and social norms (theory of planned behavior) can be used to help individuals move from the stage of "deciding to act" to the stage of "acting." If an individual does not know anything about an unhealthy behavior, providing base knowledge about the consequences of that behavior may be enough to facilitate the transition. However, if a person has chosen not to act, it may be more useful to address his or her perceptions of susceptibility and severity. This might entail a combination of strategies including providing knowledge, introducing well-known and respected individuals who support a behavior change, and guided practice with a behavior for the purpose of increasing self-efficacy.

Social Cognitive Theory

An interpersonal theory, **social cognitive theory** (Bandura, 1977) provides an understanding of how the social environment influences behavior. Figure 5.6 illustrates our conceptualization of social cognitive theory (SCT); the relationships depicted in the illustration have not been verified through research but they might help you clarify the theory's components.

An underlying assumption of the theory is that a dynamic relationship between a behavior, an individual, and the environment occurs. The three continuously interact with one another; as one changes, so do the others. It's fairly easy to see how the physical environment, thunderstorms for example, impacts the physical activity of a man who has started walking 30 minutes every day. What's more difficult to understand is how the emotional consequences of not walking for a few days will impact the new behavior and how that will change aspects of his environment. For example, he may not feel comfortable walking outside again. You can see how that would make a difference in the program.

According to the SCT, the (a) environment and situation, (b) outcome expectations and behavioral capabilities, and (c) self-efficacy perceptions and expectancies will influence an individual's behavior. *Environment*, as we stated in chapter 3, includes anything external to the individual, including social, cultural, and physical aspects of the person's life. The situation is an individual's perception of the environment. As you know from personal experience, perceptions are not always 100% accurate. Accurate or not, the situation influences both the environment and behaviors.

Outcome expectations are an individual's beliefs about potential outcomes of a behavior. When individuals state that they believe they will lose weight as a result of

Figure 5.6   Social cognitive theory. Social cognitive theory helps to explain why people choose behaviors. Among other things, it suggests that a person's belief about an outcome of a behavior and confidence in his or her ability to perform it will influence the frequency of the behavior. It also suggests that the environment influences a person and the behavior, which, in turn influence the environment.

physical activity, they are expressing outcome expectations. **Behavioral capabilities** are the skills and knowledge necessary to make a behavior change. According to SCT, outcome expectations and behavioral capabilities influence behavior directly. For example, a person who wants to lose weight, believes that physical activity will result in weight loss, and knows a little about physical activity is more likely to choose it as a means of weight loss than individuals who don't have the same knowledge and beliefs. However, individuals who place importance on weight loss and believe they will be successful are more likely to follow through. The belief in success is powerful. The value an individual places on an outcome is called **expectancy**, and **self-efficacy** is the belief that one can perform a specific behavior. So, an individual must value losing weight, have some knowledge and skills, and believe he or she can do it in order to have the most success.

Bandura (1977) believes that values (expectancies), beliefs (self-efficacy), and skills (capabilities) can be influenced through **observational** or **vicarious learning**. Observational or vicarious learning occurs when individuals watch someone else perform the behavior successfully. The next step would be actual practice with small elements of the final behavior until each is performed successfully.

Once a behavior is performed, consequences of the behavior will influence expectancies, self-efficacy, and capabilities. These, in turn, influence future behavior and the environment. This interactive influence is called *reciprocal determinism*. Social support from individuals in the environment can also influence the individual and behavior in a powerful way.

PEN-3

An important dimension of the health education picture is how you view your professional role in relation to it. It would be a sad mistake for you to see yourself as a "knight in shining armor" who arrives at a community's doorstep with all the answers and resources in hand. That isn't how effective community health education works. Most individuals and communities prefer to fight their own battles and shape their own futures. Ideally, your role will be to serve as a catalyst and support person rather than a bearer of all the right answers. This difference in perspective may seem slight, but making that shift can greatly influence the results of your efforts, particularly as you strive to become a culturally competent health educator.

PEN-3 (Figure 5.7) is a conceptual model designed by Collins Airhihenbuwa (1990), a leader in multicultural health education, as a guide for culturally appropriate health education. Each of the three model dimensions contains components health educators should consider when working with a particular ethnic community. In each dimension, the first letter of each component composes the acronym PEN. In the dimension labeled "Health Education," we are encouraged to consider whether our health education program is designed to reach only an individual **p**erson or the broader scope of that person's **e**xtended family or **n**eighborhood (school, community). In most instances, efforts that encompass the entire community result in more effective and long-lasting results.

In the dimension labeled "Educational Diagnosis of Health Behavior," we are encouraged to assess community **p**erceptions (such as attitudes, knowledge, beliefs), **e**nablers (that is, available and accessible resources), and **n**urturers (such as family, peers, religious leaders, health professionals) that influence health behaviors and health status within the community. This dimension was derived from a well-known needs-assessment model called *PRECEDE/PROCEED* that you will read about in the next section. Its primary precept is that few people live in a vacuum with no need for

Figure 5.7   PEN-3 model.
The PEN-3 model encourages us to consider the health-related influences of an individual person's extended family or neighborhood (health education); community perceptions, enablers, and nurturers (educational diagnosis); and positive, existential (exotic but harmless), and negative cultural norms (cultural appropriateness).

From "A Conceptual Model for Culturally Appropriate Health Education Programs in Developing Countries," by C. O. Airhihenbuwa, 1990, *International Quarterly of Community Health Education*, 11: 53–62. Used with permission from the author.

human or resource support. Most are dependent to some extent on the influence of others and the accessibility of health services. Thus, to bring about health-related improvements, our health education programs should address attitudes, beliefs, and behaviors not only of the individuals we serve but also of the people who influence them. And, of course, enhancing health service availability and accessibility is another important component of health promotion efforts.

The third PEN-3 dimension, "Cultural Appropriateness of Health Behavior," calls on us to carefully examine cultural characteristics in light of how they truly affect the health status of the community. Airhihenbuwa (1990) pointed out that culture-based knowledge, attitudes, beliefs, and practices of a group can exert positive, existential, or negative influences on the community's health. (*Existential* means "affirming existence"; existential effects are neutral or harmless, though they might seem exotic to someone from another culture.) Unfortunately, negative influences are sometimes the only characteristics of a culture that receive attention in health promotion. Although minimizing negative influences is an important aspect of promoting wellness, problems arise when all cultural influences are assumed to be negative and when positive cultural aspects are ignored.

Many cultures foster health-enhancing beliefs and practices that, when used as motivators in your health promotion program, can make your job easier. For example, traditional Chinese respect for older family members (Matocha, 1998) can foster support for health promotion programs designed for the elderly. The traditional African American belief that personal choices and behaviors affect one's destiny (Spector, 1996) can be useful when health-related behavior change is needed. The positive cultural influences of a traditional community can and should be integrated into your health education program to enhance program acceptance and participation.

Airhihenbuwa (1990) maintains that some health beliefs and practices may be existential; they may seem exotic or strange to the Western medical perspective but, in truth, are harmless. One example is the practice of "coining" in some traditional Asian communities where illness is believed to be caused by evil spirits who gain control of one's body (L. Rasbridge, personal communication, December 15, 1999). A traditional healer scrapes the skin with a coin to release illness-bearing spirits. The resulting red marks are usually harmless but can alarm an untrained school or health official, particularly when they appear on a child. Recognizing this practice as an existential influence could prevent you from reacting inappropriately and help you avoid jeopardizing community trust.

Social Capital Theory

Social capital theory refers to the resources available to an individual or a community that are driven by positive relationships between people. Communities in which members have a high level of trust for one another and means of communicating effectively with one another have higher levels of social capital than communities without these characteristics (Garson, 2006).

Social capital is made up of two dimensions: structural and cognitive. The structural dimension includes the relationships between people, and the cognitive dimension includes the trust between people and willingness to share with each other (Lee

& Kim, 2013). You may have heard of cohesive communities, which some describe as "tightly knit" (Mohnen, Bolker, Flap, & Groenewegen, 2013). Social capital actually results from cohesive or connected communities (Mohnen et al., 2012). Why is this important? Social capital has been shown to influence individual health behaviors (Mohnen et al., 2012), which impact the health of the entire community.

Health Social Network Analysis

Health social network analysis is not a theory, but it is an important theory-driven method used to explore the many complex relationships that impact health. These relationships and interactions between relationships can include people, resources, and phenomena.

Various behavioral theories could be applied to inform this type of analysis at levels and degrees determined by the specific situation. For example, social capital theory could be a useful choice because this theory speaks to the importance of examining and developing community trust and capacities (Lee & Kim, 2013). Social cognitive theory could also be useful because it suggests that behavioral outcomes are impacted by relationships with others and developed through vicarious learning, observations, and modeling. Social support is a useful theoretical construct because it posits that people who feel supported by others during a positive health-related behavior change, are more likely to make that change.

Although no single theory grounds health social network analysis, it uses distinctive methodology for collecting, analyzing, and creating a visual representation of data (Carrington, Scott, & Wasserman, 2005). Gardy and associates (2011) used health social network analysis to identify the source of a tuberculosis outbreak for which complex relationships made finding the source difficult.

PRECEDE/PROCEED Model

One of the most widely used health assessment, planning, and evaluation models, developed by Green and Kreuter (2005), is called **PRECEDE/PROCEED**. Although not specifically a theory, the model has components that provide a theoretical perspective. We will discuss these shortly, but for now, take a look at Figure 5.8. As you can see in the figure, this model is complex and can seem a bit overwhelming at first, until you realize that its purpose is not to belabor the process with needless attention to detail. Instead, it is designed to help us develop a full picture of our community of interest—its health needs and the factors that influence them. It isn't the only existing needs-assessment and program-planning model, but it is a good place to begin your exploration of needs because it offers a broad community-assessment perspective and provides a framework in which community members can participate in the process.

The model originally focused on the assessed health problems of communities and the ability of a central agency or organization to develop programs as solutions. It has been adapted, however, to promote community involvement in the needs-assessment and program-planning process and to incorporate a more positive approach through assets mapping, capacity building, and resource and policy development (Green & Kreuter, 2005). With a lot of teamwork and careful attention to a variety of contributing components, you can help a community develop a full picture

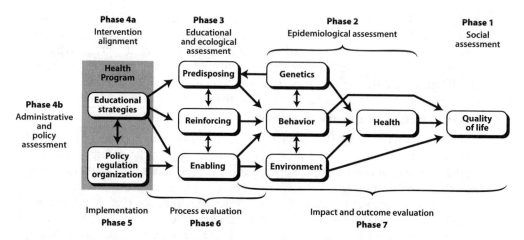

| Phase 4a | Phase 3 | Phase 2 | Phase 1 |
| Intervention alignment | Educational and ecological assessment | Epidemiological assessment | Social assessment |

Figure 5.8   PRECEDE/PROCEED model.
This model can be used to identify factors that contribute to health and quality of life within a community. The arrows depict lines of causation and how health promotion efforts can produce positive impacts and outcomes.

From *Health Program Planning: An Educational and Ecological Approach*, 4th ed., p. 11, by L. W. Green and M. W. Kreuter, © 2005 by McGraw-Hill. Used with permission of the McGraw-Hill Companies.

of the quality of life and health status of its members and develop a plan of action to enhance them.

The first four phases comprise the PRECEDE components and are implemented phase by phase, from right to left in the model. Phase 1, on the far right, entails the **social assessment** of the community's quality of life. This is the ideal place to start because the ultimate goal of health education is to foster life satisfaction and total well-being among community members. Starting here enables you to involve the community in subjectively defining the social issues of greatest importance and determining how they can be addressed for the common good (Green & Kreuter, 2005).

In the social assessment, community members are encouraged to identify **social indicators** that reflect the community's levels of satisfaction with their quality of life. These indicators vary depending on the community members' unique perspectives. FYI 5.1 provides examples of social indicators that may be identified during Phase 1 of the assessment. Assets mapping is also conducted during this phase to identify available resources and the individuals and organizations that control them (Green & Kreuter, 2005).

In the **epidemiological assessment** (Phase 2), data are collected to determine the incidence and prevalence of community health problems that affect the community's quality of life (see FYI 5.1 for indicators). These can include communicable diseases (such as measles and hepatitis), chronic diseases (such as cancer and heart disease), health-related risk factors (such as malnutrition, anemia, and hypertension), and other recognized health problems (such as domestic violence and adolescent pregnancy). **Behavioral indicators** may include compliance, consumption patterns, self-utilization, or care. The environment also impacts behavior as well as health status. **Envi-**

5.1 Examples of Social Indicators	
Community Level Indicators	**Organization Level Indicators**
Aesthetics	Absenteeism
Civil Unrest	Productivity
Comfort	Achievement
Crime	Employee Morale
Crowding	Attention
Discrimination	Property Damage

Source: *Health Program Planning: An Educational and Ecological Approach*, 4th ed., by L. W. Green and M. W. Kreuter, 2005, New York: McGraw-Hill.

ronmental indicators include such things as hazard sites, community resources such as hospitals or clinics, conditions of the physical environment such as public transportation, safe walkways, and clean air. Environmental factors may be beyond the individual's control, such as the lack of low-fat selections in fast food restaurants. If so, you may need to include long-range environmental change efforts in your action plan.

Genetic indicators were recently added to the PRECEDE/PROCEED model to acknowledge what years of scientific research have proven: that one's inherited biological code can render a predisposition to certain health conditions. For example, much has been written about the breast cancer gene and how women who have a family history of the disease may determine their course of prevention by taking a genetic test. The interactions between genetics, behavior, and environment are represented by arrows in Figure 5.8. Green and Kreuter (2005) explain these interactions by stating that "most controls on the gene-environment interactions depend on the behavior of individuals and populations in their exposure to environmental risks, so we place behavior between genetics and environment" (p. 15). By the end of Phase 2, community health professionals and stakeholders should prioritize the identified issues in terms of their degree of importance to and changeability within the community.

We stated earlier that beginning with Phase 1 of the model is the ideal. We should point out, however, that Phase 2 may be where you actually begin. Why? Because most health education jobs have a predefined focus. For example, if you were hired by the American Heart Association, you would know during job interviews that the "health problem" focus (Phase 2) is heart disease. Under those circumstances, you would first devote attention to how the community of interest perceives heart disease and its effects on community members' quality of life. Thus, in this instance, you would move from Phase 2 to Phase 1 and then back to Phase 3 (Green & Kreuter, 2005).

Phase 3, the **educational and ecological assessment**, is composed of predisposing, reinforcing, and enabling factors. Distinguishing among these three categories can be a challenge when you are first learning the model, but recognizing their different but related influences will be critical for your health education program. These factors provide the theoretical perspective to the model. You will be collecting information on the factors with the assumption that they impact health-related behaviors.

Predisposing factors (attitudes, values, beliefs, knowledge) involve those thought processes that motivate the targeted behaviors. For example, predisposing factors that sometimes influence adolescents to smoke include the belief that smoking is cool, the desire (value) to be accepted by peers, and an attitude of rebellion against authority figures who say they shouldn't. On a more positive note, adolescents may engage in physical activity regularly if they know about and value its benefits and are motivated by a desire to stay fit and trim.

Reinforcing factors are rewards or encouraging feedback (positive or negative) that community members receive from other people. In our example, smoking adolescents may receive encouragement from smoking peers, but can be positively influenced by nonsmoking role models (such as popular athletes) willing to help in your health education program. Individuals who are providing negative reinforcement may also be educated or trained through your program to shift to a more positive influence, as in the case of physical education teachers being trained to tailor their classes to the abilities and interests of their students so that adolescents develop positive attitudes about physical activity.

Enabling factors include resources and skills needed for behavior change to occur or barriers that may prevent it from happening—or both. Regular physical activity will be easier to maintain if resources, such as a safe and convenient place to jog or engage in recreational sports, are available and accessible. Because improper physical activity can cause needless muscle soreness and injury, adolescents also need training in the appropriate skills. Enabling factors that contribute to negative health behaviors may also need to be targeted, as in the case of cigarette accessibility for minors.

Now that you have collected information for Phases 1–4a, you are ready to transition into more of the planning phases, which comprise the beginning of the PROCEED portion of the model. Realize that this is the portion that comes after you have identified and prioritized needs. In Phases 4b and 5, you must determine what program components, strategies, and services are necessary to bring about the intended change. Does the program have the resources and the administrative infrastructure to make it happen? This is where assets mapping comes into play. Resources such as time, personnel, and budget are three primary considerations that can be matched at this point with identified community assets and capacities. In Phase 5, you can begin to assess barriers to implementation, such as staff commitment and attitudes or community concerns. In the policy assessment, local politics and organizational systems that may influence program implementation are also considered. This is a good place to begin emphasizing your community of interest's resources and develop community coalitions to develop solutions. Another important aspect of the PRECEDE/PROCEED model is that it emphasizes evaluation (the PROCEED portion). We will discuss evaluation in chapter 9, but Green and Kreuter make an important statement when they include evaluation as a component of program planning. Evaluation cannot be an afterthought; it should be an integral part of the entire planning process.

As valuable as the PRECEDE/PROCEED model is for broad-based community assessment and program planning, it does not address every aspect of what health professionals should know about human nature and the factors that often influence the way people think. For example, the model includes "attitudes" among the predisposing factors that often influence health behavior, but it doesn't provide detailed descriptions of the types of attitudes or perceptions that influence health most often. Other theories and models can help you further explore these psychological influences. Understanding such influences can help you be more specific in your chosen health education strategies.

≡ Selecting the Appropriate Theory

Selecting the right theory takes some time and effort on your part. The first thing to consider is the specific use for the theory. Are you preparing to conduct a needs assessment or are you ready to develop the actual prevention program? Perhaps you will be evaluating an existing program. Take time to think through what has been done and what needs to be done. You will not want to use the PRECEDE portion of the PRECEDE/PROCEED model if you are evaluating an existing program. You will not want to plan a program based on the social cognitive theory if the needs assessment was based on the health belief model. So, first be very clear on what tasks need to be completed and which theories have been used in other aspects of the program.

As you may know, all programs *should* be developed with the use of data collected in a needs assessment, if at all possible. You will learn more about needs assessment in chapter 6 but for now, keep in mind that using a theory or model as a framework for your assessment can be the best decision you make. If your needs assessment is grounded in theory, you will have a direction for your program development and evaluation.

So, how do you choose the right theory? You will first need a good working knowledge of behavioral theory gained from the professional literature. Yes, you will need to read professional journals, seek new information, and keep up with the field. You must know how to access professional literature, so if you have some confusion about that, we urge you to get some help! The selection of a theory will depend on three aspects: (a) the behavior being changed, (b) the characteristics of the participants, and (c) the environment. Each aspect must be considered and some of the best information will come from the professional literature. In studying professional literature, you will note that some models, such as PRECEDE/PROCEED, include assessments on the three aspects (behavior, participants, and environment) as part of the model.

Health-Related Behaviors

The fact that there are so many behavioral theories tells us that behaviors are not all equal. Some are deeply rooted in culture while others have a biological foundation and still others result as a reaction to another behavior. And, of course, cognition plays a powerful role in most behaviors. So, what does all this mean?

You will need to know a little about the behavior being changed in order to select the appropriate theory. If, for example, the target behavior involves a physical addiction, success is unlikely if your program is based solely on a theory that addresses only attitudes and beliefs. In fact, there may be a need to combine theoretically and medically-based program components in order to fully address the behavior. For example, some smoking-cessation programs might include strategies to change perceptions, attitudes, and skills as well as the use of a medical treatment such as the nicotine patch.

On the other hand, some theories and their relationship with specific behaviors have been extensively studied. Adolescent sexuality and social cognitive theory is an example. Studies have shown that interpersonal relationships are powerful influences on teens (Hogben, 1998). Therefore, social cognitive theory may be an excellent choice for programs working with adolescents and sexuality.

Some behaviors will require more emphasis on the process of change—taking small steps before getting to the final objective. In these cases a theory that involves change over time, such as the transtheoretical theory, might be a good choice.

How do you learn more about the behavior? As we've mentioned, reviewing what others have found through research and reported in professional literature is a good place to start. But don't hesitate to talk with other professionals and consider what you have learned through experience. Use many sources of information (unlike our elephant researchers) so you can see the whole picture. Don't forget that you also need to know something about the participant to make a good decision.

The Participant

We've already mentioned that some theories work best with individuals. These may focus on perceptions, beliefs, and attitudes. Other theories work best with behaviors highly influenced by interpersonal relationships and focus on how they interact. Still others work with community or organizational cultures and focus on belief structures of the entire community (large or small). So it will be important to understand with which you are working. Are you working with a group of individuals who, even though attending a program with others, will be working on their own beliefs, attitudes, and skills in order to make a behavior change? Or are you working with a community to help members change behaviors within their cultural beliefs? You will need to know in order to select a theory.

There are characteristics of groups that may also help guide your choice of theory. We've already discussed the mind-set of many adolescents. They often feel invulnerable to risk and are learning new things about themselves and others at every moment. Early elementary children are concrete thinkers, which means they may not understand abstract concepts about health. Individuals may have religious beliefs that preclude participation in certain activities while others have cultural beliefs that don't match some prevention plans.

Understanding the internal environments of your participants may also aid you in choosing a theory. For example, locus of control—whether an individual believes that he or she is personally in control of an outcome—could heavily influence program outcomes. For example, if individuals in your group believe incorrectly that an outside source has caused a health problem, they are not likely to change their own behaviors to make it better. Locus of control has been found to be an important predictor of healthy behaviors (Steptoe & Wardle, 2001). If control beliefs are a strong influencing factor in behavior, you will want to select a theory that addresses this issue.

How do you learn about the participants? First, you must know who they are. There is no way to plan a generic prevention program. Will it be adolescents, new mothers, or men from a senior living center? Your needs assessment, agency, funding source, or even personal interests will all play a role in determining the participants.

Just be certain that you know with whom you will be working. It may sound silly, but many programs have gone wrong because they were planned for different people than those who eventually attended the program.

You will also, as always, want to refer to the professional literature to learn more about your participants. But most importantly, learn about the participants *through* the participants. Learn by talking and asking questions. Your participants are the ones who know the most about themselves.

As you consider your participants and the target behavior changes, you will also want to fully understand the environment in which you are working. Again, all three aspects are important in your decision making.

The Environment

There are many things to consider in regard to external environment besides the evident physical aspects. These include time, money, social and political influences, and others, some of which were discussed in chapter 2. Nieuwenhuijsen, Zemper, Miner, and Epstein (2006) discuss the impact of environment on a physical activity program for a student using an electric wheelchair.

> If the student is attending a university that offers accessible sport and recreation for wheelchair users, with personal assistants and/or supportive faculty members, her chances of successfully engaging in regular physical activity will be much better than if she is attending a university with no wheelchair-accessible sport or recreation facilities; her chances grow even fewer with no accessible transportation or support from staff or faculty. (p. 246)

So, choosing a theory that involves only changing attitudes and perceptions will not work in this situation. An appropriate theory would also involve the removal of actual barriers.

It's pretty clear how money, time, and other resources impact the success of a program. If you choose a theoretical foundation that will require costly strategies and you don't have the resources, the program will not succeed, even if you understand the behavior and participants well. If you are planning a sex education program in a political environment that will not support it, you will not get far, even if you select the perfect theoretical base. Knowing the environment will help!

It might help to view the health issue you wish to address from the socio-ecological perspective. If you think back to chapter 1, you'll remember the socio-ecological model, which illustrates how many layers impact health and health behaviors. Viewing the health issue from this perspective provides a good starting place. Unfortunately, there are times when extensive reviews of literature, communication with other professionals, and talking with participants doesn't point you in a definite direction for choosing a theory. Combining theoretical components may be the best choice if a behavior is complex or a good match to an intact theory can't be found. Christine Jackson (1997) developed eight principles that might assist you in combining theories. In summary, the principles describe behavior change as a process that is powerfully influenced by attitudes, beliefs, and values. They remind us that a rewarding experience is more likely to be repeated and that the experience will influence future values, beliefs, attitudes, and behaviors. Jackson's principles suggest that participants should drive the behavior change and that health educators should understand the magnitude of influence wielded by important others in the lives of those participants. It's also important to understand the concept of reciprocal determinism, in which changes in values and beliefs change behavior, which, in turn, changes values and beliefs. The final principle returns to the idea that programs should be based in research and evaluated for effectiveness.

We know that studying theories and models for the first time can be frustrating and overwhelming. However, if you think about it, you are already using theories on a daily basis. After all, why do you do the things you do? Talk to other practitioners, practice using the theories, and read the literature. Before long it will all make more sense than you can imagine.

≡ In Conclusion

Theories help us analyze why people behave the way they do and provide models or frameworks for action. Keep in mind that some theories are best used with individuals, others with small groups, and still others with entire communities. The basic tenets of theories vary also. For example, some theories use attitudes and beliefs as the foundation for behavioral change and others include time and practice as important elements. Some theories are fear-based while others involve cues to action. As a community health professional, you will need a firm understanding of a variety of behavioral theories and planning models. You will also need to know how to assess the individuals and groups with whom you will work. This knowledge will help you build successful health education and behavior change programs.

REVIEW QUESTIONS

1. Describe the primary components of the health belief model, theory of planned behavior, and transtheoretical model.

2. Discuss how the precaution adoption model differs from the transtheoretical model.

3. Explain how the PEN-3 model can be used to distinguish between positive, existential, and negative cultural influences on health.

4. Detail how the social capital theory could be applied to inform social network analysis.

5. Diagram the PRECEDE portion of the PRECEDE/PROCEED model and explain how its components can influence community health.

6. Analyze how theories and models influence public health.

FOR YOUR APPLICATION

Draw a figure that illustrates how constructs, concepts, theories, and models relate to one another. To give you an idea of what we mean, let's say that the assignment asked you to *build* a structure that showed how constructs, concepts, theories, and models related to one another. You might use tinker toys and indicate that theory is represented by the base of the structure and the model is the structure as a whole. We are asking you to put your ideas on paper. Be sure to include constructs and concepts too.

PART II

THE PROCESS OF HEALTH PROGRAMMING

6

Needs and
Capacity Assessment

It's your first week in your role as a health educator at a county health department in Rural, USA. You've been given the directive from your supervisor to develop a tailored HIV/AIDS prevention curriculum for adolescents that can be implemented in the area's middle and senior high schools. Your supervisor informs you that the school district's superintendent is supportive of the initiative but has asked that you meet with members of the district's Health Advisory Committee before developing the curriculum. Although the county epidemiological reports show a rise in HIV/AIDS cases within the last five years, the committee is quick to inform you that there isn't really a problem with HIV/AIDS in "their schools" and what the kids really need is a healthy eating program. You sense some tension in the room and realize that there may be a discrepancy between the perceived and actual needs among the community members. Now what do you do?

Chapter Objectives

1. Describe why needs assessment is an important first step to designing effective community health programs, activities, and initiatives.

2. Explain why it is useful to assess both objective and subjective needs of an intended audience.

3. Review the four phases of needs assessment and the steps involved with each phase.

4. Contrast individual versus group strategies for needs assessment data collection.

5. Identify community assets.

6. Apply the PRECEDE portion of the PRECEDE/PROCEED model to identify factors that influence an identified health issue.

7. Conduct a needs assessment within your own community.

≡ Needs-Assessment Concepts and Definitions

Now that you have a general picture of health issues and determinants that impact communities in the U.S., it is time to consider the process through which those problems were identified. In chapter 1, we introduced the concept of quality of life and highlighted the importance of assessing community health needs, a primary competency for health promotion professionals. In this chapter, we will introduce you to methods and tools common to the assessment process and essential for tailoring health promotion to a variety of populations. In addition, it is our hope that the content we present will expand your understanding of the purpose and importance of needs assessment, how it is evolving, and how it relates to other assessment and community organization terms and principles.

Health education and promotion programs are most impactful when we base them on accurate needs-assessment data, provide careful interpretation of their meaning, and involve community members and stakeholders as partners in the process. The primary goals of **needs assessment** are: (1) to identify gaps between what exists and *what ought to exist* so that you can design a program to reduce those gaps; and (2) to use data you obtain from a number of sources to tailor the program, strategy, or initiative to those whom its intended to serve (Gilmore, 2012).

Objective and Subjective Needs

Gilmore (2012) defines needs assessment as "a planned process that identifies the reported needs of an individual or a group" (p. 9). He explains that two important groups of people are expected to provide input in needs identification: (a) health professionals and (b) community members. Ideally, both groups will be involved in planning and implementing the proposed community health program. The needs identified by these groups may be described as **objective** (needs based on evidence of incidence and prevalence data) or **subjective**, perceived needs (what individuals report based on their personal experience and views). These two types of needs sometimes differ, but they are both important pieces of assessment information.

Why Both Are Important

Why would subjective needs be as important as objective needs? The answer can be readily understood if you picture, like the introductory example, a community in which a high rate of HIV infection has been documented, although most community members deny that the problem exists. Health professionals would likely suggest you implement an HIV/AIDS education program to address this objective need, but community members might be less than cooperative. The community might be more concerned about a recent, single, well-publicized incident of school violence and prefer a violence prevention program rather than an HIV/AIDS education program. The more information you have about objective and subjective needs in the community you serve, the more equipped you will be to educate the community and work with others to prioritize program goals.

A slightly different scenario could exist if the community actually wished to address both health concerns but was still more concerned about violence (subjective need) than HIV/AIDS (objective need). Finding the common ground where data-based evidence and community concerns match is an ideal place to begin community health promotion efforts, but it doesn't always exist. When this convergence doesn't occur, it helps to respectfully acknowledge subjective needs, promote community awareness about real needs, and work within a partnership format to build and maintain a collaborative effort.

≡ What Type of Information Should You Collect?

When conducting a needs assessment, it is important to understand the different types of data available about your community, county, state, or country and how to collect this information in order to prioritize health needs. Archival documents, county or country reports, testimonials, pictures, registration logs, attendance records, budget spreadsheets—all of these are examples of data. As mentioned in chapter 3, **primary data** refers to information that stems from its original source, such as a first-hand account in a diary or a taped interview. Other examples of primary sources are letters, autobiographies, interviews, focus groups, blogs, speeches, stories, photographs, and survey responses. **Secondary data** refers to information that is not first-hand; in other words, it is information drawn from an unoriginal source. Examples of secondary data include county health reports, hospital discharge data, and national databases such as the Healthcare Cost and Utilization Project (from the Agency for Healthcare Research and Quality) and DATA 2020, a database relating to *Healthy People 2020*. Both primary and secondary data are instrumental in assessing a community's perceived and actual needs.

Collecting Secondary Data

National and international databases and sources are valuable because they can help you determine how the nature and extent of needs identified in your community compare to those of other communities. From these sources, you can learn which approaches were effective or ineffective in other locales and you may gain insights you would otherwise have missed. You can then consider the specific characteristics and needs of your community and adapt what you learned from those secondary sources.

Other important secondary sources are organizations and groups that have worked or are presently working in your community of interest. Although leaders of some organizations may view you as competition and respond in a territorial fashion, others will likely welcome your efforts and be willing to share what they know. Tapping into these local secondary sources before you begin any primary data-collection efforts can save you time and resources by avoiding needless duplication. It can also be a useful way to learn from the experience of other professionals about the culture, history, and characteristics of your community—who the real leaders and gatekeepers are, and how to best establish trust and mutual respect between you and community members. These secondary source connections can develop into future collaborative relations that will broaden and strengthen your efforts.

Collecting Primary Data

Primary data collection is a critical component of the needs-assessment process because it helps accomplish two things: First, it can provide accurate, community-specific data about problems, influences, and potential solutions to health issues. Second, if conducted appropriately, collecting primary data can help you establish important relationships with community members. Involving them in the early stages of your work helps develop community ownership. From this joint effort you can gain an insider's perspective on community culture and characteristics and the degree to which members will respond positively to your work. Their input will help you incorporate perceived needs into your program planning. It will also help you determine the best methods to collect primary data and the types of questions to ask. Primary data-collection methods are usually categorized as individual or group assessments; these will be discussed later in the chapter.

≡ The Four Phases of Community Needs Assessment

Conducting a community needs assessment is a lot like working a jigsaw puzzle with a group: there are myriad pieces of information scattered around your community that, when put together, help form a vivid picture of the quality of life that exists in that corner of the world. As you begin the process of collecting these "pieces," and involve others, you will continue through four stages of needs assessment: (1) gathering preliminary data and generating assessment questions, (2) collecting community data, (3) analyzing the data and interpreting results, and (4) prioritizing needs, identifying assets, and providing recommendations. You will move through the phases of needs assessment by completing 13 steps. These phases and steps are illustrated in Figure 6.1.

Phase 1: Gather Preliminary Data and Generate Assessment Questions

You are ready to begin the vital first step in planning an effective, evidence-based program that will improve the health and/or quality of life of members of your targeted community. Before you try to go at it alone, it's worth repeating here that the most impactful health promotion programs and initiatives involve community members: Assessment and program planning is not a solo endeavor. You, as a health pro-

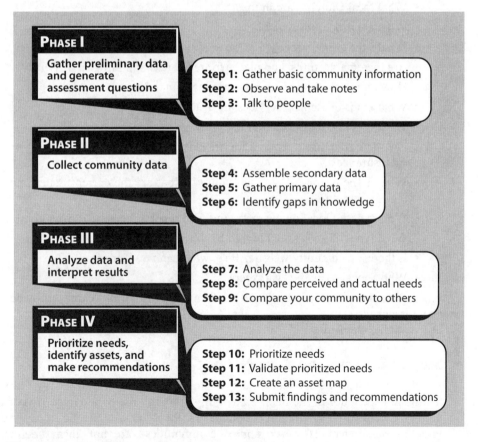

Figure 6.1   Four phases of needs assessment.

motion professional, may be helping to "steer the ship," but ideally, community members and an advisory team reflective of various groups within the community are involved and adding their voices and insights to this process.

Step 1: Gather Basic Community Information

Start by collecting some basic resources such as maps of the area, phone books, and Chamber of Commerce information (such as brochures or welcome packets)—or find this information online. Keep in mind that the Chamber of Commerce materials will read like a travel brochure, so be sure to read past the propaganda and focus on the facts. You may want to check websites, visit the local library and health department, and speak to individuals within the community to gather the following information:

- What are your community's demographics (i.e., characteristics of a population such as mean age, average family size, ethnic group composition, median yearly salary, etc.)?
- How many schools and universities are within the area?
- What is the average level of education?
- What local churches are in the area?
- What are property values?
- What's the crime rate?
- Are there parks, trails, and places for recreation and physical activity?
- How many fast food restaurants are in business?
- What kinds of medical services are available?
- What is public transportation like?
- Are there supportive services for the elderly or those without housing or medical insurance?
- What is the history of the community? What are the current issues impacting the community?
- What types of local media exist, and who reports the news in your community?
- What types of stories are covered by this media?
- Is there a community website? If so, what can you learn from it?
- Who appear to be the "gatekeepers"?

Examining the pieces of community information listed above may provide clues about the health status of your community and lead you to explore factors that impact its overall health picture.

Step 2: Observe and Take Notes

While gathering secondary data is important, you will learn best through first-hand experience in the field. Take a drive through the community. If your community is defined by geographical boundaries, then you will be able to easily determine its parameters. However, some "communities" are not always defined by geography. For example, if you're working with a refugee Hmong group in your region of the state, find out where people within this population gather, such as refugee centers, neighborhood gardens, grocery stores, churches, community clinics, restaurants, and so forth. Talk to the people within the community to decide which sites are most relevant.

In addition, pay attention to environmental cues. For example, what areas might be potential hazards? Is there a lack of pedestrian walkways? Is there graffiti on buildings, and if so, what does it say? Are lawns well kept? What types of stores and advertising surround the community? Is alcohol sold in the area? You may want to write your observations in a notebook or record audio notes on your phone or another audio voice recorder. Taking photos of various public places will reinforce your memory and enhance your field notes. Your observation notes offer yet more pieces of the community "puzzle" you are assembling.

Step 3: Talk to People

After you've taken the time to collect your own field notes, it's time to talk to members of the community to gain their perspectives. You will want to talk to an array of individuals, from those who hold powerful leadership positions to those who vote for the leaders (and of course those who do not vote at all). **Gatekeepers** are members of the community who hold some position of influence. Examples of gatekeepers are listed in FYI 6.1. It's also important to converse with individuals who live within the

FYI

6.1   **Examples of Community Gatekeepers**

- The mayor and city officials
- School officials and PTA leaders
- Ministers and religious leaders
- Realtors and other business people
- People who work in social service agencies
- Representatives from nonprofit organizations and grant-funded programs
- Community activists
- Physicians and health professionals
- Local health educators and epidemiologists
- Rotary or Kiwanis Club presidents
- University professors or school teachers
- Presidents of neighborhood associations
- Members of Congress
- Local journalists and members of the news media
- Law enforcement officials
- Town historian
- People who are well-respected and lead informally

community and who are served by some of the services and individuals mentioned below. Community perspectives differ according to the roles people play within the community, so listening to multiple voices is essential to gaining a broader perspective.

When you contact gatekeepers and members of the community, what should you say? You might start with some general questions, such as "How long have you been a member of the community?" and "How do you feel about the community overall?" If the individual is a long-standing resident of the area or a member of a target group, you might ask about some historical events that have impacted the community. You might then transition into more health-related questions, not giving any probes (such as facts or statistics), but allowing the individuals to voice their own perceptions about quality of life. You might ask, "What health issues are most pressing?" and "Why do these health issues exist?" You can follow up with questions about issues that are not health related (chances are, these are related to health anyway). Keep in mind that everyone will have their own interpretation of what is "pressing," another reminder of why it is important to gain multiple perspectives from people in a variety of community roles.

After you've interviewed these members of the community, be sure to thank them for their time and insight, and follow up with a thank-you note or a token of appreciation. It leaves a good impression and speaks to your level of professionalism. Remember, too, that networking within the community is key to developing "buy in" and to building support for future health education or public health initiatives.

≡ Phase II: Collect Community Data

Now that you've gained some subjective viewpoints from local community members and leaders, it's time to seek out facts and figures that will add to the store of puzzle pieces you've already collected.

Step 4: Assemble Secondary Data

There are myriad resources at your disposal. The Community Toolbox, an online resource that promotes community health and development (http://ctb.ku.edu), offers the following examples:

- The state or county health department can help you determine health indicators on a variety of issues.

- The state human services department should be able to tell you the number of Medicaid recipients and food stamp program participants.

- Hospital admission and exit records can give you information on issues such as teen births, causes of deaths, etc. Depending on the community, some of the data may not be part of the public record, but it may be possible to purchase or arrange to use it in some form.

- Census data and demographic information are available for your community and the United States as a whole. This information is found in the *Statistical Abstract of the United States* on the Census Bureau website at http://www.census.gov. Many states have similar information on their own websites, and state departments of health may also have links to the census on their sites. One note of caution about using census data: It has not always proven reliable. For example, lack of documentation of nonnative immigrants, homeless persons, or those who simply refuse to participate in the census survey can influence the accuracy of census data.

- Police records can give you crime rates and the incidence of problems such as domestic violence or motor vehicle accidents.
- Chamber of Commerce data include statistics on job growth, unemployment rates, and property values.
- Nonprofit service agencies, such as the United Way or Planned Parenthood, generally have records on a variety of different issues. These agencies may have already conducted surveys and found the information you need.
- School district reports may include demographic information, graduation rates, test scores, rates of school violence, and truancy rates for local schools. For comparative figures across school districts, check with your community's state department of education.
- Centers for Disease Control reports national information on rates of many diseases, such as HIV/AIDS and diabetes. Access this at http://www.cdc.gov.
- HealthyPeople.gov can provide progress reports about areas of priority for U.S. health initiatives.
- The Bureau of Health Statistics and Research of the Pennsylvania Department of Health provides you with the capability of compiling reports on a number of health issues from adolescent health to yellow fever. Visit the site at http://dsf.health.state.pa.us.
- A reference librarian at a public or university library can point you to valuable local resources.
- Specialized local, statewide, or national organizations may help. For example, if you were interested in substance abuse or diabetes, you would want to track down and consult an organization specializing in that topic. You may want to look in *Gale's Encyclopedia of Associations* as a resource. In addition, most organizations have their own websites with abundant topic-specific information.

Step 5: Gather Primary Data

In addition to the informal interviews you conducted in step 3, you may want to gain more detailed information about community members' knowledge, attitudes, behaviors, and perceptions of various health issues. You may need to use a survey to collect this type of data. As you will learn later in this chapter, this type of data is only as good as the survey you use to collect it. Therefore, search out existing community health surveys for sample questions and formats. You might also check the Internet, your health texts, and professional journals (Are there specific survey titles listed in articles related to your subject matter?). Chat with the local health department staff, or contact representatives from professional organizations related to your topic. Be sure that the survey is culturally relevant as well as conducive to the reading level of your community members. If you cannot find an existing survey that "fits," it might be necessary for you to prepare your own. The important steps in this process are detailed in chapter 10.

Other strategies for collecting primary data from your community include facilitating focus groups, conducting interviews, moderating town meetings, and using **Photovoice** (a process by which community members take pictures reflecting their unique perceptions of community needs and assets). FYI 6.2 includes a more complete list and description of these data-collection strategies.

INDIVIDUAL ASSESSMENTS

FYI 6.2 includes an overview of the four types of individual survey methods. The information provided there is described in great detail by Gilmore (2012), a well-respected authority in needs assessment. He defines a **survey** as "a structured process for gathering information directly from individuals by asking questions" (p. 46).

The type of survey you choose will depend on a number of factors, including who and how many people you are trying to reach and how much time and money you have to put toward the effort.

Mailed surveys.   Mailed surveys have the potential to reach large numbers of individuals and may generate thoughtful replies (since participants have time to complete the survey at their leisure). The expense involved varies, depending on postage and the cost of the survey itself. If you are using an existing survey, there may be a fee associated with its use. You may also have to pay for the mailing list. Mailed surveys can reduce the bias and influence that interviewers may exert in telephone or face-to-face surveys; however, you cannot always verify if the person completing the mailed survey is the individual intended to receive it. Gilmore (2012) suggests using a mailed survey if the type of information you need could be considered private and more personal contact would seem threatening to survey participants.

Telephone surveys.   Telephone and face-to-face surveys usually result in higher response rates than do mail-outs; and face-to-face surveys in particular can be more effective among those with low literacy or minimal English. Telephone surveys can be conducted more quickly, but face-to-face interviews are best for open-ended questions.

Face-to-face surveys.   A face-to-face survey is the best way to distribute a lengthy questionnaire (Fowler, 2002, p. 71). More complex questions are best handled with face-to-face surveys because follow-up questions are more easily asked. Also, those without access to a phone or the Internet would be better reached through a written, face-to-face survey. However, there are several drawbacks to this format. First, anonymity may be sacrificed. Second, participants may answer a certain way because you are present. Third, face-to-face surveys can be expensive because those distributing and collecting the surveys must travel. Fourth, the interviewee may talk longer in person than by mail, e-mail, or telephone, and large projects could require several interviewers. Fifth, interviewers may need to be trained beyond the scope of those who survey by e-mail or phone because the interviewers may have to make decisions in the field without the benefit of consulting with a supervisor. Finally, as modern living has gotten busier and concerns with security and privacy are increasing, it may be harder to reach participants through face-to-face methods than by other delivery modes.

FYI

6.2 Overview of Individual and Group Data-Collection Strategies for Needs Assessment

Individual Assessments	Advantages	Disadvantages
Mailed surveys	Low cost, wide distribution possible, valid information (allows time for thinking before answering)	Lengthy process, low response rate, limited questions, no control over answers (no clarification possible), mailing list required
Telephone surveys	Shorter process than mailing, better response rate, more/different questions possible, better control over answers (can ask for clarification)	More costly than mailing, less valid information (may receive socially desirable answers)
Face-to-face surveys	Best opportunity for questioning, most control over answers (can read nonverbal expressions), effective for low-literacy individuals	Most costly (time and travel expense), least valid information (socially desirable answers), access to participants may be difficult (privacy and security issues)
Online surveys	Potential to collect a large amount of data in a short period of time; flexibility; convenience for participants; ability to garner participation across the globe; ability to reach unique populations; has equal or better response rate than mailed surveys if incentive is provided; allows for anonymity; may be less expensive than paper format	May not reach individuals from older or lower socioeconomic groups; technological errors can occur while individuals are completing the survey; hard to verify whether individuals from intended sample are actually the ones completing the survey or are only completing it once
Group Assessments		
Nominal group	Direct involvement, planned interactivity, allows for diverse opinions, full participation of all group members, creative atmosphere, recognition of common ground fostered	Time commitment, competing issues may slow process, participant bias can emerge, segmented planning involvement
Focus group	Low cost, convenient, creative atmosphere, ease of clarification, high flexibility potential	Qualitative information only, limited representativeness, dependence on moderator skill, preliminary insights only, some group members dominate
Community forum	Allows a large number of people to assemble in one setting (one-time effort vs. repeated attempts); encourages a diversity of perspectives; may allow for community "buy in" and support from community members and leaders	Requires time to plan and advertise; facilitation skills are essential in order for forum to remain orderly and effective; may result in backlash
Photovoice	Imbues community members with ownership in the process; uses photography to reflect community members' perspectives of community barriers and assets; initiates discussion for community members; creates awareness	Can be time intensive; participants must be trained; may be expensive depending on type of equipment used; qualitative information only; may require a translator

Online surveys.   Online surveys are gaining momentum as a popular survey mode because they allow for a larger participant sample, convenience, and anonymity (Wright, 2005). However, technological errors can occur, and this mode is not appropriate for those without access to computers. Also, there is a risk that those completing the survey are not really part of the intended sample or that people will complete the online survey more than once. It is important to carefully consider all of these factors—type of information, audience, money, time, and personnel—in order to choose a method that will work well for your purposes (Wright, 2005).

Another individual assessment method that bears mentioning is the **Delphi technique**; it is used when objective information is not available from other sources and generates "a consensus through a series of questionnaires" (Gilmore, 2012, p. 68). It is often used to identify goals and establish priorities, brainstorm possible alternatives, or gather information about group values and perspectives. The process usually involves three to five rounds of mailed questionnaires in which participants are first asked to respond to a few broad questions; from those responses, more specific questionnaires are developed to further clarify and specify the information. Although this approach can be useful in clarifying important issues, it is more likely that you will be involved in various local survey methods when you first enter the profession.

GROUP ASSESSMENTS

Advantages and disadvantages of the nominal group, focus group, community forum, and Photovoice are also outlined in FYI 6.2.

Nominal group.   As can be deduced from the description there, the nominal group process is more structured than the focus group process. In the nominal group process, five to seven individuals who are knowledgeable about community issues meet to address a particular issue. In the beginning, each member is asked to write down, without discussion, personal responses to a single question (such as, "What do you think are the most pressing health concerns in our community?"). Each written response is shared with the group in round-robin fashion, until every response is recorded. The group then discusses and clarifies items on the list and ranks them according to what is considered most important. The process continues until a prioritized list is agreed on, through a vote if needed. This high-structure approach is designed to foster equal input for every member.

Focus group.   The focus group process is a much more relaxed approach in which 6 to 12 fairly homogenous group members answer questions asked by a trained moderator. The moderator's role is to help the group stay focused, stimulate interaction, and encourage clarification and expansion of ideas without biasing the results. These sessions are usually taped so that ideas expressed in this free format will not be lost or forgotten. This format is designed to encourage spontaneity in generating ideas through the process of free expression. It is particularly useful in collecting qualitative information for a preliminary assessment of community opinions and goals. It does, however, require a well-trained, experienced moderator who will remain impartial and focused on the assigned group task.

Community forum.   Of all the individual and group strategies mentioned here, the community forum is the least structured and can involve the greatest number of participants. Community forums, or public meetings, are often used to distribute information but can also be helpful in gaining initial feedback from any community member who wishes to voice an opinion about a particular health issue. Although it is not considered the most rigorous approach to community assessments, it does allow all community subgroups or segments to voice their views and can be a positive communication channel when carefully planned and implemented. The key is to maintain a positive, objective tone during the meeting and avoid possible degeneration into a gripe session.

Photovoice.   This method employs a participatory action technique that allows individuals to photograph their everyday realities and highlight factors that may enhance or diminish their individual health status or that of the community. As Baker and Wang (2006) explain, "It [Photovoice] is also structured as a mechanism to engage participants in group discussions about their images and to present these images in public forums" (p. 1408). Photovoice is gaining momentum as an empowering strategy in public health. The technique has been used to "capture" health issues among diverse and unique populations. Some of these examples include a clinical and nonclinical sample of older adults in Michigan who chronicled their daily pain levels; factors impacting inner-city adolescents' health and well-being (Strack, Magill, & McDonagh, 2003); health and community issues of rural Chinese women in the Yunnan province (Wang & Burris, 1997); quality of life among rural African American breast cancer survivors (Lopez, Eng, Randall-David, & Robinson, 2005); men's experiences with prostate cancer (Oliffe & Bottorff, 2007); perceptions of safety among battered women (Frohmann, 2005); socio-ecological factors that influence health and development of orphaned and abandoned children in Sierra Leone (Walker & Early, 2009); the dilemma of "to be seen or not to be seen" among queer and trans youth (Holtby, Klein, Cook, & Travers, 2015); and the cultural and social context of physical activity and dietary intake among U.S. Hispanic women (Keller, Fleury, Perez, Ainsworth, & Vaughan, 2008). The main goals of Photovoice are to engage people in active listening and dialogue, create a safe environment for introspection and critical reflection, and move people toward action (Baker & Wang, 2006). There is a specific protocol when using Photovoice, and these steps are listed in FYI 6.3.

When choosing data-collection methods for assessing community needs, remember that each alternative has pros and cons. We suggest you consider using multiple strategies, depending on your available time and resources. The nominal or focus group can be a good way to get started because each provides insight into community values and concerns in a relatively short amount of time. We recommend, however, that information gleaned from small-group processes be used to develop surveys or questionnaires for implementation among larger representative groups within the community. An appropriately balanced collection of group and individual assessment data can help you develop a truer picture of your whole community.

Keep in mind that you need to set limits on how much information you will collect. Too much information will be just as much of a problem as not enough. You can easily become overwhelmed. Consider what is feasible—given your time frame—and then establish your limits.

6.3   Using Photovoice to Assess Community Needs

Photovoice is a component of participatory research that uses photography to create and encourage social change. Caroline Wang (2006) and Mary Burris (Wang & Burris, 1997) present a nine-step methodology to successfully carry out the goals of Photovoice.

1. Recruit Photovoice participants. Wang and Burris recommend that a Photovoice group should include six to ten people. This provides efficiency in collecting data and adequate discussion.

2. Select a target audience of policy makers or community leaders. The participants select this group based on the target audience's ability to make decisions that will improve the problems identified through Photovoice activities.

3. Introduce Photovoice to the participants. The researcher must conduct a workshop or training session to explain Photovoice and to demonstrate proper use of the cameras. This session is also used to educate the participants about obtaining consent when photographing others.

4. Obtain informed consent. The researcher must obtain informed consent from each participant. This is typically completed during the training session.

5. Brainstorm with participants. A brainstorming activity is highly recommended to familiarize the participants with initial themes for taking photographs. This helps facilitate the Photovoice activity because participants will gain a clearer focus to guide their picture taking. Brainstorming can be done at the training session.

6. Distribute cameras. This is done at the training session. Each participant will need a camera to complete the Photovoice activity. The facilitator (researcher) will decide which type of camera to distribute to participants.

7. Provide time for participants to take pictures. The most commonly allotted time frame for picture taking is seven days. This provides each participant enough time to take a sufficient quantity of pictures related to the research project.

8. Meet to discuss the photographs. After the seven days, the participants are asked to return with the cameras and their images to discuss the photographs taken. This can be done as a group or individually. Each participant will review his or her photographs with the facilitator and select the photographs that best tell the story. The facilitator will then work with participants to contextualize their photographs using the SHOWeD Method. Common themes are identified and discussed with participants.

9. Plan with participants a format to share photographs and stories. The facilitator and participants will choose the best medium to present the photographs and descriptions to the target audience. Formats used in the past include websites, slide shows, and exhibits.

Sources: "Photovoice: Concept, Methodology, and Use for Participatory Needs Assessment," by C. C. Wang and M. Burris, 1997, *Health Education and Behavior*, 24(3): 369–387; "Youth Participation in Photovoice as a Strategy for Community Change," by C. C. Wang, 2006, *Journal of Community Practice, 14*(1/2): 147–161.

Step 6: Identify Gaps in Your Knowledge

This is where you begin to put the puzzle together. Go back to the questions you generated in Step 1 and use the data you've collected to answer them. What pieces are missing? What information might help you form a complete picture? You may need to extend the data collection at this point or decide it's time to stop gathering information. Try to fill in the knowledge gaps as best you can with solid information—remember what happens when we assume anything. It sometimes helps to invite others who have not been involved in the process to join you at this point to view the overall set of information you have gathered so far. The fresh perspective of people who have not been closely involved in the process can help you identify what's missing. They may also help you discover new ways to use the data you have collected to more fully answer your assessment questions.

≡ Phase III: Analyze Data and Interpret Results

Collecting community data can be hard work that takes both time and patience. However, once the information is collected, knowing how to interpret this data can also be a challenge.

Step 7: Analyze the Data

Data analysis, the process of examining and interpreting data, can be either formal (as in using computerized statistical analysis) or informal (eyeballing the data in search of obvious differences between what is and what should be). If your community's perceived needs match obvious gaps in health education or services, the less formal approach will suffice. For example, during a town meeting you may learn that community members are concerned about alcohol-related traffic accidents in the area. Local police and hospital emergency room records confirm that alcohol-related accidents are a frequent problem, with often tragic results. Further, a review of community settings in which the much-needed education could occur reveals inadequate efforts. All of this information combined points to an obvious need; therefore, more rigorous data collection and analysis may not be necessary because the prioritized need is obvious.

Step 8: Compare Perceived and Actual Needs

What if data about the community members' perceived needs, local secondary data, and available services or education don't match? Or, what if several needs from each of these sources are evident and the results are mixed? There are no foolproof solutions to this common dilemma, but there are some steps you can take to help clarify the issue. The first is actually preventative. By working with members and organizations within the community to start, engaging them to think about their own experiences in relation to available data might actually get everyone closer to being on the same page. Second, you may need to collect more data. If local records indicate a high incidence or prevalence of a health risk, you may need to go back to community members for more primary data about their perspectives and experiences with that specific issue. If a particular health issue is evident in the primary data but is not showing up in secondary data, you may need to consult local health professionals and community members to determine why the issue is not evident in local records. These decisions about "what is" should be driven by input from all stakeholders, with the desired end result being a list of identified problems, their nature, and their extent.

To further illustrate what we mean by working with both perceived and actual needs, consider the following story about an international public health group that decided to build a hospital in a very remote region of a developing country. The group decided to build the hospital because of the high rate of maternal and infant deaths in childbirth in that region, a problem attributed to the scarcity of trained physicians and appropriate medical facilities. So the group diligently raised the money needed, built an amazingly modern facility in view of the surrounding conditions, and flew in well-trained professionals to do the work. But after some time, childbirth death rates remained high and few local people had even visited the new facility. Someone decided to ask "Why?" and learned from the people who lived there that they trusted the local midwives and preferred to remain in their familiar home surroundings to give birth rather than move to a new and unfamiliar building to be cared for by strangers. The public health group realized it had failed to accurately assess the situation. It decided to try again, this time armed with needed information about the local community, its interests, and perceived needs. With time, the health group was able to reach out to the locals by inviting their midwives to train in the facility and work in the birthing room along with the "imported" professionals. Had someone fully understood the need to assess the whole picture before the plan was implemented, things might have progressed quite differently.

Step 9: Compare Your Community to Others

It is important to put the information you have collected into a context, either positive or negative. For example, pinpointing that the rate of HIV/AIDS in your area is ten times higher than the national rate could have a significant impact on whether grant-funding organizations decide to fund your proposed HIV/AIDS awareness program.

☰ Phase IV: Prioritize Needs, Identify Assets, and Make Recommendations

Now comes the hard part, deciding which needs to address first. This important step determines the direction your health education program will take. Often, there are several important needs on the list and people disagree about which should receive immediate attention. Yet limited resources and time rarely allow you to address them all at once. You have to start somewhere.

Step 10: Prioritize Needs

McKenzie, Neiger, and Thackeray (2013) suggest that you evaluate each listed need in light of four questions:

1. What is the most pressing need?

2. Are resources adequate to deal with the problem?

3. Can the problem best be solved by a health promotion intervention, or could it be better handled through administration, politics, or changes in the economy?

4. Can the problem be solved in a reasonable amount of time?

Reality dictates that you have to consider questions 2 through 4 due to time and resource constraints imposed by your employer or by funding sources who have agreed to support your efforts. Green and Kreuter (2005) would likely categorize these four questions under the heading of how "changeable" the health situation is. They suggest you assign each of the identified needs to one of four areas (FYI 6.4). These categories weigh levels of pressing need (importance) with the potential for change (changeability) as a result of health education efforts. Any decision-making process should also consider the degree to which other community agencies and organizations are providing similar programs. This can help you avoid duplication of existing services and minimize potential territorial issues with leaders of other organizations.

FYI

6.4   Prioritizing Health Needs

A community's health needs should be prioritized according to their importance and changeability as determined by community members and the health professionals who serve them.

	More important	**Less important**
More changeable	Needs that are highly *changeable* and *important*	Needs that are highly *changeable* but are less important
Less changeable	Needs that are highly *important* but are less changeable	Needs that are neither changeable nor important

Adapted from *Health Program Planning: An Educational and Ecological Approach*, 4th ed., by L. W. Green and M. W. Kreuter, 2005, Boston: McGraw-Hill.

Step 11: Validate Prioritized Needs

After putting all of the puzzle pieces together, an image of your community will emerge. How do you know, however, that your picture is accurate? Validating needs may seem unnecessary because it calls for a return to previous steps, such as conducting focus groups to determine the community's reaction to the prioritized needs or gaining second opinions from other health professionals. If careful groundwork has been laid, this step may be less important. However, because so many people have likely provided input to the process, some may have lost sight of the final goal along the way. If the needs are not properly validated, you could possibly proceed with costly programs that are less effective than expected. For that reason, we suggest you consider this step as an important reminder to constantly validate your prioritized needs as you proceed. You can confirm your decisions through careful, consistent communication with community members and collaborating health professionals as you move from the assessment to the program-planning stages.

Even if you arrive in a new employment situation where much of the data collection and prioritizing groundwork has been completed, we encourage you to at least spend time establishing personal relationships with primary and secondary data contacts to foster your awareness of the situation.

Step 12: Create a Community Asset Inventory or Map

After prioritizing needs, it is important to identify existing community resources that may help address those needs. For example, if the data you've collected and the responses you've received from community members indicate that obesity is the health priority for this community, you should next determine what services, organizations, and resources relating to obesity already exist in the community and may be included as part of the solution. For example, is there an obesity task force already in place in a local school district? Identifying existing resources allows for greater community involvement, prevents replication of services, and allows for more efficient allocation of funding.

Health programs and services that are built upon **community assets,** or existing resources, are more effective because they already have roots in the community. The process of identifying community assets is also known as **community capacity building** because it encourages program planners to build upon community strengths, not deficits. Specifically, **capacity-focused assessment** identifies capacities, skills, assets, or contributions that can be provided by community individuals, associations, and institutions (Gilmore & Campbell, 2004). FYI 6.5 provides examples of community assets. The information collected in capacity assessment (or assets mapping) can be used later to form community coalitions and advisory panels for program planning and implementation (see chapter 7). All of this can lead to community empowerment, which is the ideal. As we explained in chapter 2, community health professions have moved toward a community empowerment approach that involves community members in the health education process.

As defined in chapter 2, community empowerment is a social-action process by which individuals, communities, and organizations gain mastery over their lives, change their surroundings, and improve their overall quality of life. In other words, community empowerment is about helping people help themselves in a way that encourages them to take ownership of their health problems and use their abilities and resources to develop solutions. By having a stake in assessing, planning, and implementing health programs, community members are more likely to accept, participate, and adopt health interventions and behaviors that support a healthier community overall.

Step 13: Report Findings and Make Recommendations

As you've noted from the prior 12 steps, completing a thorough community needs assessment takes time, diligence, and collaboration. After you and your assessment team have validated your findings and have included community members in the prioritization process, it's time to compile a report and provide suggestions for addressing these needs. Consider your audiences when preparing this report. Keep in mind,

6.5 Types of Community Assets

A community's health needs should be prioritized according to their importance and changeability as determined by community members and the health professionals who serve them.

Individual Assets	**Organizational Assets**	**Physical and Land Assets**
Individuals and their	Community centers	Agriculture
• Skills	Radio/TV stations	Emergency resources
• Talents	Small businesses	Forest
• Experiences	Large businesses	Industrial areas
Consider:	Home-based enterprises	Lakes, ponds, streams
• Professional	Religious organizations	Mining
• Personal	Nonprofit organizations	Natural resources/
• Resources	Clubs	landmarks
• Leadership	Citizen groups	Parks/recreation areas
Institutional Assets	Business associations	Vacant land
Churches	Transportation networks	Waste resources
Colleges and	Cable and phone companies	
universities	**Governmental (State and Federal) Assets**	**Cultural Assets**
Elderly care facilities	City government	Historic/arts groups
Fire department	State capital	Ethnic/racial diversity
Hospitals and clinics	Bureau of Land Management	Heritage
Mental health facilities	Economic development departments	Crafts, skills
Libraries	Forest service	Cultural traditions
Police department	Military facilities	
Schools	School service center	
Utilities	Small business administration	
	State education agency	
	Telecommunications agency	

for example, that you want to engage others and make this information seem relative to them as well as pressing. When writing the formal needs assessment report, be sure to include the following components: (a) introduction and community description, (b) methods for data collection, (c) data analysis, (d) findings, (e) implications for health education and program development, and (f) conclusion. FYI 6.6 includes a detailed description of each component.

≡ Using a Theoretical Lens to Assess Community Needs

So far, we have discussed how needs-assessment data are collected and how that information is combined with a capacity assessment to develop a health education program plan. What we haven't addressed is what to look for in those assessments or how to use a theoretical lens. As we discussed in chapter 5, applying a theoretical basis to program development is necessary if you want the program to be relevant to the community and have a significant impact.

FYI

6.6   Components of a Formal Community Needs Assessment Report

Title Page	Title of your assessment project, name of author/s, and date.
Executive Summary or Abstract	A brief (250 words or less) summary of the purpose of the assessment, methods used, and findings.
Table of Contents	List all of the paper content sections with appropriate first page number.
Introduction & Community Description	Overview of the community (history, demographics, geographic boundaries, etc.). Provide facts collected through secondary data.
Data-Collection Methods	Discuss the data collection strategy used along with the step-by-step protocol.
Data Analysis	Explain how the collected data was analyzed.
Findings	Illustrate and discuss results from the data analyses. Include graphs and charts to display your findings.
Community Assets	Identify community assets that would be helpful in program development, coordination, implementation, evaluation, and maintenance.
Implications for Health Education and Program Development	Discuss the implications of what you found, explain emergent health priorities, segment health needs by group, provide suggestions for health education and health interventions, and suggest guiding theoretical frameworks.
Conclusion	Provide a few summary statements and offer some of the limitations of the needs assessment. Explain how the results of the study will help plan or assist programs within the community.
References	Be sure to list all references in a format such as APA and provide parenthetical reference citations throughout.
Appendixes	You may want to include copies of the surveys or questions you used for data collection; articles or handouts relating to the community and any miscellaneous documents you feel enrich the community assessment.

How can we approach the assessment process with any assurance of knowing what to look for? This is rarely a simple process because each community has its own unique characteristics and a variety of influences that have shaped it (see chapter 2). However, some helpful guidelines and models used in the health education profession can increase our chances of identifying a full assessment picture. One of the models we find most helpful for community needs assessment is the PRECEDE portion of the PRECEDE/PROCEED model described in chapter 5. An explanation of how to use the constructs of this model for community assessment and asset mapping follows.

You may recall from chapter 5 that the PRECEDE/PROCEED model can seem a bit overwhelming at first, until you realize that its purpose is not to belabor the process with needless attention to detail. Instead, it is designed to help you develop a full picture of your community of interest—its health needs and the factors that influence them. It isn't the only needs-assessment and program-planning model, but it is quite useful for your exploration of needs because it offers a broad community-assessment perspective and provides a framework in which community members can participate in the process.

Applying PRECEDE to Community Needs Assessment

In chapter 5, we presented the history and purpose of the PRECEDE/PROCEED model and discussed the various phases that comprised its framework. Now it's time to apply it! Figure 6.2 presents a sample PRECEDE assessment of adolescent smoking. The words or phrases in each PRECEDE box represent factors we might identify and target if we were conducting a needs assessment among adolescents in a local school system. We invite you to use this visual as a guideline to create your own PRECEDE assessment of a similar adolescent health issue, such as drug abuse. FYI 6.7 lists needs-assessment strategies you might employ as you move through the four phases of the PRECEDE model.

To begin, draw a small "quality of life" box on the far right side of a sheet of paper. Record in it social indicators you think would emerge from a needs assessment about high school drug abuse. Draw a "health" box to the immediate left of the qual-

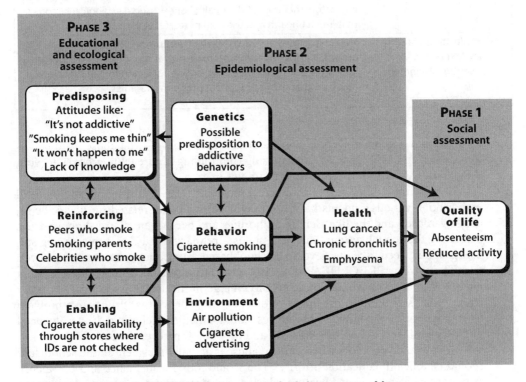

Figure 6.2   A sample PRECEDE assessment of adolescent smoking.
Based on Green and Kreuter's (2005) PRECEDE model, this example shows selected factors known to influence smoking behavior and its long-range effects as outlined using the first three phases of PRECEDE.

FYI

6.7   Needs Assessment Strategies Using Phases 1–4 of PRECEDE

Phases	Strategies
1. Social Assessment (Quality of Life)	Observe and take field notes, use photos or facilitate Photovoice, interview community gatekeepers and residents, conduct public forums and/or focus groups.
2. Epidemiological Assessment (Health, Genetics, Behavior, & Environment)	Collect secondary data such as reports from the state health department, county health department, and hospital data. Other sources include police records; school district reports; CDC data, reports, and publications; Center for National Health Statistics data; nonprofit organization data, reports, and publications. Use Photovoice; conduct geographic information system mapping (GIS); review or distribute community surveys to collect primary data.
3. Educational and Ecological Assessment	Review existing research from credible sources; develop and/or implement community surveys; conduct interviews, focus groups, or public forums to assess the predisposing, enabling, and reinforcing factors that impact the health issue; observe ecological factors that impact health and use field notes; take photos.
4. Administrative and Policy Assessment & Intervention Alignment	Map community assets; use Delphi group, nominal and/or focus groups, and/or public forums to discuss and prioritize community needs; review media and public policies; select theory or theories to guide program; list appropriate program strategies.

ity-of-life box and list in it some possible health indicators of drug abuse. Add behavioral, environmental, genetic, predisposing, reinforcing, and enabling boxes to your drug abuse model and insert relevant examples in each.

Suppose there have been a number of incidents related to drug abuse in a local high school; various students have been involved in alcohol-related traffic accidents, drug overdoses, and the like. School authorities and parents are alarmed about drugs pervading the school system, and the issue is a primary discussion topic among students. You've been asked to develop a school-based drug education program and you wish to apply the PRECEDE/PROCEED model to assess influencing factors. What quality-of-life factors would you expect to emerge in the social assessment? In other words, what social indicators might be detected as evidence that drugs are a problem in the school? Any number of indices could emerge, including drug-influenced domestic problems, school absenteeism and dropouts, and even arrests.

How would you know whether drug abuse is actually prevalent in the school and should be a health education priority? You would look for incidence and prevalence rates of specific drug-related health problems. Examples of indicators you could name include the frequency of alcohol-related traffic accidents, drug overdoses, and diagnosed drug addictions recorded over the past year. These statistics could be compared to other possible health problems such as injuries or sexually transmitted diseases to validate drug problems as an important priority.

With drug problems confirmed as an important target, what behavioral and environmental factors might you find to be contributing to the drug problems? In an educational and ecological assessment, what predisposing, reinforcing, and enabling factors might emerge? Individual surveys and group assessments could reveal important answers, such as the need to address social drinking and drug experimentation (behaviors) commonly practiced at parties and sporting events (a social environment factor). Common adolescent attitudes, values, misconceptions, and beliefs about drug and alcohol use (predisposing factors) might be similar to those associated with cigarette smoking, and just as damaging. Your needs assessment might reveal that a well-designed health education campaign could counter the usual negative peer pressure if it involved recognized role models and school heroes (reinforcing factors). The assessment could also help you understand drug accessibility issues and identify the skills needed to refuse drugs in a social setting (enabling factors).

The PRECEDE assessment results we just described could serve as a visual framework for a needs-specific drug abuse prevention program. Specific aspects of program development, including goals, objectives, and implementation, will be addressed in chapter 7. Then, in chapter 8, we will revisit the model to discuss program evaluation plans and strategies.

≡ In Conclusion

As mentioned throughout this chapter, assessing community needs and assets is a vital first step for those planning health-related programs or services. It is important for health education specialists and other health professionals to understand the unique characteristics and health needs of each community in order to provide effective and relevant health education and services. In order to achieve this, the process itself must be collective in nature. In this chapter, we presented a number of needs assessment and community-capacity-building concepts and methods that we hope will serve you well in the future. We outlined steps in the assessment processes and highlighted a way to map community assets. Planning models are helpful when developing programs and the PRECEDE/PROCEED model is one of the most comprehensive tools of this kind. In chapter 7 you will have the opportunity to learn how to use the model to move from needs assessment to program development.

REVIEW QUESTIONS

1. What is a community needs assessment and why is it important?

2. Discuss the difference between objective and subjective needs and explain the value of assessing both.

3. Explain why involving community members as part of the needs assessment process from the beginning may enhance community engagement, authenticity, and sustainability.

4. Outline the benefits and drawbacks of using various types of data-collection methods in community needs assessment.

5. Explain how models and theories can be useful in the needs-assessment process.

6. Draw the PRECEDE portion of the PRECEDE/PROCEED model and analyze how its components can influence a community's health.

7. Justify why community asset mapping and community empowerment are important for program development.

FOR YOUR APPLICATION

Develop a PRECEDE Assessment

1. Choose a specific health problem within your zip code. Use the PRECEDE/PROCEED model and data available to you to identify multiple factors contributing to the health problem and subsequent quality-of-life issues prevalent in your area.

   A. Draw the same PRECEDE boxes you see in Figure 6.2 on a sheet of notebook paper. Write the PRECEDE labels (quality of life, health, behavior, and so forth) at the top of each box.

   B. Write your chosen health problem inside the "health" box. (If it's a behavior, such as smoking, enter it in the "behavior" box instead.)

   C. Move to the right and enter some quality-of-life issues that might arise in your chosen community as a result of this health problem. (If you began with a health behavior, complete both the "health" and "quality-of-life" boxes.)

   D. Now move back toward the left. Fill in each box with factors you think contribute to the problem. Try to be specific to your chosen community.

   E. Make a list of potential community resources, capacities, and solutions.

2. Apply the four phases (and 13 steps) of community needs assessment to your chosen community. Practice using some of the data-collection strategies outlined in this chapter, analyze the results, and create a formal report to submit to your instructor and peers.

Use Photovoice in Your Community

Ask a couple of your friends, work colleagues, or a few individuals in your family to take pictures (using a digital camera or cell phone camera) of what they perceive to be community barriers or assets that impact quality of life and overall health within the area. Use the steps of Photovoice (FYI 6.3) and analyze the results. Prepare a presentation of your findings to share with your classmates and members of the community.

Create Assessment Opportunities

Contact a local health department or health agency that provides health education programs. Ask about health issues and programs the agency is planning to address in the future. Volunteer to conduct a literature search to (a) clearly define the health issue, (b) identify factors that could potentially influence the targeted health problem, and (c) locate existing needs-assessment survey instruments that could be used by the agency. Use the PRECEDE model as a guide, and create a brief report of your findings. Give one copy to the agency and place one in your portfolio. Create a folder in your portfolio labeled "Needs Assessment (Responsibility I)." Ask an agency representative to write a brief evaluation of your efforts to include in that portfolio folder.

7

Planning Processes for Evidence-Based Programs

You are invited to serve on a planning team to develop a wellness promotion program for students on your university campus. The task seems easy enough until your planning team discovers that students are too busy with course work, jobs, and personal lives to squeeze in time for regular physical activity. Conversations with coordinators of student health services, the campus wellness center, and the academic department that offers wellness courses reveal that students don't effectively use these resources to their full advantage. You discover that a number of students struggle with health-related issues that are seriously impacting their quality of life and placing their futures at risk. Where do you begin in your attempt to make a difference?

Chapter Objectives

1. Describe benefits and general characteristics of the planning process.
2. Explain how the various phases of the PRECEDE/PROCEED model can be applied to the planning process.
3. Outline the phases of the MAPP model.
4. Describe the general components of a grant proposal or program plan.
5. List steps commonly used in the planning process.
6. Provide examples of a program vision, mission, goal, and objective.
7. Contrast process, impact, and outcome goals.
8. Develop a measurable objective.
9. Conduct a SWOT analysis for program planning.
10. Describe common budget categories.

≡ Planning Concepts and Strategies

"So, what's the plan?" This is a common question in everyday life. Whether it is asked among friends putting together a last-minute social event or among coworkers responding to an emergency, the general assumption is that a good plan can be useful. Our goal in this chapter is to equip you with basic planning concepts and strategies that can help you develop good planning skills. We begin with a general description of planning concepts.

Planning Benefits and Characteristics

Success in community-based health promotion can be thwarted by complex health issues, conflicting opinions, and shifting community dynamics. Trying to overcome these challenges to achieve long-range goals can feel like aiming at a moving target from a rocking rowboat. The precious commodities of time, momentum, funds, and other resources can be wasted when no clear sense of direction is in place. A well-designed plan can serve as:

- A communication tool to help partners focus on established goals, minimize unrealistic expectations, understand roles, and build trust.
- An action guide to streamline efforts, use resources effectively, and foster productivity.
- An evaluation guide for measuring progress and success.

Effective planning calls for patience, diligence, flexibility, and the realization that few plans are ever perfect or finished. Planning is an ongoing process.

Planning partners from different backgrounds sometimes struggle to find a common language to use in the process. Some groups stall over confusion about whether they are planning a "program" or an "intervention." Green and Kreuter (2005) defined a **health program** as "a set of planned and organized activities carried out over time to accomplish specific health-related goals and objectives" (p. 1). McKenzie, Neiger, and Thackeray (2017) defined an **intervention** as a "the planned actions that are designed to prevent disease or injury or promote health in the priority population" (p. 192).

Though these terms are often used interchangeably, when used together, "the term *intervention* will usually refer to a specific component of a more comprehensive *program*" (Green & Kreuter, 2005, p. 192). We have included in this chapter a sequence of planning steps that you can use to design an intervention. This intervention could be the only program component or could serve as one of several components of a large program.

A Model-Based Approach to Planning

Planning models can be useful planning guides. McKenzie, Neiger, and Thackeray (2017) identified more than a dozen program planning models, most of which contain five common elements: "(1) assessing needs, (2) setting goals and objectives, (3) developing interventions, (4) implementing interventions, and (5) evaluating results" (p. 42). The PRECEDE/PROCEED model (Green & Kreuter, 2005) described in chapter 5 is one of the most widely used planning models in public health and health education. As illustrated in Figure 7.1, needs assessment data collected in Phases 1–4 can be used by a planning group to set priorities, develop a vision, create goals and objectives, and align the planned intervention with available resources and administrative support. Phases 5–8 can be used to plan implementation and evaluation strategies.

An online strategic planning guide called the *MAPP Tool* may serve as a useful resource as you develop your planning skills. The tool is based on the Mobilizing for Action through Planning and Partnerships (MAPP) model created by the National Association of County and City Health Officials (NACCHO, 2017) to help "communities apply strategic thinking to prioritize public health issues and identify resources to address them" (para. 1). In Phase 1 of MAPP, Organize for Success, collaborative groups discuss partnership benefits and barriers, identify and organize participants, design the planning process, assess resource needs, secure commitments, assess readiness for planning, and develop needed tools for a successful planning process. In Phase 2, Visioning, the group discusses current and past community visions and develops a shared vision for the next 5 to 10 years. In Phase 3, Assessments, the group conducts assessments (see chapter 6) and/or examines findings through the lens of the

Phase 4:
Administrative and policy
assessment, PROCEED to
action, formative evaluation

Phase 2–3:
Epidemiological,
educational, and
ecological assessments

Phase 1:
Social and quality-of-life
assessments and situation
analysis

Phase 5: Implementation
Pretest Methods
Activate timelines for
training interventions

Phase 6: Evaluation ⟶ **Phase 7:**   **Phase 8:**
. . . of methods   . . . intermediate objectives   . . . ultimate goals

Figure 7.1   PRECEDE/PROCEED model: Three levels of analysis for planning.

From *Health Program Planning: An Educational and Ecological Approach*, 4th ed., p. 65, by L. W. Green and M. W.
Kreuter. © 2005 by McGraw-Hill. Used with permission of the McGraw-Hill Companies.

vision statement. In Phase 4, Strategic Issues, the group identifies and prioritizes strategic issues that emerged from previous phases. In Phase 5, Goals/Strategies, the
group creates goals and feasible strategies based on these priorities and available
resources. In the final MAPP phase, Action Cycle, the group creates measurable
objectives and an action plan for implementation and evaluation.

A Proposal Framework for the Planning Process

In public health and health promotion, planning usually includes the development of a document that contains a rationale, goals and objectives, activity descriptions, timeline, and other elements needed to develop, implement, and evaluate a
program or intervention. This document may be called a program or intervention
plan, an action plan, or a work plan. It may be called a proposal if you plan to submit
it to decision makers from whom you are requesting resources (e.g., a grant proposal
or service contract), administrative approval (e.g., a service plan for an agency), or a
formal partnership agreement (e.g., with other organizations or community groups).
Common components of a plan or proposal (FYI 7.1) usually reflect the basic planning elements of assessment; goals and objectives development; and intervention
design, implementation, and evaluation.

If you are creating a grant proposal to submit to a specific funding agency, you
will likely need to adapt your content and format to requirements described in an
application guide. This application guide is usually called a **funding opportunity**

announcement (FOA) or a request for proposals or applications (RFP/RFA). An FOA usually includes extensive requirements for format and content that should be precisely followed. Some funding agencies offer grant-writing workshops for a specific FOA and have staff members available to help guide the process.

Most funding agencies have a cover page or application form that must be submitted with the proposal. This page can be accessed through the FOA and usually requires the name and address of the responsible individual, sometimes called the **principal investigator**. It will also require the name and address of the person or orga-

7.1   General Outline for Plans and Proposals

A proposal or program plan often contains sections similar to those listed below. You will also need a cover page/application form (for grant proposals), an executive summary (1-page overview of all components), and a table of contents. Adapt the following outline to meet specific proposal guidelines and/or your specific planning needs.

Statement of Need or Problem Statement
- Thorough discussion of problem the intervention will address
- Recommended components:
  - Review of the literature to quote national or global statistics related to the need
  - Findings from assessments conducted in local priority population
  - General living conditions, challenges, and capacities of priority population
  - Summary statement of what is needed based on information provided

Mission, Goals, and Objectives
- Program mission statement
- Program goals and measurable objectives
- Narrative if needed to explain context of proposed intervention within broader programmatic efforts

Intervention Description (Methods/Procedures)
- Overview of intervention scope and rationale
- Work plan (detailed descriptions of activity methods/procedures)
- Administrative plan (roles, responsibilities, expertise)
- Intervention timeline (Gantt chart)

Evaluation Plan (Data Collection/Analysis)
- Overview of evaluation scope and rationale
- Evaluation methods and procedures
- Evaluation timeline

Budget
- Summary table and brief narrative
- Item-line budget

Appendixes
- Reference list for all sources cited in document
- Assessment reports or summaries
- Intervention materials (marketing flyers, session/lesson plans, instruments, etc.)
- Vitas/resumes of personnel/consultants identified in administrative plan

nization responsible for fiscal management of the grant, the amount requested, the time period for the project, and a brief description of the agency. You will likely need to obtain signatures from designated officials in your workplace for this form, so be sure to learn about proposal-routing procedures for all organizations involved and allow time to obtain signatures prior to submission.

Some FOAs require a brief overview or **executive summary** of the entire proposal presented on one page or less. Because the executive summary is often the first (or only) part of your proposal that some decision makers read, we cannot overstate its importance. It should capture the reader's attention with a strong rationale for the need and value of the planned intervention. It should include a complete, yet concise, overview of the entire project (e.g., goals, strategies, time frame, capacities, needed resources, costs, benefits, expected outcomes), and should highlight the plan's strengths and innovative elements.

The more detailed sections of the proposal should contain information that answers the following questions.

1. What is the need in your priority population? (statement of need/rationale)
2. What is the mission of your planned intervention? (mission statement)
3. What specific changes are expected as a result of the intervention? (goals and objectives)
4. What is the general rationale and design of the intervention? (scope and sequence)
5. What specific activities will occur? (work plan methods/protocols)
6. Who will do the work? (administrative plan)
7. How will you know that you have met your goals? (evaluation plan)
8. What resources are needed to make it work? (budget)
9. How will this effort make a difference? (expected benefits and outcomes)

Some guidelines for developing a proposal are integrated into the recommended planning steps that follow.

Planning Steps

In an ideal world, all planning groups would work through a series of stress-free steps to a successful end. In the real world, that rarely happens. However, some common planning activities, when adapted and sequenced according to your specific needs, can help streamline the process, enhance productivity, and increase your chances for success. The planning steps described below and outlined in Table 7.1 can serve as a general guide. It is highly possible that your planning group will need to adapt these steps to your specific situation as part of Step 1.

Step 1: Establish a Shared Vision and Organize Planning Groups

Partnerships and a shared vision may have already been established when planning begins. However, in some cases, those partnerships and vision may need to be more fully developed as part of the early stages of planning. Bypassing this critical step can result in lost opportunities and closed doors.

Table 7.1   Planning Guide

Step 1: Establish a Shared Vision and Organize Planning Groups
1.1 Form planning and advisory groups
1.2 Develop a shared vision
1.3 Establish communication and decision-making structures
1.4 Develop work scope and action plan

Step 2: Assess Needs and Capacities
2.1 Identify existing and needed information
2.2 Collect and synthesize information
2.3 Determine priorities
2.4 Write rationale or statement of need

Step 3: Develop a Mission, Goals, and Objectives
3.1 Create a mission statement
3.2 Write goals and objectives

Step 4: Design the Intervention
4.1 Create a logic model
4.2 Select intervention strategies
4.3 Develop an intervention guide
4.4 Identify and develop needed resources
4.5 Create a budget

Sources: Green and Kreuter, 2005; KU Work Group, 2018c; McKenzie, Neiger, and Thackeray, 2017; NACCHO, 2017.

1.1 FORM PLANNING AND ADVISORY GROUPS

We recommend **participatory planning** in which "everyone who has a stake in the intervention has a voice, either in person or by representation. Staff of the organization that will run it, members of the target population, community officials, interested citizens, and people from involved agencies, schools, and other institutions all should be invited to the table" (Kansas University Work Group for Community Health and Development [KU Work Group], 2018d, para. 1). The nature of the planning groups formed and the extent of participants' contributions will depend on interest levels, time availability, relationships between groups/organizations, and the scope of needed work.

It may be helpful to organize a **coalition**, "A group of individuals and/or organizations with a common interest who agree to work together toward a common goal" (KU Work Group, 2018a, *What is a coalition?*, para. 1). To keep your coalition vibrant and productive:

- Communicate openly and freely with everyone
- Be inclusive and participatory
- Network at every opportunity
- Set reachable goals, in order to engender success
- Hold creative meetings

- Be realistic about what you can do: don't promise more than you can accomplish, and always keep your promises
- Acknowledge and use the diversity of the group (KU Work Group, 2018a, *In summary*, para. 5)

Continually report and celebrate progress and successes along the way so that all coalition members and the community at large are aware and appreciative of the work invested.

When no coalition exists or when your planned intervention is one of several coalition projects, you may need to form a smaller planning group of 5–12 members. This group may consist of a subset of coalition members; other stakeholders; and experts who possess needed insights and skills, will be trusted by stakeholder groups, and will work collaboratively and efficiently. McKenzie, Neiger, and Thackeray (2017) recommend that you include **doers**, "people who will be willing to roll up their sleeves and do the physical work needed to see that the program is planned and implemented properly" (p. 34), and **influencers**, "those who with a single phone call, e-mail, or signature on a form will enlist other people to participate or will help provide the resources to facilitate the program" (p. 34). This planning group can also consult with an advisory panel of experts for technical assistance and/or a community advisory group for input about population-based needs and perspectives.

1.2 DEVELOP A SHARED VISION

A unified vision within and across groups can serve as a solid foundation for all planning activities. This vision can emerge from an examination of previously collected and/or newly implemented assessments (see Step 2) and from the collective experience and wisdom of the partnership group. Your group's **vision statement** should be futuristic and reflect a conceptualized ideal for the priority population.

1.3 ESTABLISH COMMUNICATION AND DECISION-MAKING STRUCTURES

Groups work more effectively when communication and decision-making structures are clearly understood. Group leaders, decision-making rules, and communication channels should be designated before the work begins. Decision-making procedures can include group consensus, a formal vote, or a designated executive committee that makes final decisions when consensus cannot be reached. Be consistent in how decisions are made and, whenever possible, openly communicate decision-making processes, outcomes, and rationale with all partners.

1.4 DEVELOP WORK SCOPE AND ACTION PLAN

Members of the planning group should agree to serve based on a clear understanding of roles and expectations. When inviting individuals to join the planning group, provide a written description of the purpose, work scope, and expected outcomes of the planning process. The established group should then refine the action plan to include planning goals and tasks, decision-making and communication channels, and other details that will guide the planning process.

Step 2: Assess Needs and Capacities

Though much of the needs and capacity assessment work may have already occurred before your planning group is formed, your group will need to examine this information in light of your planning goals. The goal of this step is to validate the need for your planned intervention.

2.1 IDENTIFY EXISTING AND NEEDED INFORMATION

The MAPP and PRECEDE/PROCEED (Phases 1–4) models can be used to determine the information and resources you will need to plan and implement the intervention. Your group should create a list of existing and needed information, the sources from which they have been or will be obtained, and how that information will be used in the planning process.

2.2 COLLECT AND SYNTHESIZE INFORMATION

The assessment methods described in chapter 6 can be used to collect any additional information that may be needed. Synthesizing all information into a concise and useful format is an important part of the planning process. This synthesized information should be used to determine priorities for your planned intervention.

2.3 DETERMINE PRIORITIES

Your group can use a prioritization matrix (see chapter 6) to identify important and changeable factors to be addressed in the intervention. A SWOT analysis (KU Work Group, 2018f) can also be used to develop a matrix of strengths, weaknesses, opportunities, and threats (SWOT). The upper half of the matrix (see Figure 7.2) should contain internal strengths and weaknesses of your partnership group or organization (the group that will develop and implement the intervention). These strengths and weaknesses can include a variety of elements such as existing or needed resources (e.g., equipment, supplies, and materials), levels of personnel expertise and experience, organizational structures and policies that can enable or hinder progress, or the degree to which all partners possess the needed vision and commitment.

The lower half of the matrix represents external opportunities and threats in the environment or setting in which you plan to implement the intervention. For example, a recent community event that has intensified interest in issues related to your program mission could be viewed as an external op-

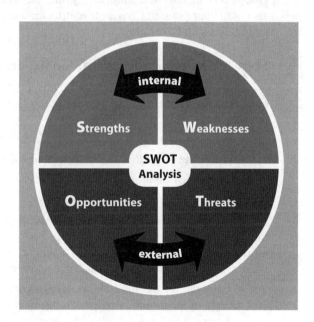

Figure 7.2   SWOT analysis matrix.

Adapted from *SWOT Analysis: Strengths, Weaknesses, Opportunities, Threats*, ch. 3, sect. 14, KU Work Group for Community Health and Development, 2018f, Lawrence, KS: University of Kansas.

portunity for your intervention to be well received. New leadership, changes in policies or laws, or the development of new funding sources or partnering organizations can serve as external opportunities that can increase your chances for success.

It is important, however, to weigh these opportunities in light of potential threats in the environment that could hinder your progress or negatively impact your intended outcomes. In the business world, the paradigm in which the SWOT analysis concept was first developed, an external threat is often another business that competes for the same customers. In public and community health promotion, it is important to identify potentially competing programs and services and avoid unnecessary duplication. External threats can also include "competing messages" or other elements that counter or distort your health message and intended outcomes. For example, unhealthy weight-loss programs, fast food restaurants, and tobacco stores can serve as external threats to a program with a health promotion mission. Social norms that embrace risky behaviors such as unsafe sex and alcohol abuse can also be external threats. A SWOT analysis should enable your group to enhance and capitalize on internal strengths and external opportunities and address or minimize the impact of internal weaknesses and external threats.

2.4 WRITE RATIONALE OR STATEMENT OF NEED

A written rationale or statement of need that summarizes your findings in Steps 2.1 through 2.3 can serve as a useful communication tool for interested stakeholder groups. It can also be included in grant proposals and plans. The statement should also help your planning group develop a mission statement, goals, and objectives that match needs and capacities.

Step 3: Develop a Mission, Goals, and Objectives

Most program or intervention plans include a mission statement, goals, and objectives that frame the intervention design and planned activities. These three components should:

- Reflect prioritized needs and capacities in your priority population
- Frame the scope and specific elements of your planned intervention
- Guide the evaluation process to monitor progress and outcomes

3.1 CREATE A MISSION STATEMENT

A **mission statement** is a "short narrative that describes the purpose and focus of the program" (McKenzie et al., 2017, p. 134). Where the vision statement describes a future ideal condition, the mission statement clarifies the purpose of the program or what will be done through the program to achieve that vision. Examples are listed below.

- The mission of the *BU-LiveWell Program* is to promote total well-being and health-related quality of life among Baylor University students.
- *BodyWorks* is a program designed to help parents and caregivers of teens and preteens improve family eating and activity habits (Office of Women's Health, 2014, *BodyWorks*, para. 1).

Every goal, objective, and strategy of your planned intervention should be designed to help your group achieve its stated mission.

3.2 WRITE GOALS AND OBJECTIVES

Your program goals and objectives should serve as the guide for designing, implementing, and evaluating your intervention. The first step in creating them is to clarify what your group plans to call them. In this chapter, we use the term *program mission* to refer to the overall purpose of the program. Any goal (e.g., health goal, behavioral goal) associated with your program is referred to in this chapter as a *program goal.* A **goal** is commonly a short, general statement that indicates what will change and the individuals or groups expected to be affected by the change. An **objective** contains detailed criteria needed to measure the degree to which you have achieved that goal (CDC, 2015; Green & Kreuter, 2005; McKenzie et al., 2017). Because goals and objectives are so critical to effective planning, we have provided some detailed information about how to create them.

Writing goals. A goal can be written as an incomplete sentence that begins with the word "to" as in "To reduce the incidence of teen pregnancies in McLennan County" or "To increase physical activity among Baylor University students." Notice that these goals do not include details that would be needed to measure these intended changes. Your objectives will contain the details.

Also notice that each of our example goals focuses on only one specific change (reduced pregnancies, increased physical activity). There is a practical reason for this singular approach. When you begin to evaluate your program and interpret results, you will need to clearly determine and report whether you did or did not achieve each goal. If you combine two or more targeted changes in the same goal (for example, "To increase *physical activity* and *healthy eating* behaviors . . ."), interpreting and reporting results can become a bit confusing, particularly if you observe an increase in one behavior but not the other. It is also easier to create measurable objectives for a goal that contains only one intended change.

There is no rule about the number of goals you will need. However, most planning groups create too few. If your planned intervention is intended to be part of a long-range community building effort, multiple goals that systematically connect the immediate results of your intervention to that broader long-term mission can be very useful.

In the following paragraphs, we will use the PRECEDE/PROCEED model to present a systematic approach to goal development that you may find useful. However, before we begin, we believe it is important for you to be aware that uses of the terms *impact* and *outcome* can differ when referring to program goals. Leaders in some organizations refer to short-term and immediate changes that can occur as the result of a program or intervention as *outcomes* that can then lead to more long-range *impacts,* such as improvements in health and quality of life. By contrast, these two terms are reversed in the PRECEDE/PROCEED model. We encourage you to learn both perspectives and adopt the approach that works best for you and your community partners.

We now invite you to consider Phases 1–4 of the PRECEDE/PROCEED model as a framework for goal development. The factor or object of interest assessed in each of those phases can be used to develop a related program goal for that factor. Figure 7.3 contains an example of possible program goals that could be developed using these four PRECEDE phases if your planning group was developing a physical activity promotion program for university students. A long-range **quality of life goal** to

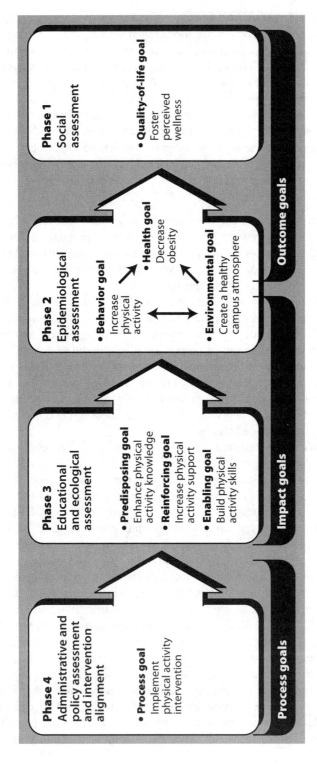

Figure 7.3   PRECEDE Phases 1–4: Examples of program goals.

Adapted from *Health Program Planning: An Educational and Ecological Approach*, 4th ed., PRECEDE/PROCEED model, by L. W. Green and M. W. Kreuter, 2005, New York: McGraw-Hill.

promote wellness among students could be at least partially achieved if increased physical activity (behavior goal) and reduced obesity (health goal) were achieved through the intervention.

To create and implement a comprehensive physical activity promotion program, your planning group would likely need to create several physical activity-related **health goals** (statements of intended changes in mortality, morbidity, disability, or physiological risk factors or health status indicators such as blood pressure or body fat percentage). Health goals represent "health outcome measures" that are often considered an essential measure of success among health care professionals and health service administrators. Our sample health goal in the figure targets an intended change in the physiological risk factor of obesity as an expected outcome of our physical activity intervention. But we could also have targeted changes in health problems that are commonly associated with lack of physical activity and obesity such as diabetes or heart disease. We focused on obesity, a health indicator, because our program is designed for college students who may not begin to experience the chronic illnesses associated with obesity until later in life.

In the PRECEDE/PROCEED model, quality of life and health goals are generally referred to as **outcome goals,** statements of intended changes that are often long term and far reaching. When these goals focus on long-range outcomes such as decreased mortality and morbidity rates, the emergence of observable changes can take years. To maintain morale and support for your intervention, goals that reflect more immediate successes can be an asset.

Impact goals, in the PRECEDE/PROCEED model, are statements of intended change in the factors identified in Phases 2–3 of the model that impact health and quality of life. The behavioral goal (increased physical activity) in our example (Figure 7.3) is a type of impact goal. Our sample **environmental goal** (create a healthy campus atmosphere) can result from an intervention that contains other goals and activities designed to impact the physical, social, and/or economic environment on campus. Figure 7.3 also contains samples of other types of impact goals designed to address the predisposing, reinforcing, and enabling factors that may influence physical activity and/or the campus climate. Figure 7.4 contains more complete versions of our sample impact and outcome goals, along with some example objectives linked to each goal. We describe how to create measurable objectives in the following section.

Once your planning group knows *what* you want to change (stated in your impact and outcome goals), you can create goals that state *how* you will make those changes happen. These **process goals** can focus on the development, delivery, and/or quality of your planned intervention. Some process goals target the completion of specific tasks (e.g., testing educational materials, distributing a newsletter, or conducting an orientation meeting) and the delivery of health promotion sessions or services (e.g., attendance or participation). Other process goals target perceptions of program quality among program participants, staff, and other stakeholders. For goal-writing purposes, we refer to these factors that often serve as the measurement targets in process goals as **program delivery factors** and **program quality factors.** We included examples of these two types of process goals, along with some related objectives, in Figure 7.5 on p. 169.

Impact	Outcome

Impact

* **Predisposing Goal:** To increase physical activity-related knowledge among program participants (*KNOWLEDGE*)

O-1: By the end of Week 1 of the program, at least 80% of program participants will be able to list at least 3 types of aerobic activity.

O-2: By the end of Week 2 of the program, at least 60% of program participants will be able to describe three essential criteria (intensity, duration, frequency) for an aerobic activity.

Reinforcing Goal: To increase support for program participants

O-1: By the end of Week 2 of the program, all program participants will have received guidance in developing personal physical activity goals.

O-2: By the end of Week 3 of the program, at least 40% of program participants will report having a partner for physical activities.

Enabling Goal: To increase physical activity skill levels among program participants (*SKILL*)

O-1: By the end of Week 2 of the program, at least 80% of program participants will demonstrate an ability to accurately measure their heart rate at the end of a three-minute step test.

O-2: By the end of Week 6 of the program, at least 60% of program participants will demonstrate an ability to monitor goal achievement.

Behavioral Goal: To increase physical activity among program participants

O-1: By the end of Week 3 of the program, at least 60% of program participants will report engaging in physical activity at least 3 times per week.

O-2: By the end of Week 3 of the program, at least 40% of program participants will report engaging in physical activity for a minimum of 40 minutes in each exercise session.

Outcome

Health Goal: To reduce the prevalence of obesity among program participants (*RISK FACTOR*)

O-1: Within 6 months of program initiation, at least 10% of program participants with overweight baseline measures will have reduced their body fat percentage by 5%.

O-2: Within 6 months of program initiation, all program participants with normal weight baseline measures will still be in the normal weight category.

Quality of Life Goal: To enhance perceived wellness among program participants

O-1: Within 6 months of program initiation, at least 10% of program participants who indicated low levels of perceived wellness in a baseline survey will have reported moderate or high levels of perceived wellness on a follow-up survey.

Short-term Outcomes** ⟶   Mid-term Outcomes   Long-term Outcomes ⟶

* Based on PRECEDE/PROCEED model terminology (Green & Kreuter, 2005).
** Logic model terminology (W. K. Kellogg Foundation, 2004).

Figure 7.4   Impact and outcome goals and objectives.

Sources: Green and Kreuter, 2005; W. K. Kellogg Foundation, 2006.

PROCESS

Program Delivery Factors

Number of sessions or services delivered, participants, tasks completed

Process Goal 1: To implement the *BU-LiveWell* program

> **O-1:** By the end of Week 1 of the program, at least 70% of program participants will have completed all baseline assessments.
>
> **O-2:** By the end of Week 6 of the program, at least 70% of program enrollees will have attended all weekly meetings.

Inputs

Program Quality Factors

Peer review, quality control, accreditation, audit, certification

Process Goal 2: To enhance the quality of the *BU-LiveWell* program

> **O-1:** By the end of the first year of the program, at least 70% of program participants who completed a participant satisfaction survey will have rated the *BU-LiveWell* program as "high" in overall program quality.
>
> **O-2:** By the end of the third year of the program, the *BU-LiveWell* program will have received a rating of *excellent* on overall program quality by an outside program review team.

Outputs

Figure 7.5   Process goals and objectives.

Source: *Logic Model Development Guide*, W. K. Kellogg Foundation, 2006.

Program objectives.   Each program goal you create should be accompanied by a set of measurable objectives similar to the examples in Figures 7.4 and 7.5. These objectives can be used to help you determine the degree to which that goal has been accomplished. For the same reason that each goal should state only one change, each objective should be designed to measure only one aspect or component of the goal. For example, if your behavioral goal is "To increase physical activity," you may need separate objectives to measure changes in different types of physical activity such as aerobic, strength-building, and flexibility activities.

Regardless of the type of objectives you write, every objective should be **SMART**: **s**pecific, **m**easurable, **a**chievable, **r**ealistic, and **t**ime bound (CDC, 2015). In general, an objective should contain at least four elements that are described below (Green & Kreuter, 2005).

1. *Who* will change or benefit from the planned intervention?
2. *What* will change or what benefit will they receive?
3. *How much* will change or how much benefit is expected?
4. *By when* will the change or benefit be evident?

Figure 7.6 illustrates needed components of a SMART objective with an example objective designed to measure changes in reported frequency of physical activity

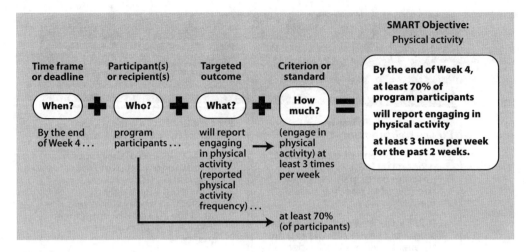

Figure 7.6   Elements of a SMART objective.

Sources: CDC, 2015; Green and Kreuter, 2005.

(what) among college students enrolled in a physical activity program. In the sample objective, we refer to this group as program participants (who).

Who will change? Be careful and precise in naming the "who" of your intended change or benefit. This "who" will normally be members of a specific subgroup of your priority population whose knowledge, behaviors, or health status, for example, you intend to change. However, consider the implications of naming your entire priority population as the "who" in your objective. If, for example, you name the entire target population (e.g., members of McLennan County, Baylor University students), in the objective, you just committed to measuring or having access to measures of the targeted knowledge, behavior, or health status of the entire population. In some cases, such widespread data does exist, particularly in the form of epidemiological data maintained by a government health agency, for example. But in other cases, it may be more realistic for the "who" of your objective to be defined as actual participants in your intervention so that immediate and, perhaps, long-term changes can be monitored. Either approach (a broad population group or only program participants) may be appropriate depending on your planning group's situation.

What will change? This component of the objective should state the exact factor or object of interest you plan to measure. The more specifically you describe this factor, the easier it will be to measure it. When writing a predisposing objective to measure changes in knowledge or attitudes, make sure that the verb you use to describe "what" you'll measure is observable.

For example, the two objectives listed in Figure 7.4 under the predisposing goal are knowledge objectives. These objectives are designed to measure changes in knowledge by measuring the participant's demonstrated ability to "list at least 3 types of aerobic activity" (objective 1) and "describe three essential criteria for an aerobic activity" (objective 2). Note that you could observe this knowledge change by listening to the participant verbally describe the targeted knowledge or reading the participant's written description. This is what we mean by "observable" measures. Even though it may seem logical to write an objective that says participants will "understand" this information, no one can truly measure or observe what a person understands until that person demonstrates that understanding by describing or applying it in some way. The words listed in FYI 7.2 are but a few observable action verbs you can use to write objectives.

FYI

7.2   Measurable and Observable Behaviors

Cognitive (with increasing levels of cognitive ability)

Count	Express	Apply	Analyze	Assess
Define	Locate	Examine	Calculate	Judge
List	Review	Practice	Debate	Evaluate
Identify	Compute	Illustrate	Compare	Revise

Affective

Accept	Seek	Display		
Observe	Complete	Discriminate		

Psychomotor

Taste	Position	Copy	Create	Walk
Place	Repeat	Build	Produce	Climb

Another way to write the "what" of the objective in measurable terms is to provide more specific details about the exact type of action or behavior you will be evaluating to determine whether the objective was achieved. In our example of a SMART objective (Figure 7.6), the object of interest is "reported physical activity frequency." The words "at least 3 times per week" could be viewed as further clarification of what will change in that only those participants who report exercising at least 3 times per week (not one or two) will be counted as having achieved this objective. This clarifying condition for inclusion could also be considered part of the "how much" component of your objective (described below).

How much will change? As already stated, the condition of having to report a frequency of "at least 3 times per week" could be considered part of the criterion or standard of achievement in your objective. Examples of other number-based measures of "how much" include percentages (e.g., 20% increase in physical activity frequency), scores (e.g., minimum score of 50 points), averages or rates (average resting heart rate below 70 beats per minute). However, this standard does not necessarily have to relate to the object of interest (what) that is expected to change. In some cases, a number or percentage of the people (who) expected to change or benefit can serve as your standard for "how much" or, in this case, "how many." If it is unlikely that every participant in the intervention will achieve the stated objective, it may be more realistic for you to name a number or percentage of participants (e.g., at least 70%) as your criterion for achieving the objective.

By when will the change or benefit occur? The time frame component of your objective should serve as a benchmark or "deadline" for when your objective should be achieved. The time frame can be stated as an exact date (e.g., by February 10, 2020), a specific time period in the program or intervention (e.g., by the end of Week 4), or a time frame attached to initiation or completion (e.g., within one year after program completion).

These stated time frames are helpful when it is time to schedule your intervention activities or plan of action on a timeline. For example, for our SMART objective example (Figure 7.6), a primary intervention activity could be a group session of physical activity three times per week. The planning group could assume that it may take a couple of weeks for all participants to adapt to this thrice weekly routine. The sample objective reflects the planning group's expectation that most participants (at least 70%) will be on track by the third week of the program. The sample objective would indicate a plan to survey all participants at the end of Week 4 to determine participation levels. Activities needed to help participants meet this objective on time and a description of the actual survey event would be included in the intervention plan and timeline.

Step 4: Design the Intervention

With goals and objectives in place, your planning group is now ready to design the intervention. Decisions about the type of intervention strategies and materials used should be based on information obtained from assessments and your mission, goals, and objectives. To more readily match these elements, we recommend creating a logic model (Step 4.1) and adding relevant information resulting from Steps 4.2 and 4.3. The model can then be used to guide the development of your budget (Step 4.4) and intervention guide (Step 4.5).

4.1 CREATE A LOGIC MODEL

A **logic model** is "a picture of how your effort or initiative is supposed to work . . . Effective logic models make an explicit, often visual, statement of the activities that will bring about change and the results you expect to see for the community and its people." (KU Work Group, 2018c, para. 1). A logic model generally illustrates the connection between your group's available resources, planned activities (your intervention), and expected outcomes (W. K. Kellogg Foundation, 2006).

Logic models come in a variety of forms and are used for a variety of different purposes. The PRECEDE/PROCEED model, for example, is a type of logic model that can be used for assessment, planning, and evaluation of programs and interventions. Our logic model development guide in Figure 7.7 contains the generic terms often used in logic models (top row of visual), with PRECEDE/PROCEED phases and terminology inserted beneath them. In this planning step, your group could create a similar visual to brainstorm and illustrate connections between your intervention goals and planned intervention. To do so, you would replace content in the "Standards or categories" row with your actual process (Phase 6), impact (Phase 7), and outcome (Phase 8) goals. The remaining two boxes on that row ("Inputs" and "Activities") would be completed through Steps 4.2 and 4.3. The resulting intervention logic model could be similar to our sample in Figure 7.8 (on p. 174).

Logic Model Terms*	Inputs	Activities	Outputs	Short-Term Outcomes	Mid-Term Outcomes	Long-Term Outcomes	
PRECEDE/ PROCEED Phases†	Phase 4 Educational strategies, policy, regulation, organization	Phase 5 Implementation	Phase 6 Process evaluation	Phase 7 Impact Evaluation		Phase 3 Outcome Evaluation	
Objects of interest in evaluation†	Needed resources/ conditions in community to operate program**	Planned strategies/ intervention components**	Health program or intervention	Predisposing, enabling, and reinforcing factors	Protective behavior or environment	Health status	Societal benefit
Standards or categories†	• Funding • Equipment • Supplies • Personnel • Policies • Organization/ Community support	Strategy Types:‡ • Health communication • Health policy/ enforcement • Environmental change • Health-related community service • Community mobilization	Peer review, quality control, accreditation, audit, certification	Changes in knowledge, attitudes, beliefs, skills, resources, social support, policy	Changes in frequency, distribution, timing of behavior, or the quality of the environment	Changes in mortality, morbidity, disability, or risk factors	Changes in quality of life

Figure 7.7   Logic model development guide.

* Logic model terms from Logic Model Development Guide, W. K. Kellogg Foundation, 2006, Battle Creek, MI: Author.

** Not usually included in PRECEDE/PROCEED evaluation.

† Logic model terms from PRECEDE/PROCEED evaluation.

† Adapted from *Health Program Planning: An Educational and Ecological Approach*, 4th ed., Figure 3-16, p. 140, by L. W. Green and M. W. Kreuter, 2005, New York: McGraw-Hill.

‡ Strategy types from *Planning, Implementing, and Evaluating Health Promotion Programs: A Primer*, 5th ed, by J. F. McKenzie, B. L. Neiger, and R. Thackeray, 2009, San Francisco: Pearson Benjamin Cummings.

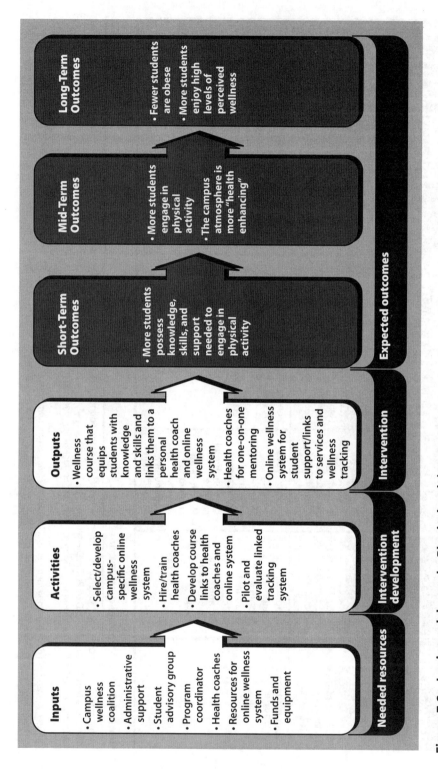

Figure 7.8   Logic model sample: Physical activity program.

Sources: Green and Kreuter, 2005; McKenzie et al., 2009; W. K. Kellogg Foundation, 2006.

4.2 SELECT INTERVENTION STRATEGIES

An intervention strategy is a type or category of activities designed to achieve program goals and objectives. Use your program goals and objectives and the output and outcome sections of your logic model to select the strategies needed to achieve your intended changes. These strategies can be listed as "activities" in your logic model and serve as the framework for your **intervention scope** (the breadth and depth of your intervention).

As you select intervention strategies and develop the scope, we recommend that you practice the **principle of multiplicity and comprehensiveness** (Green & Kreuter, 2005) by combining "interventions that address at least three theoretical constructs implicated in the change process: predisposing factors, enabling factors, and reinforcing factors" (p. 195) and include "educational, organizational, economic, regulatory, and other environmental change components" (p. 195). In other words, your scope of intervention strategies should be broad enough to allow you to address all of the types of program goals recommended in the PRECEDE/PROCEED model.

McKenzie et al. (2017) provide a detailed description of the six strategy types listed under "Activities" in the logic model development guide (Figure 7.7). These six categories serve as a general guide for selecting strategies to be used in your intervention (see chapter 8 for more details about intervention development). Health communication strategies are often developed based on four common communication channels: intrapersonal channels (e.g., one-on-one interactions), interpersonal channels (e.g., small groups and classes), organizational and community channels (e.g., organized social and religious groups, organizations, agencies), and mass media channels (e.g., print and electronic messages and campaigns). Health education strategies promote "voluntary behavior decisions conducive to health" (Green & Kreuter, 2005, p. G–4), through structured learning experiences such as classes, workshops, and learning programs. Examples of health-related community service strategies include health screenings, treatment, and referrals provided through community-based clinics and health fairs.

Health policy/enforcement strategies include "executive orders, laws, ordinances, judicial decisions, policies, regulations, rules, and position statements" (McKenzie et al., 2017, p. 206). Laws or ordinances that make it illegal to drive intoxicated or smoke in public places and policies related to health service eligibility are examples. A related type of strategy, environmental change strategies, can promote or enable healthy choices and behaviors (e.g., building recreational parks, providing healthy choices in cafeterias) or protect communities from environmental hazards (e.g., environmental waste regulations, smoke-free ordinances).

Community mobilization strategies are commonly used in public and community health education to equip community members with leadership skills and resources needed to promote personal and community health (see chapter 2). Health advocacy activities aimed at health-enhancing social and political change are also examples of this type of strategy (see chapter 12).

The challenge lies in selecting or developing strategies that will work for your priority population. When considering the quality and utility of an intervention, Green and Kreuter (2005) recommend that you consider:

- **Best practices** (sometimes referred to as evidence-based practices): interventions that have been proven effective in multiple settings and populations.
- **Best experiences:** "the prior experience of other practitioners, communities, states, or national programs in addressing the same issues. Best experiences can come from prior or existing programs and from the indigenous wisdom of the local community in which the program would be implemented" (p. 206).
- **Best processes:** proven methods and strategies used to assess the population and local situation to select appropriate interventions.

Though evidence-based practices are commonly valued in clinical settings where rigorous control can produce research-based evidence, best experiences and best processes are more feasible criteria for selecting interventions in community settings (Green & Kreuter, 2005).

Green and Kreuter (2005) recommend that you "match, map, pool, and patch" (p. 125) selected strategies to integrate them into a comprehensive program that fits the needs, interests, and capacities of your priority population. In brief, this process includes matching intervention strategies to individuals or group leaders at various ecological levels (e.g., individuals at risk, organizations, communities, governments); mapping or linking proven interventions to your specific program goals (particularly, predisposing, enabling, and reinforcing); and pooling existing interventions, community-preferred interventions, and your selected/proven interventions to patch or fill gaps in current efforts.

This intervention you develop should be given a test run (see chapter 8); you can then apply the **principle of intervention specificity** to adapt the full intervention and each component to fit the unique aspects of your priority population. This adaptation process is called **tailoring** when you adapt interventions or materials for individuals and **segmentation** when you do so for specific groups within a larger population (Green & Kreuter, 2005).

4.3 DEVELOP AN INTERVENTION GUIDE

We use the term **intervention guide** in this chapter to refer to a description of the general rationale and scope of the planned intervention (a general overview of strategies), a timeline for implementing all activities, and detailed descriptions of specific activities (protocols/methods, sequences, needed materials/equipment, etc.). These activities may encompass preparatory work like training personnel, developing materials, creating marketing and participant recruitment plans, orientations, and so forth, as well as activities that are actually part of your intervention strategies (e.g., awareness-building events, educational and training activities, mass media events, etc.). Though an evaluation plan is sometimes provided in a separate proposal section, the scope, methods, and instruments should be developed during this planning step and included either in the intervention guide or a separate section of your full plan or proposal.

A detailed timeline for all activities (preparation, implementation, evaluation) can be represented in one or more visuals. One of the most effective charting methods for timelines is called a Gantt chart (Figure 7.9). This type of chart helps you visualize when an activity will start, how long it will last, and which activities are overlapping.

An administrative plan with descriptions of roles and responsibilities related to tasks should be included in your intervention guide. Actual or sample materials such

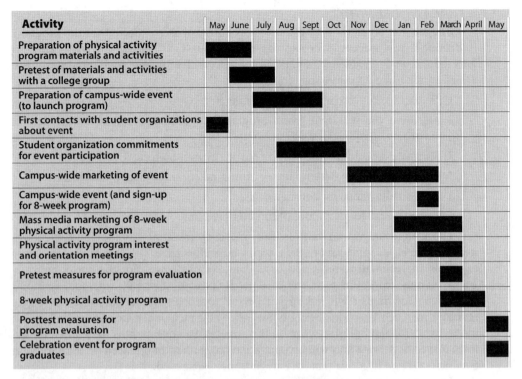

Figure 7.9   Gantt chart for a physical activity program.
Although projecting an accurate timeline can be a challenge, it is a vital part of program planning. It influences all aspects of the program from start to finish.

as marketing flyers, educational materials and lesson/session plans, and evaluation instruments should be included in an appendix of the guide or full proposal. Chapters 8 and 9 provide additional information that will help your group develop these plans and components.

4.4 IDENTIFY AND DEVELOP NEEDED RESOURCES

With your strategies selected and intervention guide in place, your planning group can now brainstorm a list of needed and available resources for the intervention. These needed resources, often referred to as *inputs* in a logic model, can include funds, equipment, supplies, personnel, and facilities. The time needed to implement, monitor, and evaluate each strategy is also considered a resource that can help shape your descriptions of roles and responsibilities in the intervention guide (Step 4.3) and determine personnel costs for the budget. Other inputs identified in this step may include administrative support, structure, and policies as well as various types of community support and commitments needed for program development, implementation, and evaluation. A thorough approach to this step will enhance your ability to obtain all that is needed for effective implementation.

4.5 CREATE A BUDGET

Budgets are predictions of the revenues and expenses expected for the program. Budgeting is the process of developing the budget. That process includes gathering information and reviewing similar programs to identify potential program costs. There are six basic steps in budgeting:

1. Select the cost categories for your budget.
2. Decide if you will divide your program budget into sections by time slices or phases.
3. Estimate costs for all the cost categories in your budget.
4. Document anticipated monetary or in-kind contributions to the project.
5. Add an allowance for contingencies.
6. Calculate the total amount of funding needed.

The sample budget summary in Table 7.2 contains some common budget categories: personnel, supplies, services, travel, and indirect costs. Correctly categorizing expenses and estimating projected costs can be a challenge. For the personnel category, you must determine the number of people needed, their roles and qualifications, the amount of time it will take each person to do his or her job, and the wages required for each position. Benefits are generally included if personnel will spend more than 50% of a full-time wage on the project. If a consultant is to be hired to perform a specific service and will be paid a flat fee (rather than placed on a salary with benefits), a separate consultant fee category may be needed.

The equipment category is usually reserved for durable items specifically needed for the planned intervention (e.g., blood pressure monitors, educational puppets). Some organizations separate equipment categories by cost ranges or types of equipment (e.g., computers or telephones that require ongoing service fees or technical support). Consumable supplies can include any item (e.g., paper, food items) or service (e.g., printing costs) that will be "used up" during the funding period. Some durable equipment also involves an expense for consumable supplies such as ink cartridges for computer printers or individual testing strips for glucometers (machines that measure blood glucose levels).

Depending on the budgeting practices of the organizations involved, fees charged for communication (postage, telephone services) and facility rentals may be placed in separate categories or included under consumable supplies. Travel expenses for program implementation or conference presentations are usually categorized separately and, in government-funded agencies, travel rates may be negotiated at the state level.

All of the costs previously mentioned are sometimes referred to as **direct costs** because they are specifically associated with a program and will be paid for directly with the requested grant funds. But there are also indirect costs to an institution or agency receiving funding that are not included in those direct cost categories. **Indirect costs,** also called facilities and administrative costs, include the less obvious expenses of maintaining the agency's infrastructure such as electricity and building maintenance. It is possible that the agency for which you work will have specific policies related to the addition of indirect cost coverage in a proposal budget.

If a program-planning project is large, it may be easier to break it into phases. For example, you might want to have three divisions: planning, implementing, and evalu-

Table 7.2 Sample Budget for a College Physical Activity Program

Budget Items	Hours	Rate	Totals
Personnel			
Health education specialist	960	$ 30	$ 28,800
Program assistant	800	20	16,000
Subtotal			$ 44,800
Personnel benefits (fringe) @20%			$ 8,960
Total personnel costs			**$ 53,760**
Supplies			
Printing brochure			$ 4,000
Postage (20,000 × .50)			10,000
Office supplies			500
Physical activity equipment			5,000
Total supplies			**$ 19,500**
Services			
Telephone			$ 1,000
Photocopying			600
Consultants			
Data processing	25	$ 17	$ 425
Marketing consultant	62	125	7,750
Graphic artist	16	25	400
Total services			**$ 10,175**
Travel			
National conference ($800 air; $300 per diem)			$ 1,100
Total travel			**$ 1,100**
Total direct costs			**$ 84,535**
Indirect costs (20% of direct costs)			**$ 16,907**
Total budget estimate			**$101,442**

ating. Some projects for which multiple funding years are awarded require a breakdown of expenses by funding year.

Budgeting can be both fun and challenging if you approach it with a positive attitude. Because adequate funds are often essential to intervention success, we strongly encourage you to be thorough and as detailed as possible in developing a workable budget plan. Model budgets for similar projects can be a useful resource. The individuals responsible for budgets, personnel, and other fiscal management activities should be able to help you develop a budget plan.

≡ In Conclusion

Though the steps provided in this chapter are presented in a linear sequence, in reality the planning process is rarely linear. In large-scale projects, for example, a planning group may use a linear sequence to initiate a smaller component of the intervention while continuing to collect additional assessment data to fill in information gaps. Some aspects of evaluation (discussed in chapter 9) actually occur during the planning and early implementation stages. And, no matter how hard you try to keep things organized, few interventions happen exactly the way they were planned. For these and other reasons, the key to effective planning is to use models and planning strategies as a general guide but remain flexible and fluid as the work progresses. Stay focused but do not be afraid to be creative and innovative when the situation calls for it. In the end, it is the quality of life of the people in your priority population—not the plan—that matters most.

REVIEW QUESTIONS

1. Describe the general benefits and characteristics of the planning process.

2. Explain the similarities and differences between a program and intervention.

3. Provide examples of a program vision, mission, goal, and objective.

4. Explain how Phases 1–4 of the PRECEDE/PROCEED model can be used in the planning process.

5. Describe the general components of the MAPP model.

6. Name the four planning steps described in this chapter. Provide examples of tasks a planning group might be doing in each step.

7. Explain the differences between and utility of process, impact, and outcome goals. Provide an example of each.

8. Write a SMART objective.

9. Describe the components of a SWOT analysis and provide a brief example for how it could be used.

10. Outline the general components of a proposal or program/intervention plan.

11. Create an example of a Gantt chart that would accompany a program plan.

12. Describe the categories that are commonly used in a health program budget.

FOR YOUR APPLICATION

Writing Goals and Objectives

Practice creating goals and objectives using the PRECEDE/PROCEED model as a guide. Use a model template or create your own on a blank piece of paper by sketching the boxes of Phases 1–4 of the model (use Figure 7.3 as a guide). Choose a health problem or behavior in a specific population about which you have some knowledge (e.g., teen pregnancy, diabetes among older adults) and proceed as if you were going to develop an intervention to address that problem or behavior in that population. Refer to Step 3.2 of the recommended planning steps in this chapter to create one goal for each box in the model (e.g., quality of life goal, health goal, behavioral goal). Then use Figure 7.6 (elements of a SMART objective) as a guide to create one sample objective for each goal. Ask a friend or colleague to check your work to ensure that you have applied the steps to create feasible goals and measurable objectives.

8

Implementation Processes

You are excited about getting started with the new program you developed for pregnant teens. You have taken all of the right steps. You conducted a needs assessment and carefully planned your program based on the perceived and documented needs of the population or partner community. You are ready to go! But wait, there are still a few missing links. You find that you need more money than expected to conduct the program and you need to make certain that information about the program reaches the people it is meant to serve. You also have materials to develop and schedules to create. Don't let the excitement wane; the success of the program you implement will be tied to the time you take to address these issues.

Chapter Objectives

1. Detail sources of external financial support for health promotion programs.
2. Describe methods of social marketing.
3. List ways of assessing marketing effectiveness.
4. Discuss key considerations in the hiring and training of individuals who will deliver the health education programs.
5. Identify teaching methods that employ experiential or critical thinking activities.
6. Describe appropriate program record keeping.
7. Practice developing an action or lesson plan.
8. Detail tips for training program implementers/staff.

Necessary Skills for Health Promotion Program Implementation

As you might guess, implementation processes involve putting the program into action. These processes require giving attention to everything we've already discussed, including assessing health education needs; planning an effective data-driven program; and strengthening the assessment, planning, implementing, and evaluating processes by grounding them in theory. Implementation processes also include marketing the program, using strategies that will provide the best opportunities for learning, monitoring the implementation plan, making changes to the plan as necessary, training program staff, "monitor[ing] adherence to ethical principles in the implementation processes" and "ensur[ing] compliance with legal standards" (NCHEC, 2015, p 4).

Supplementing Funds for the Program

Important implementation issues range from crucial concerns like money to smaller problems like projection units that don't work correctly. Of course, money is one of the largest concerns because all programs require funding to some degree.

Adequate resources, including personnel, materials, equipment, the site, and so forth, can make or break the program. Although these issues must be addressed early in your planning, they make such an impact on program implementation that we want to discuss them a bit more in this chapter. The adequacy of program resources will depend on the available money. You learned about grant writing in the last chapter and, ideally, you will receive grants large enough to fund all of the programs you will run. If not, you may need to supplement from local funding sources.

Seeking Donations or Sponsors

If no grants are available for a specific program at a particular time, you might seek a **corporate sponsorship** or pursue donations from individuals who are likely to support your objectives and are in a position to help. According to Ken Tysiac, "To attract donations, they [non-profits,] need to create value for donors in the form of events and perks, explore partnerships with for-profits, use technology to explore new avenues for fundraising, [and] tell their story in an engaging way" (2016, p. 35). As you can probably imagine, there is no single method for seeking donations. Sometimes you write a letter; other times, you make personal contact via a face-to-face meeting, with a telephone call, or, for many donors, through social media (Tysiac, 2016). However, there are some important things to remember, regardless of your method. For example, check with your agency about policies regarding donations. In some circumstances you won't be able to accept donations at all. In other circumstances, you will be able to receive donations but will be required to follow a well-defined set of guidelines.

If you receive approval to seek donations, make certain that other divisions in your agency aren't seeking donations from the same company or individual at the same time. It is unwise to overwhelm a corporation or individual who has been generous in the past with numerous new requests for money. If you request funds from a corporation, ask about the procedures you will be expected to follow. Most donate money frequently but have specific procedural requirements (such as submission of documents similar to a grant proposal).

Regardless of whether you will be writing letters, making phone calls, or developing a Web-based donation request, put thoughtful preparation into the project. Proofread your letters, have others read them for clarity and flow, and revise accordingly. In the case of telephone contacts, develop a script and practice before you make the call. Be sure to test your Web-based donation request and have others operate the site under the directions you will provide to ensure they are effective. And, of course, if you receive a donation or sponsorship, give appropriate acknowledgment. In addition to written thank-you notes, you might consider thanking donors on program handouts; this may be part of the value marketed to donors mentioned earlier.

Special Event Fund-Raising

Almost any activity can be a fund-raiser. Some of the most common today include fun runs, golf tournaments, and silent auctions; some organizations think outside the box and offer events such as quidictch matches, monster marches, and golden crown (painted toilet) sales. Of course, funds are raised through entrance fees or product sales.

Wood, Snelgrove, and Danylchuk (2010) suggest people participate in fund-raising events for varying reasons including finding the cause meaningful, enjoying the specific fund-raising activity, and liking the social aspect of the event. Fund-raising events should involve elements that reach out to all three categories of participant.

Fund-raisers have great potential, but they can also cause headaches if the planners are not experienced. For example, one of our local service clubs planned a chili supper fund-raiser. The planners understood promotion but did not grasp the total marketing picture. They advertised very effectively. In fact, approximately 500 people attended. However, the organizers did not assess the effectiveness of their promotion or the likelihood that so many people would attend. They cooked for only 100. Can you imagine the chaos?

Although this mistake was somewhat humorous, some planning errors can be dangerous to participants. What if you planned a 6-mile run but did not offer runners water or first aid? You could easily put participants in danger. Our suggestion is that you involve an experienced special-events planner on your fund-raising committee.

≡ Social Marketing

You may want to launch the implementation of your program with a **social marketing** campaign, which is a process of "influencing human behavior by creating, communicating, and delivering products and services to target audience members for the purpose of advancing (public health) objectives rather than for commercial profit" (Maibach, 2003, p. 41). A similar concept is **prevention marketing,** which is "CDC's adaptation of social marketing in which science-based marketing techniques and consumer-oriented health communication technologies are combined with local community involvement to plan and implement prevention programs. Essentially, prevention marketing equals social marketing plus community involvement" (CDCynergy, n.d., p. 5).

Understanding Social Marketing

Social marketing evolved from the strategies of commercial marketing. In social marketing, decisions must be made about the product, price, place, and promotion, often called the four Ps of commercial marketing. Other Ps to consider include partnership, policy, and politics. Philip Kotler and Gerald Zaltman (1971) conceived the idea of social marketing when they realized that traditional marketing principles could apply to attitudes and behaviors that influence social issues. Prior to the development of social marketing, large social campaigns often succeeded only in increasing people's awareness of a specific health issue. On the other hand, large advertising campaigns for new products continued to effectively increase use of specific products. Today, social marketing uses the methods of commercial marketing, with differences in content and objectives.

PRODUCT

Your **product** has actually been determined before you implement your program. In social marketing, the product can range from an actual product (a physical object) to a health-related service (like your teen pregnancy program) or even an idea. Keeping this in mind, you can see that the product is actually developed during program planning. For example, some products you could market for a smoking-cessation program include a device or invention to help individuals stop smoking (like a patch), the idea that smoking is not healthful even for teens, or an actual smoking-cessation program (service).

PRICE

By **price** we mean more than just money. Although monetary cost is one aspect of price, other intangible things like time, effort, and risk of embarrassment must also be considered. In general, people will weigh the benefits of the product against the costs. Their use of the product will depend on a perception that benefits outweigh the costs.

PLACE

The means of distribution for the product defines **place**. In the traditional form of marketing, you might decide that your product would be distributed from a warehouse via trucks to retail stores. In social marketing you make decisions about the channel of communication. The channel of communication might be a newspaper, a television show or commercial, a counseling session with a physician, or face-to-face interviews.

Social media may be the route that best matches your target population. As you know, people are more connected than ever before through this channel. A good portion of our population is sifting through huge amounts of information on social media on a daily basis (Ryan, 2014). Technology continues to progress at a remarkable pace, so stay abreast of the changes and if you find that your target population is using a new media type, don't be afraid to try a new strategy. No matter what channel you choose, be sure to take time to match your message to the media type. Every type of media requires you to shape the message in a different way. Using social media and technology for developing health messages is discussed more fully in chapter 11.

PROMOTION

It is easy to confuse promotion and place in social marketing. **Promotion** deals with keeping consumers interested and motivated to use the product. It might also involve news and telephone media. But, whereas place would refer to the channel or mode of communication you choose (such as a newspaper ad), the promotion aspect refers to how your message is worded to motivate or persuade the reader. The purpose differs from place; you might think of promotion as advertising and place as the medium you choose for your advertisement.

PARTNERSHIP

Health-related social problems are complex. In most cases, partnership requires collaboration among health agencies. Partnerships between agencies facilitate effective decisions about price and place. However, the most important partnerships are with people from all aspects of the community.

POLICY

According to Weinrich Communications (1999), "Social marketing programs can do well in motivating individual behavior change, but that is difficult to sustain unless the environment they are in supports that change for the long run. Often, **policy** (a planned course of action to guide decisions) change is needed, and media advocacy programs can be an effective complement to a social marketing program" (p. 3).

POLITICS

Your social marketing plan will require making decisions about the political environment. Suppose the product involved is controversial—for example, discussing birth control methods in public high schools. Unless an assessment is made of the politics surrounding the product, difficulties can snowball. Politics can destroy even the most beneficial program. There are times when it is best to wait until the political environment is more conducive to successful completion of the program.

Developing a Marketing Plan

Creating a marketing plan requires focusing on the people who will be using a product rather than on the product itself. Research and evaluation are the keys to developing an effective plan (CDCynergy, n.d.). Keeping in mind that the product has already been determined, planners must establish marketing objectives, assess the target audience, develop pricing and placing that correspond with the target population needs, and conduct promotion or advertising campaigns. Once a product has been identified during planning, we think of the acronym MAPP (Figure 8.1) as a guide to developing a marketing plan. This process of developing a marketing plan should remind you of the PRECEDE portion of the PRECEDE/PROCEED model. As you know, assessments come first, followed by planning, implementing, and evaluating. In fact, if you have used PRECEDE, writing a marketing plan will be much easier.

WRITING MARKETING OBJECTIVES

Marketing objectives relate directly to the program objectives. As we stated earlier, the product is determined during program planning; therefore, those very program objectives are part of the marketing objectives. Other marketing objectives specifically address promotion. Let's look at an example of a promotion objective. "During the year 2018, center staff will improve potential participants' perception of the program by creating updated brochures with the assistance of a graphic designer." As you can see, the objective contains all of the components of program planning objectives. The difference is in the focus on place and promotion rather than actual programming.

Figure 8.1   The MAPP approach to marketing. The MAPP acronym is a simple way to remember the steps to marketing a program. Some form of marketing will be necessary for any program to be a success. Having at least a rudimentary grasp of marketing will improve your chances of success.

ASSESSING THE TARGET AUDIENCE

This aspect of the marketing plan includes knowing the demographic makeup of the audience, such as the economic status, education levels, and age structure. It also includes psychosocial information such as attitudes and beliefs. Cultural and religious beliefs and behaviors are important to understand when you are creating a social marketing plan. Fortunately, you can achieve an understanding of your target audience for marketing purposes at the same time you conduct the initial needs assessment for program planning.

Both qualitative and quantitative methods of audience assessment can be used. A combination of methods might be best. Surveys, a frequently used quantitative method, can be mailed, conducted via the telephone, or conducted in face-to-face settings. Focus groups and interviews, commonly used qualitative methods, also involve primary data collection. Can you name some secondary sources of data that might be helpful in your needs assessment and marketing research? You might have considered reviewing the professional literature or accessing previously collected morbidity and mortality data.

DETERMINING DISTRIBUTION CHANNELS, OR PLACE

Communications media are the most commonly used channels for distribution in social marketing. Media include television, Internet, radio, newsprint, magazines, billboards, and cinema. Other types of distribution channels are personal face-to-face communication, telephone contact, posters, direct mail, direct sales, and distribution of brochures and other written documents. The selection of the appropriate channel depends on both the target audience and the product. For example, you won't choose the business section of a local paper to provide program information that you want teens to read. Again, you must know your audience before you can determine the appropriate channel. An important theoretical basis from which to identify an appropriate channel is the theory of the diffusion of innovation.

The **theory of the diffusion of innovation** describes the ways that an innovation spreads through a population. An **innovation** can be anything from a product (like new athletic shoes) to an idea (like the belief that smoking kills). In marketing terms, this is considered the product. Understanding the theory can help you determine what channels to use to advertise your innovation (health program). As you can see from Figure 8.2, the theory can be depicted as a bell shaped curve. Theorists believe that consumers can be categorized into five groups by the rate at which they adopt an innovation. As you read through this information, think about where you fit along the curve. You may find that it is not easy to determine your exact speed of adoption. Each of us adopts innovations according to the type of innovation and the current environment. In other words, the speed of adoption is not necessarily a stable characteristic; however, most of us fall into patterns of adoption. As you read, keep in mind that innovations can spread across organizations as well as among individuals (Dearing, 2015).

Innovators adopt change easily. In general, they are highly educated and can be reached through mass media channels. If they determine that an innovation might benefit them, they will change quickly. Suppose, for example, that we are promoting a new, effective stress-reduction strategy across the United States. For innovators, we could put an article in a national publication like *USA Today* or *Newsweek*. Innovators would be more likely than others to read the article and choose to try the new plan as a result. **Early adopters** are often public leaders and highly respected in communities. Others

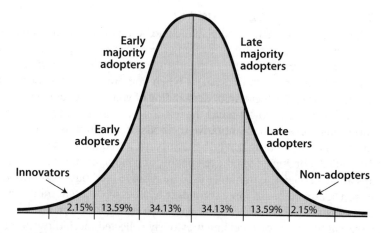

Figure 8.2   Diffusion of innovation theory.
This theory describes acceptance of change as following a bell-curve pattern. It also suggests that innovators will accept a new product or program much more quickly than individuals who are late adopters or non-adopters.

often follow their adoption patterns. Like innovators, they can be reached via mass media, although state or regional channels may be more effective. Again, a newspaper might be the appropriate place for dissemination of our stress-reduction plan; but, instead of an article, we might want to place an advertisement that suggests how effective the plan has been with individuals who have tried it. **Early majority adopters** accept innovations once they determine that others they respect have done so. Demonstrating the adoption patterns of innovators and early adopters is often the most effective way to reach most of the early majority adopters. For the promotion of our stress-reduction plan, we might use the same strategy that we used for early adopters, except that we would place our advertisement in a regional or local newspaper. **Late majority adopters** are somewhat skeptical of change. They will adopt an innovation most readily when they are required to do so (public law) or they believe that the change will benefit them dramatically. In order to reach late majority adopters, we might work directly with leaders in corporate worksites. Our goal would be to encourage corporations to require use of our stress-reduction plan. **Non-adopters**, historically known as hard-to-reach and even laggards, include individuals who choose not to make a change when most people—even late majority adopters—have already done so. The decision not to make a change may be a result of interwoven social determinants such as education and income, but it might also simply represent a point-of-view that must be respected. One-on-one, face-to-face communication about the innovation may help a health educator understand a non-adopter's perspective. For our stress-reduction plan, we might have other adopters, who were initially doubtful about the plan, make personal contact with non-adopters.

The relative advantage, complexity, compatibility, testability, reversibility, and observability of an innovation also influence the rate of adoption (Glanz, Rimer, & Viswanath, 2008). FYI 8.1 defines some of the terms associated with the theory of the diffusion of innovation.

8.1   Diffusion of Innovation Terms

According to the theory of diffusion of innovation, there are seven characteristics of an innovation. Each will be important for you to understand when projecting how a new program or product will be accepted by the target participants.

Compatibility   When innovations are consistent with the economic, sociocultural, and philosophical value system of the adopter, adoption is more likely to take place.

Flexibility   Innovations that can be unbundled and used as separate components will be applicable in a wider variety of user settings.

Reversibility   If for any reason, the adopting individual or organization wants to revert to its previous practices, it is desirable that an innovation be capable of termination. Innovations that are not are less likely to be adopted.

Relative advantage   If an innovation appears to be beneficial when compared to current and previous methods, adoption is more likely.

Complexity   Complex innovations are more difficult to communicate and to understand and are therefore less likely to be adopted.

Cost-efficiency   For an innovation to be considered desirable, its perceived benefits, both tangible and intangible, must outweigh its perceived costs.

Risk   The degree of uncertainty introduced by an innovation helps determine its potential for adoption. Innovations that involve higher risk are less likely to be adopted.

From "Implementing Comprehensive School Health Education: Educational Innovations and Social Change," by L. J. Kolbe and D. C. Iverson, 1981, *Health Education Quarterly*, 8: 57–80. © 1981 by Sage Publications. Used with permission.

PRICING THE PRODUCT

Although seemingly simple and easy to define, pricing is complex. On the one hand, price determines the accessibility of the service or product; on the other hand, price can imply credibility or quality (Alward & Camunas, 1991). People often believe that a product is not worth much unless it is associated with a high price. In order to determine the price, you must consider your objectives. FYI 8.2 (on the following page) discusses pricing objectives for tangible products. For further information on this subject, reference *How Customers Perceive a Price Is as Important as the Price Itself* by Sandeep Heda, Stephen Mewborn, and Stephen Caine.

Assessing Marketing Effectiveness

In chapter 9, you will read more extensively about evaluation research. We hope it is evident to you now, however, that you must always check to see if your plans are working. One of the biggest wastes of time and money comes from continuing with activities that don't work. You will learn about a number of research and evaluation methods in chapter 9; for now, we would like to suggest a few questions to ask about your marketing plan to assess its effectiveness:

8.2   Using Pricing Objectives for Tangible Products

The price of your product or program will be determined by the type of outcome desired. The following provides suggestions for determining price.

Goal of Marketing	Pricing Activity	Consequence of Activity
High percentage of target population to accept health product or service	Offer product or service at a low cost	Potential perception of a product or service of low worth
Equal distribution of health product or service	Offer product or service at a flexible price structure	Individuals with high income pay more, potential perception of inequality
Expense and income are balanced	Offer product or service at a price that defrays the cost	Cost may be too high at first
Maximizing profit	Offer service or product at a price that improves the demand	Cost may be too low at first
Minimizing excessive demand of an unhealthful service or product	Offer service or product at a very high price	Negative perception of pricing

From *A Short Course in Social Marketing*, Novartis Foundation for Sustainable Development, 1999.

- Does the product meet the needs of the population? Or, in other words, are the participants making the planned change? Do the participants perceive the program to be useful? Are people healthier as a result of the program?
- Can the population access the product? Or, are people attending the program? Do participants perceive the price of the program to be appropriate? Do participants perceive the benefits of the program to outweigh the barriers to attending?
- Are the distribution channels effective? Or, do participants report hearing about the program through your selected channels of advertising? How did participants hear about the program?
- Do policies and politics serve as barriers or boosters to the product? Or, how do agency politics affect the program? How do local politics affect the program?

≡ Other Aspects of Implementation

Effective implementation requires that you attend to every aspect of the program, not just money and marketing. Going with the flow, or simply letting events unfold, is not appropriate. Other aspects of program implementation that you need to address include selecting and training staff and or volunteers, developing curricula and teaching methods, identifying equipment and facilities, determining program logistics, preparing materials, and program follow-up.

Selecting Staff and Volunteers

Randy Pennington, owner of a leadership consulting firm in Dallas, states that an effective way of viewing staff is to consider them as essential volunteers (personal communication, November 8, 1999). Adopting this attitude requires you to spend adequate time training your employees and demonstrating to them that they are valued. This approach is as necessary for retaining good employees as it is for keeping volunteers.

You must also strive to create an ethical work climate in order for employees to identify more strongly with your organizations (DeConink, 2013) and make ethical, work-related decisions. Also, "it is reasonable to expect that diverse groups with inclusive climates may benefit not only from lower levels of conflict but also from better performance" (Nishii, 2013, p. 1768). An inclusive climate that requires ethical work creates a strong and healthy organizational culture.

New employees should understand the organizational culture you have worked to create, have experience working with the target audience, demonstrate professionalism, and have content expertise and skills (Carnevale, Gainer, & Metzler, 1990). That said, how do you find people who fit these criteria?

Begin the process of selecting employees by asking for a portfolio and continue by interviewing those who demonstrate the knowledge and skills that you require. Many professional preparation programs encourage students to develop portfolios. As the potential employer, you can judge the potential employee's work for yourself. For example, if the individual will be asked to write pieces for a newsletter, you will want to read sample articles or other written documents that demonstrate effective written communication skills.

Begin the interview process by modeling professionalism. Be on time, prepare in advance, select appropriate attire, communicate effectively, and act with integrity. Your first meeting with the prospective employee will be your first training session. If you demonstrate a lack of preparation or ineffective communication, you are essentially giving permission for the individual to act in the same manner if hired. Remember that new employees want to do a good job and they will follow your lead.

We suggest that you ask potential employees to demonstrate their skills. If you expect your new employee to make presentations to small groups, ask applicants to do so as part of their interview. If they will be conducting program evaluations, give them an actual scenario to discuss. We also encourage you to wait for the right person rather than resorting to panic placement (selecting anyone just to get someone in the position). It may be a relief just to hire someone; but you will ultimately spend a lot more time, effort, and money if you have to start over because the individual did not match the position.

If you are seeking volunteers rather than paid employees, you should still ask for information about their educational background and skills. You want to place volunteers in an area that fits their skills and desired type of work. Unlike job applicants, volunteers are not usually turned away. But most agencies and organizations have many types of work that can be performed by volunteers, so it's wise to ensure that a volunteer's skills match the job requirements.

It addition, you need to make sure that prospective employees or volunteers do not hold beliefs that are contrary to the philosophical foundation of the agency. For example, an individual who does not approve of abortion may not support a policy that requires women to be given information about abortions. You will have the responsibility of making certain that the individuals you hire or invite to volunteer support the agency's philosophies.

Training New Employees

We asked people who had recently started new jobs to comment on their training needs. Several themes appeared in their comments. Every person noted that clear and honest descriptions of expectations were vital. Some also stated that they needed to know the extent to which they could develop their own goals. The people in our small survey indicated in various ways that they needed to understand the agency mission as well as the purpose of the specific job they would be performing. Some mentioned that explanations of their employee benefits and important agency policies were necessary. Others also valued the identification of available resources and acknowledgement of resources that were not available. Last but not least, all of the individuals mentioned that they needed training for new skills as well as feedback on the acquisition of those skills.

Interestingly, the people we talked with regarded the training process as a reflection of the philosophical basis from which their employer worked. In other words, agencies that offered appropriate training were more likely to value their employees. And agencies that value employees provide opportunities to help them succeed rather than focus on performance problem areas. Even though our study was small, we feel that the participants targeted the major points of effective training: (a) a clear job description, (b) guidelines for developing personal professional goals, (c) guidance in following the agency mission and policies, (d) an account of available resources, (d) methods for accessing resources not readily available, (f) training for new skills, and (g) feedback meant for growth not punishment.

Planning training workshops or sessions involves most of the same tasks as planning a health promotion program and a marketing campaign. An assessment of training needs should take place, training goals and objectives based on the assessment should be written, clear and useful training materials should be developed, and the logistics of the training sessions should be carefully planned. Don't forget to recruit participants, create a positive learning environment for participants, practice effective presentation skills, use technology successfully, and evaluate the health education program as it relates to aspects of the training workshops if needed. And of course, the training workshops and sessions themselves should be evaluated and modified before the next training sessions.

Facilities

The physical environment can make a major difference in people's ability to learn. Have you ever attended a lecture in a room that was very hot or very cold? How did the temperature affect your ability to listen? Room temperature, sound levels, amount of light, colors, room setup, room size, and type of furniture work synergistically to impact participants. The success of your program will be determined partially by the environment, so consider your options carefully and plan in advance.

CHOOSING THE SITE

Health programs can be conducted in many types of locations. If you do not have space available in your agency, other choices might include hotels, conference centers, universities, ships, resorts, other public buildings, and corporate settings. Your choices will depend on your budget, program objectives, size of audience, and location of potential sites. Table 8.1 provides a comparison of different types of sites.

Table 8.1   Comparison of Site Types

The type of site you select for your program will make a difference in attendance and participant satisfaction. However, the type of site also influences the cost of your program, so you will want to compare and contrast the advantages and disadvantages of different types of sites before you make a selection.

Site	Description	Advantage	Disadvantage
Hotels	Buildings that provide sleeping rooms, meeting rooms, and restaurants	Staff available to help coordinate Needs are met in one location	Possibly expensive
Convention centers	Special facilities that provide meeting rooms and resources	Able to host large groups of people Resources readily accessible	Hotels and restaurants may not be within walking distance May be expensive
Universities	Institutions with a primary purpose of educating	Rooms of various sizes available May be less costly	Distance between rooms may cause difficulties Meeting equipment may not be as readily available
Resorts	Sites designed for recreation	Provide other activities for participants	Participants may not attend meetings May be expensive

ROOM SIZE AND SETUP

Don't forget to plan how the tables and chairs will be placed. It may sound like busywork, but think again about your own learning experiences. Have you ever attended a small-group discussion in a classroom where you could not move the chairs? The room setup probably caused a barrier to both the discussion and the learning. Room setup should be determined only after you have decided on the method of instruction for each program. Remember the discussion of methods in chapter 7? If your program requires face-to-face interaction, you will want to make decisions about whether individual rooms are needed for each face-to-face meeting, if a table will separate you and your participants, and how many people will be able to attend. In the case of presentations to a group of individuals, there are numerous ways to set up the room. Figure 8.3 illustrates some of the most common.

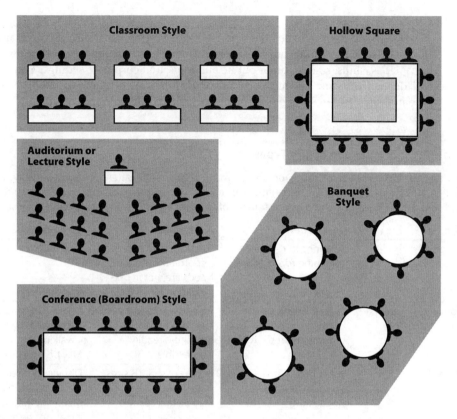

Figure 8.3   Common room setups.
Rooms can be arranged in a number of different ways. Careful consideration of the type of presentation or activity should be made before the room setup is selected.

Adapted from *Case Western Reserve University Room Setup Styles*. Retrieved from http://studentaffairs.case.edu/thwing/facilities/setups.html

The Content

In all educational environments, there are two types of curriculum: planned and unplanned. According to Doll (1992), a **curriculum** is "the formal and informal content and process by which learners gain knowledge and understanding, develop skills, and alter attitudes, appreciations, and values" (p. 6). A curriculum pertains to all programs, not just those in an educational institution. As a health professional, you will need to purposefully and thoughtfully develop your health program curriculum—this is where you build upon your planning efforts by adding substance and detail.

DEVELOPING CURRICULA

There are three paths you might choose for curriculum development. You might select a new idea (innovation), continue with what has been previously used in the agency, or revise the old curriculum. Make this decision early enough to allow you plenty of time to develop the content. Consider the learning tips in FYI 8.3 to help you make decisions about curriculum development. Also, pay attention to the scope (depth of coverage) and sequence (order of presentation) for each content area covered in the curriculum.

8.3   Learning Tips

Learning is an integral part of the process of making healthy behavior changes. Just as many aspects of a person's life affect health and wellness, many things influence learning. This list provides a few suggestions for making learning successful.

• Each person is unique.

• High stress affects learning negatively.

• Strong emotions change an individual's perceptions.

• All aspects of an individual's life influence learning (food, sleep, and physical activity).

• Assistance can be given to improve information retrieval.

• Individuals learn differently; include methods for varying intelligences.

• Most individuals learn best by experiencing.

• Individuals learn from everything that happens in their environment.

BLOOM'S TAXONOMY: THE COGNITIVE DOMAIN

It has long been known that providing information is not enough to promote behavior change for most people. Every education session should be based on an understanding of Bloom's taxonomy (Bloom et al., 1956), which distinguishes levels of learning. The original taxonomy contained three overlapping domains: the cognitive, psychomotor, and affective, but we are most interested in the cognitive domain. In the cognitive domain, Bloom listed six levels: knowledge, comprehension, application, analysis, synthesis, and evaluation. If you look at the words, you will note that each level requires an increasing amount of critical thinking. Anderson and Krathwohl made understanding the taxonomy easier by converting the terms into verbs:

• **Remembering:** Retrieving, recognizing, and recalling relevant knowledge from long-term memory.

• **Understanding:** Constructing meaning from oral, written, and graphic messages through interpreting, exemplifying, classifying, summarizing, inferring, comparing, and explaining.

• **Applying:** Carrying out or using a procedure through executing, or implementing.

• **Analyzing:** Breaking material into constituent parts, determining how the parts relate to one another and to an overall structure or purpose through differentiating, organizing, and attributing.

• **Evaluating:** Making judgments based on criteria and standards through checking and critiquing.

• **Creating:** Putting elements together to form a coherent or functional whole; reorganizing elements into a new pattern or structure through generating, planning, or producing. (2001, pp. 67–68)

The most effective educational programs will help participants go beyond gaining knowledge or remembering facts. The way in which information is presented to program participants will make a great difference in their level of understanding and future use of what they learn.

MULTIPLE INTELLIGENCES

As a student, you are well aware that there are many ways to impart information. Many teachers use lectures alone, while some supplement lectures with graphics on PowerPoint slides or videos. There is certainly nothing wrong with lecture, especially when topics are highlighted through visual aids; but lecture generally works best when used in combination with other methods. Just as there are many ways to teach, there are varied ways to learn. One theory that has been useful in many educational settings is **multiple intelligences (MI)** (Gardner, 2003). This theory suggests that many types of intelligence influence learning. Each individual will learn in different ways, depending on the dominant type of intelligence. Figure 8.4 depicts the different types of intelligences. They include being word-smart, logic-smart, picture-smart, body-smart, music-smart, people-smart, nature-smart, and self-smart (Armstrong, 1994). If after reading this section you feel that your best learning comes though the use of several intelligences, you have discovered an important point. While people lean toward one way of interacting with content, most use multiple ways or multiple intelligences (Edutopia, 2016).

Word-smart people interact with content through the use of words. They read well and understand what they read. These individuals will enjoy receiving brochures or other written material about health issues and will gather useful information from them. Logic-smart individuals use and appreciate analytical thinking in their daily lives. Understanding how health information applies to real life will help logic-smart people absorb the information you want to convey.

Picture-smart individuals have a feel for shapes, colors, and pictures. They enjoy using their hands to create visually pleasing products. Information geared to picture-smart people will incorporate visual effects. Movement is very important to those who are body-smart. They learn best if activity is part of the learning process. Music-smart individuals love sounds and learn best through auditory means. Incorporating pleasing sound as you present health information will improve the likelihood that your message will be well received.

People-smart individuals are social; they communicate and relate well with others. Providing opportunities for them to socialize while learning will enhance their learning. Self-smart individuals are strongly in tune with themselves. They understand their own feelings and express them well to others. Providing opportunities for self-smart individuals to stretch their knowledge of self while learning new information will make your program more successful. Nature-smart people relate well to their surroundings and the way their immediate environment plays a role in the larger environment (Infed Search, 2008). Nature-smart individuals will feel most successful when they participate in real-life experiences while they learn.

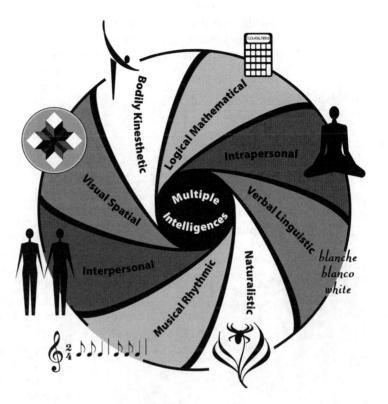

**Figure 8.4
The different types
of intelligence.**
Each person expresses
intelligence in a unique
way. An individual's
form of intelligence
influences the way he
or she will learn. It is
important to use meth-
ods that make sense to
individuals with varying
types of intelligence.

You might have heard about learning styles theory and if so, you might be won-
dering how to differentiate it from multiple intelligences theory. According to Silver,
Strong, and Perini, "learning styles are concerned with differences in the *process* of
learning, whereas multiple intelligences center on the *content* and *products* of learning"
(1997). Learning style theorists categorize styles in slightly different ways; however,
many agree on four categories. People in each category process information differently. For example, some people process information in a concrete, linear way, while
others process information in an abstract, ideologic way. On the other hand, some
people process information through feelings and emotions while others use social
relationships to assist in processing.

We encourage you to get to know your participants well enough to discover the
ways in which they learn best. If this is not possible, plan programs that involve multiple intelligences and learning styles. Use pleasing sounds or music as part of the program; provide activities with movement; give information in writing as well as
verbally; make sure that written materials are visually pleasing and use colors, shapes,
and pictures; allow opportunities for socialization within the program; and ask participants to apply the new information to real life.

EXPERIENTIAL METHODS

Think about the environment in which you live. Would you say it is fast-paced, visual, and interactive? Most of us deal with a plethora of images, activities, and ongoing

change on a daily basis. As a result, the participants in our health programs are likely to expect fast-paced programs, filled with images and activities. You will want to select methods that are creative and engaging. One of the oldest forms of teaching, providing experience, is often the most interesting and offers the greatest long-term benefit. Sometimes participants must understand a concept before they can apply it in a real-world experience. **Experiential** elements provide hands-on activities for learning concepts such as trust, teamwork, networking, and even planning.

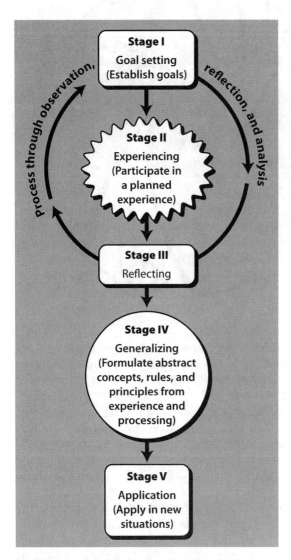

Experiential model. The basic experiential education model presented in Figure 8.5 has five stages: (a) asking participants to set personal goals, (b) engaging participants in planned experiences, (c) facilitating the processing of the experience (helping people find personal meaning), (d) helping participants develop concepts or guidelines from the processing, and (e) guiding application of the concepts and guidelines to other situations. This model is based on three assumptions:

- Learning is most effective when the learner is personally involved in the learning experience.

- Knowledge has to be personally discovered if it is to have meaning or make a difference in behavior.

- Commitment to learning is highest when the learner sets personal learning goals and actively pursues them within a given framework.

Figure 8.5   Experiential model.
Experiential learning requires more than just an experience. As this model depicts, goals must be set, the experience should be planned, and participants should be allowed an opportunity to reflect, generalize, and then apply what they have learned to the "real" world.

A quick and easy experiential activity to help people understand stressors and stress reduction uses a bowl, sponge, and water. A volunteer is asked to hold a large sponge above a large bowl. A second volunteer is asked to hold a cup of water above the bowl and sponge. The other participants are told that the sponge represents the human body. They are asked to think about things in their lives that cause stress (stressors) and then to call them out. A little water is poured onto the sponge each time a stressor is called out. The instructor stops the activity when the sponge is totally waterlogged and facilitates a discussion about the activity.

Processing the experience.   As you conduct experiential activities, remember that your role is one of **facilitator**. You will help participants navigate the challenges presented to them through planned experiences and then help them integrate the learning that results into future experiences (Henry & Ward, 1999). Assisting participants as they comprehend (reflect), internalize, and transfer (generalize) the lessons learned through these experiences is called **processing.** In processing the sponge activity, the instructor would ask something like, "What happened here?" The participants would describe what they saw and probably begin relating it to real life. They might comment on how the dripping sponge represents someone who is not coping well with stress. They might also note that squeezing the sponge would represent the effective use of coping and stress reduction strategies. Rather than lecturing, the instructor *guides* the discussion so that students understand the concepts of stressors and stress reduction.

Hundreds of books contain experiential elements and activities; we hope you will check out a few. Experiential activities designed to create the same decision-making skills used in real-life experiences can be very effective if the issues that arise during the activity are processed well. Participants should encounter challenges similar to those they might actually face and be given the opportunity to practice the same skills they will need to solve real-life problems. Processing the activities helps participants alter future behaviors. Failing to process the experience could negate the benefits of the activity. FYI 8.4 (on the following page) lists reflection questions and generalizing questions that a facilitator might ask to help participants maximize the processing of experiential activities.

Two aspects of teaching and learning become clear when using experiential methods. First, the strategies or methods used must be grounded in an understanding of teaching and learning. The Four Quadrant Model of Facilitated Learning (Greber, Ziviani, & Rodger, 2011) could serve as a stable base for planning interventions or programs even when purely experiential methods aren't being used. According to the model, learning generally follows a linear path through four quadrants, the first two are teacher directed and start with very clear instructions and demonstration, then move through asking higher-order questions and prompting action on the part of the students. The second two quadrants are learner directed and begin with giving self-clues or creating mnemonics, then address problem-solving and autonomy (Greber, Ziviani, and Rodger, 2011). The second aspect of teaching and learning that becomes clear is the importance of deep reflection. According to Tsingos, Bosnic-Anticevich, and Smith, reflection can stimulate "deep learning from past experiences" (2014, p. 18) and also assists students in developing new perspectives and insights.

THE ACTION PLAN

An **action plan**, called a **lesson plan** in an educational setting, is an important component of any program. Most programs have several parts; therefore, there may be more than one action plan. Programs might include a series of classes, or they

---

8.4 Potential Processing Issues and Questions from Processing

Allowing participants time to process their experience provides them with the opportunity to derive meaning from it. The following provide some sample questions that would maximize successful processing.

Reflection

General Opening Questions (getting the issues "out in the middle of the circle")
1. So, what just happened?
2. Tell me what you just experienced as you prepared for, moved through, this activity.
3. What were some of your thoughts and feelings during this activity?

Recognizing/Understanding/Expressing Feelings
1. Can you name a feeling you had at any point in completing the activity? Where in your body did you feel it most? Did it influence your behavior?
2. What beliefs were responsible for generating that feeling?
3. Did any of the feelings you had remind you of feelings you have experienced during stressful situations?
4. What did you do with these feelings? Were they expressed? If so, how? If not, why not?

Cooperating
1. Can you think of specific examples of when the group or specific classmates cooperated in completing the activity? Explain.
2. What does cooperation look like? Specify behaviors you saw today.
3. Were there any actions or efforts that seemed to block the group from achieving its goal? Explain.
4. What were some of the observed results of cooperating and helping others?

Appreciating Self
1. What kind of self-talk did you do during the initiative?
2. Do you sometimes put yourself down when you make a mistake? What effect might that have on your actions? On the function of the group?
3. What could you say to yourself to counteract the put-down message?

Generalizing

Transfer of Learning (essential if you want to make a difference)
1. What did you learn in this activity that you think will be helpful to you in getting through this or another class successfully?
2. Can you think of an example in school where you have faced a similar challenge as an individual? In a group situation?
3. What abilities or skills did you or your group exhibit that will help you in future courses or semesters?
4. How will you use what you learned to make school, work, and life better?

Closure Questions
1. What did you learn about yourself? What did you learn about others?
2. Was there a specific person who did something you think worthy of recognition?
3. Is there anything else you would like to say to a specific person or to the group?
4. What was the highlight of the day for you?

From "The Art and Science of Health Education," by J. Henry and S. E. Ward. Unpublished paper.

might include discussion groups as well as face-to-face meetings. An action or lesson plan would be developed for each component of the program. Action plans are not lengthy; they provide just enough information to guide each part of the program. We strongly encourage you to develop them even if others in your agency don't use them. Many sample forms exist for action/lesson plans; see Figure 8.6 for one example.

Activity:			
Instructor:			
Date:			
Description of participants:			
Objectives:			
Schedule	Description of activity	Content to be covered	Resources

Figure 8.6   Sample action plan.
As with every other aspect of program planning and implementation, individual lessons or contacts with participants should be well planned. Most professionals find it easiest to use a consistent planning tool like the action plan shown in this illustration.

Program Logistics

Careful attention to program logistics helps the health education program run smoothly and ensures that results are accurate. Program logistics tasks include record keeping and scheduling.

RECORD KEEPING

Record keeping is both painful and joyful. Accurate records help you document that your program is working and that you are managing the funds adequately. This is only the case, however, if your records are consistent, accurate, and accessible. We encourage you to use a computer for your record keeping. A number of software programs provide effective tracking and organization of program data. The types of records you must keep are related to process, impact, and outcome (see chapter 7) and will relate directly to your objectives. In regard to process, you will certainly keep attendance records, but you may want to collect information about the participants' perceptions of the program, content, and learning environments. Statistical software, such as the IBM Statistical Package for Social Sciences Software (www.spss.com), allows you to enter and store data easily and will produce descriptive statistics (frequencies, averages, and percentages) at a click of a button. These same programs will help you store and analyze your impact and outcome information. These are the data that will document the effectiveness of your program, so they become, in a sense, the lifeblood of the program.

SCHEDULES

Another aspect of the program is the timing or scheduling of the activities. As always, there are a number of ways that you can illustrate and distribute your schedules. One of the most common methods involves the use of a monthly calendar as a flyer. The program activities are simply placed on the correct day of the month. Participants can then post their monthly schedules in an easily accessible location. Another method is a program-like document that lists the days and times of upcoming events. Participants receive a brochure or small booklet that provides a quick look at upcoming events. Calendars and programs can also be put on Web pages or sent in e-mails. The key is to carefully plan your schedule with regard to the characteristics of your intended participants. Keep in mind that if a schedule isn't working, it should be changed.

Creating Materials

Every detail of a program must be planned and implemented with care. Creating materials seems straightforward—just put a few words on paper or on the Internet and present it to the participants. But to do the task well, you must take into consideration such variables as language disorders and literacy levels as well as the appearance of the materials.

Language Disorders and Literacy Levels

"The ability to read and write is strongly influenced by the ability to understand and use language. Individuals who are good listeners and speakers tend to be strong readers and writers" (American Speech-Language-Hearing Association, 1999). The term **language disorder** refers to any impairment in form, semantics, or pragmatics (American Speech-Language-Hearing, 1999). At one time or another you will have program participants with some degree of language disorder. An individual who has difficulties with form might misunderstand the information provided by word endings. Individuals who have difficulties with semantics may not understand *idiom* (a phrase or expression that cannot be understood from the ordinary meanings of the words in it); for example, describing something as the "nuts and bolts" of the program. The meaning of "nuts and bolts" in such usage is not explained by the definition of the two words as pieces of hardware. Other examples of idiom include "butterflies in the stomach," "kick the bucket," and so on. Pragmatics means using the same phrases or words for different purposes; for example, the word *cool* might indicate temperature or it might indicate a value judgment. You will need to prepare materials that are accessible to individuals with language disorders.

You will also encounter individuals with varying **literacy levels** in your programs. "How well adults can use printed and written information to function in society, to achieve their goals, and to develop their knowledge and potential is the definition of literacy" (Educational Testing Service, 2008, p. 1). Although it may not seem so, health literacy is more complex. The National Library of Medicine and National Institutes of Health define health literacy as "the degree to which individuals have the capacity to obtain, process, and understand basic health information and services needed to make appropriate health decisions" (n.d., *Quick Guide*).

If you are working with college students, you know that the **readability** level of your materials can be high; but for the general population, you will want to keep your materials between the fourth and sixth grade levels (National Library of Medicine and National Institutes of Health, 2007). Readability refers to reading ease as well as the difficulty of the material. There are many methods for determining readability, but one common procedure is the SMOG index (McLaughlin, 1969). This index assigns a grade level for written materials. Fortunately, many word-processing programs have readability indexes built into them. Unfortunately, health literacy is not so easily programmed. Keep in mind while you prepare materials that you should differentiate between medical terms that might be known to the participants and those that are unfamiliar. While difficult medical terms may raise the reading level as measured by a test like SMOG, this won't be an issue if participants are familiar with the term. For example, using the word *diabetes* might increase the reading level of a document, but if you are working among individuals with diabetes, they are less likely to have difficulty with the word (Zeng, Eunjung, & Tse, n.d.). Familiarity with a word, however, does not necessarily translate into a full understanding of it. Many people will recognize the word *diabetes* but even some individuals with the disease won't truly understand it. According to the National Library of Medicine (2006), "Health information needs to be designed, written, formatted, and communicated in such a way that it is executable by the end user, including multi-media and interactive materials" (p. 9).

There are several actions you can take to develop materials that are accessible to individuals with language disorders or low literacy levels. See FYI 8.5 for a list of tips. As you can see from the list, including words with fewer syllables, writing shorter sentences, and using pictures will increase comprehension.

8.5   Tips for Developing Materials

The characteristics of the materials you select or develop will influence learning. This list will help ensure that your materials are appropriate for the audience.

- Keep the readability level between the fourth and sixth grade unless you know the specific level of your audience.
- Use pictures to supplement text. Make certain that the pictures are relevant to your audience.
- Unless the members of your audience have medical backgrounds, assume that they are not familiar with medical terms.
- Ask a member of the target population to check the language and adjust it. It should be meaningful to the people who will read it.
- Ask a second member of the target audience to read the adjusted material and describe the content. Make certain that the adjusted material still means what you intend it to.
- Provide examples that are relevant to your audience.
- Field-test your material by asking several members of the target audience to preview the materials and provide feedback.

Creating Web Pages

Web pages are excellent resources for your program. A Web page is an online informational brochure or flyer that is posted for all to see. The good news about developing Web pages is that, like other aspects of implementation, computer software makes it easy. Keep in mind that your Web pages exist to communicate information. Color, font, and format are important—but the message must be paramount. Answer the following question to get started, "What is the purpose of the website?" Then derive your content from the information your participants need and want.

Once your content has been selected, consider the design. The best Web pages are simple, which means they are easy to read. According to Roger Parker, the author of *Web Design and Desktop Publishing for Dummies* (1997), nine guidelines assist in Web design:

1. Design should be purposeful.
2. Design should simplify complicated information.
3. Design should provide visual contrast.
4. Design should make your program competitive.
5. Design should show how the program pieces fit together.
6. Design should help the participant know what is important.
7. Design should involve a few effective font and color changes.
8. Design should save the participant time.
9. Design should involve editing.

Individuals with special needs can have difficulty with a poorly designed Web page. FYI 8.6 provides tips for creating Web pages for individuals with special needs.

8.6 Creating Web Pages for Individuals with Special Needs

Some individuals have special needs that will require changes made to the materials they use in a program, including Web-based programs or pages. Following are some ideas for meeting the needs of individuals with barriers to Web access.

Visual Barriers
• Eliminate screen cluttering.
• Design high-contrast texts and backgrounds.
• Provide text-only options and text descriptions of pictures.

Hearing Barriers
• Explain sound clips using text.
• Provide text descriptions for all video clips that include sound.

Learning or Cognitive Barriers
• Have lots of descriptive pictures.
• Have step-by-step explanations for all instructions and commands.

Physical Barriers
• Provide compatibility with mouse substitution software such as touch screen or touch board.
• Provide compatibility for voice recognition software.

Economic Barriers
• Provide text-only options for use with slower computers.
• Provide paper alternatives.

Adapted from "Web Accessibility," Alliance for Technology Access. Retrieved from http://www.ataccess.org/rresources/webaccess.html

Keeping the Program Alive/Ethics in Implementation

One aspect of programming helps ensure its ongoing existence—ethical practices. Ethics comprises a whole host of issues, some of which we will discuss further in chapter 9. For now, think about the following characteristics of ethics: honesty, integrity, confidentiality, and communication. Honesty involves acting truthfully, integrity requires basing one's actions on a set of principles, confidentiality means ensuring that only authorized individuals have access to private information, and communication entails creating shared meaning by sending and receiving messages. When combined, these characteristics describe the basis for almost all codes of ethics. You can find the Code of Ethics for the Health Education Profession from the Coalition of National Health Education Organizations (CNHEO) online. Almost all professions and most agencies have codes of ethics. They have similar content, so read through one for the general feel. You will see as you read that honesty, integrity, confidentiality, and communication are reflected in every section.

≡ In Conclusion

After completing the legwork involved in needs assessment and program planning, implementation may at first seem like the "easy" part. But it must be approached with an understanding of its importance. Ongoing funding for the program is necessary and you may need to seek supplemental funds through donations or special events. Once appropriate funding is secured, your next goal will be effective marketing. Social marketing encompasses much more than advertising. You'll revisit the needs assessment to define the market audience, address issues of place and price, and develop promotion strategies. You will also want to consider partnering with other agencies, and you'll need to review current policies and politics.

The nuts and bolts of the program will be fine-tuned in program implementation. Appropriate program materials and schedules should be developed with the target population in mind. Record keeping, although not always fun, will document your ability to manage the program and produce positive impacts and outcomes. Treat program implementation seriously.

REVIEW QUESTIONS

1. List and describe the Ps in social marketing.
2. Detail the strategies you might use to select a new employee and justify your choices.
3. List tips for developing effective materials.
4. Discuss why experiential and critical thinking methods are important.
5. Describe ways to help individuals with barriers use the Web.
6. Analyze ways in which to improve health literacy.
7. Explain why ethical practice keeps a program alive.

FOR YOUR APPLICATION

Select or create a format for a lesson plan. It should include space for the following categories: descriptions of the topic and target population, objectives, projected schedule, content to be covered, and needed resources. Once you have selected the format, complete the plan for one session in the program you are developing in your project. If you are not doing a project, just select a topic and target audience and develop a lesson plan for one session. Ask your instructor to review the plan and provide feedback. If you are creating a portfolio, be sure to include the updated version of your lesson plan.

9

Research and Evaluation

You developed a program for teen mothers in your community. You assessed their attitudes, beliefs, and perceived needs and based the program development on the assessment. Lots of teens attended the program. Everyone seemed to be having fun. Does that mean the program was effective? Can you assume that the program accomplished what it was supposed to? Did you check to see if the program had been studied in action before you used it?

Chapter Objectives

1. Describe the process of research.
2. Discuss developing research objectives, questions, and hypotheses.
3. Detail selected quantitative and qualitative research designs.
4. List the purposes of evaluation.
5. Create an evaluation plan.

What Is Research?

Research is a process. It provides a means for examining the reality of a circumstance, establishing patterns and relationships in aspects of a situation, or even satisfying curiosity about something. The difference between research and a casual inspection of a topic is the systematic nature of the process. Research involves a clearly defined process delineated prior to starting. There are many types of research, each involving a wide choice of study designs; all of which can be clearly defined, described, and planned in advance. Even studies that use emerging designs (such as some qualitative research designs) are planned in advance to the extent possible.

In the past, you might have been asked to write a research paper. It's important to note that research is not solely getting information from the library and writing a paper about it. A literature review—seeking information from articles written by professionals—is only one part of the research process, not the entire endeavor. The first step in the research process is to create a plan of action, sometimes called a *proposal*.

The Research Plan/Proposal

The research plan confirms the systematic nature of the process. In other words, the process is not one of "going with the flow" or "taking it as it comes." The plan should include carefully defined procedures that you will follow in order to conduct an effective study. It is almost like a recipe, but more prescriptive. Recipes can be adjusted to fit an individual's taste, but a research plan should be followed carefully so that others who wish to replicate the study can do so. The steps for creating a research plan and thereby fulfilling the research process involve critical analysis and include, but are not limited to, the following:

1. Determine the problem to be solved.

2. Identify information currently available about the problem (literature review).

3. Write objectives, research questions, and hypotheses.

4. Select a study design.

5. Create a timeline.

6. Establish a budget.

7. Select measurement instruments.

8. Set up implementation plans.

9. Formulate data-analysis strategies.

10. Determine a research dissemination plan.

Determining the Problem to Address

It is fairly easy to identify health-related problems throughout the world: read the newspaper, watch television, search the Internet, or simply look around. However, determining the issue to be studied in a research project requires more than just selecting a problem on which to focus. It includes analysis, prioritization, and justification. There are many considerations to resolve, not the least of which are the time and money available for the project. There is no use even contemplating a project without adequate resources. If resources are available, you can proceed to select a problem to address in a research project.

If you work for a nonprofit or voluntary health organization, research will be guided by the organizational mission. Public health agencies may be limited to programming and research that matches the national funding streams. In other words, the federal government will make monies available for selected public health issues, some of which have been determined to be national public health concerns and others that are of interest to politicians and lobbyists. In the best of all worlds, research would be determined by a partnership between community members and professionals. The problem would be analyzed and aspects of the issue would be prioritized through assessments, literature reviews, and collaborations between members of the partner community and various professionals. Justification for conducting the research would be created through the analysis and prioritization. Later in the chapter, we'll talk more about community-based participatory research, which is a process that involves the community in every phase. We will also discuss evaluation as a type of research in more detail. As in the beginning of the chapter, the research example presented in the next sections will be composed of program evaluation.

Writing Objectives, Research Questions, and Hypotheses

The quality and success of a research project depends on planning. Once the research problem has been identified, the planning begins with the development of objectives, research questions, and hypotheses.

WRITING OBJECTIVES

Hopefully, you have already learned the fundamentals of writing objectives and understand their importance. Basically, research objectives state what you hope to achieve with the study. There may be both general and specific objectives—that is, a broad overriding objective and several detailed objectives that when combined address the overall objective and research problem. Writing these objectives entails steps similar to those discussed in the program planning chapter. In some ways, creating research objectives is like writing a newspaper article: they should answer who, what, where, and why. For example, a broad research objective might be "To determine the effectiveness of the teen pregnancy program (we'll call our example program *Rising Star*) provided by the health education section of the local public health department." The word *effective* is not defined in this broad objective so it must be clarified in the more detailed objectives linked to it. These linked objectives might include:

1. To determine if the financial needs (what) of teen participants (who) were met through the program's social services offerings (where), for the purpose of examining the deficits (why).

2. To identify the costs incurred (what) by the public health department (who) to conduct the program (where) in order to relate the costs to the benefits of the program (why).

3. To measure the participants' (who) satisfaction (what) with the program (where) to determine if it is appropriate for them (why).

4. To compare the number of future pregnancies (what) of program participants and nonparticipant teens (who) to determine if the problem is truly being addressed (why) by the program (where).

5. To use the findings of the study (what) to improve future teen pregnancy programs (why and who) through dissemination of the results (where).

Each of these linked objectives measures a different component or aspect of the effectiveness of the program.

WRITING HYPOTHESES AND RESEARCH QUESTIONS

You may hear the term *research question* used in two ways. It is often used as an umbrella term for any of the questions that will be addressed in a research project, whether quantitative or qualitative. The broad questions are developed directly from the objectives that we described in the previous section. For example, one of our objectives stated, "To compare the number of future pregnancies of program participants and nonparticipant teens to determine if the problem is truly being addressed by the program." A research question based on this example objective might ask, "What are the differences in second pregnancy rates between Rising Star participants and control participants?"

The next step after writing your research question will be to develop a prediction or hypothesis regarding the question. A **hypothesis** is a prediction of the results of the study. The hypothesis will then be tested using an appropriate research design and statistical test. The hypothesis (prediction) should not be based on your hopes for the program. Instead, it should be based on your previous experience with the same program, research or program evaluation done by others using the program, or results of other programs that are similar in nature.

You may also hear the term *research question* used in qualitative research as a specific title for the questions that will be addressed in that type of study. (See the explanations of qualitative versus quantitative in the next section.) Though it is appropriate to use the term *research question* in a qualitative study, it is not appropriate to use the term *hypothesis* for this type of research. The specific title for questions in a quantitative project is *hypotheses* because a hypothesis can be tested. Hypotheses generate the use of inferential statistics (quantitative), which we discussed briefly in the epidemiology chapter. Because qualitative research questions generate words, phrases, and explanations from individuals, the results do not produce the numbers needed to test a hypothesis. So, when conducting qualitative research, you will generate research questions but not hypotheses.

Developing a Study Design

The study design will serve as a guide for data collection and analysis. Note that there is a difference between study design and data collection strategy. You must know what type of data you will be collecting in order to select your study design. The type of data needed will depend on your study objectives and research questions or hypotheses. First let's review the definitions of the broad types of data, quantitative and qualitative. **Quantitative** data consist of numbers. A number may be a frequency count (i.e., there are 15 men and 12 women), a score (i.e., 87 out of 100 points), the result of a mathematical computation (87%), a code to signify membership in a specified category (1=male and 2=female), or another numerical representation. **Qualitative** data are words and phrases because the researcher wants to understand "why" something is happening. So, even though words represent the data, the meaning of the words and phrases is what is important.

Let's look at some examples of hypotheses and research questions and their relationship to types of data. Suppose your hypothesis states: "Participants in the Rising Star class will score higher on the post-program survey than control participants." This hypothesis provides three important pieces of information. First, because this is a hypothesis or a prediction that can be tested, the data will be quantitative. Second, there will be an intervention (something that will be tested, such as the program) and third, because a comparison will be made, there will be a control group. At a minimum, measurements will be taken post-intervention; preferably, pre and post. As you can see, this study design must be quantitative in nature.

However, suppose your research question asks: "What perceptions about the Rising Star program do participants hold?" It's difficult to make a prediction about this research question. In fact, it can best be answered by talking to participants and learning from their words, body language, and facial expressions. After all, think about the reason this question has been asked. You want to know what participants like or dislike and why. Knowing why people feel the way they do can help you adapt the program to their needs and interests. The data and the study design will be qualitative.

When you have determined the research questions and hypotheses, you will be able to select your study design. Your proposal or research plan should describe, in great detail, the activities that make up the design, including the data-collection strategies and the way in which study participants or study sample will be selected.

QUANTITATIVE DESIGNS

There are more quantitative designs and their variations than we can cover in this chapter. However, we will describe a few basic designs to give you an overview. If you select an **experimental design** for your research project, you will first need to carefully identify who could be part of the study in a broad sense (teen women in your community who have been pregnant). This group will be the study population. Then, you will *randomly select* a predetermined number of individuals who will be invited to actually participate in the study, based on how many you can feasibly involve. Those who agree to participate (they must agree voluntarily) will be *randomly assigned* to one of two groups, control or intervention. If you remember, random selection means giving every person in the population the same chance to be selected for the study; computer programs can be used to ensure randomness. Random assignment means that, once in the study, all participants will have equal chances to be put in the intervention or the control group. An **intervention** can be an educational program, medical treatment, marketing effort, one aspect of a program, or something else that you would like to study. One way to prove that your intervention works (or doesn't) is to use an experimental design in which two comparable groups of people receive different programs or different parts of the program (the intervention). In some cases, one group (the control group) will receive no type of programming; instead, they will complete only the pretest and posttest.

The specific behavior, knowledge level, attitude, or medical outcome that you hope will change for your participants after the intervention is the **dependent variable.** Some examples might be knowledge score, attitude rating, smoking frequency, blood pressure, and in our example, second pregnancies. The dependent variable will be measured in both groups of people (those who received the intervention and those who did not) at two times (before and after the intervention). The degree to which members of each group changed their behavior will be compared. Of course, you hope that the group that received your intervention will have the most favorable results.

If the experiment has been carefully conducted, you will be able to say that your intervention made a difference. If an intervention truly causes the effect desired, it is said to have **internal validity** (Godwin et al., 2003). In a carefully designed experiment (one that uses random selection and assignment), you can also claim **external validity**; that is, results can be generalized to other people in the population.

You will have to determine if the experimental design is appropriate and feasible for your research project. Will you be able to assemble intervention and control groups? Will you be able to make certain that the participants in each group don't talk with one another and contaminate the results? Will there be factors in the community that influence one group of participants but not the other? Experimental designs are not easy to carry out; however, the superiority of this method should encourage its use where practicable.

Some research designs that are weaker but have potential include a one-group posttest study, one-group pretest/posttest study, and post-only comparison study. Just as its name suggests, a **one-group posttest study** involves only one group and one measurement of the target behavior. All participants would be in the intervention group and would be tested after the intervention has occurred. If you select this type of research design, you look for the target behavior to be healthier after the intervention. Unfortunately, this design has some problems; can you see the flaws in it? There are many reasons, other than the intervention, for the behavior of interest to be improved after the program. The program participants might have had positive behaviors before the program even began, but you would not know because they weren't measured. Some other stimulus, like a TV show or movie, might have precipitated a change in behavior. You would never really know if your program was responsible for the positive behavior because you had no measurement of the behavior before the program started and no comparisons with individuals who did not receive the intervention.

A pretest is added in the **one-group pretest/posttest design.** With this design, you are able to measure changes in the behavior because you take measurements both before and after the intervention. But you would still not be able to say with certainty that the program itself was responsible for the change. Can you see why? Again, some other stimulus in the environment might have prompted the change. Suppose some participants read a self-help book during the same time they attended the program. Behavior change might be a result of the reading, not the program.

In the **post-only comparison**, you are able to measure differences in the target behavior between two groups, control and intervention, that are both tested after the intervention. Only one group has received the program, and neither has been pretested. You would find out if the post-program behaviors were healthy and how the behaviors differed between intervention and control participants. But what if the intervention group had healthier behaviors than the control group in the first place? You would not be able to determine the impact of the intervention with this study design. Figure 9.1 on the next page provides schematics of the quantitative study designs discussed in this chapter. Keep in mind that there are many more quantitative research designs, as well as variations of the ones we have already discussed. We encourage you to take a research design class to enhance your knowledge of this valuable and interesting topic.

QUALITATIVE DESIGNS

In general, qualitative research is an in-depth review and analysis of the meaning of documents, settings, relationships, and verbal communications. Like quantitative research, there are numerous qualitative designs and varied data-collection strategies that fit into those designs. We'd like to present a few broad qualitative approaches to give you an introduction to this type of research.

Ethnography. This type of research takes place in the field, not a laboratory. Detailed descriptions are made of people, places, customs, cultures, and societies with emphasis on one group of people and their culture. Nothing is studied independently; rather, the emphasis is on determining how people, places, beliefs, and behaviors fit together and influence one another (Trochim, 2006). The researcher often becomes immersed in a culture in order to study it in a technique called **participant observation**. The researcher is always an integral part of this research process because his/her analysis of the meaning of the observations ultimately tells the story of the culture.

Grounded theory. Researchers use this qualitative approach to create theory from preliminary data collection, which in turn, guides further research. This approach is an *emerging design*, a phrase mentioned earlier that means data collection and analysis decisions occur while the study is progressing. Content and communication analyses are used in all phases of data collection in order to find theoretical concepts and links between them. The purpose in the end is to create a new theory that is grounded in systematic observation.

Phenomenology.   Determining the lived experience of individuals regarding a specific phenomenon is the goal of this approach. Researchers conduct in-depth interviews with a number of individuals who have a shared experience; for example, very young teens who have given birth. Researchers will then look for commonalities across the interviewees in order to understand the collective lived experience with the event or phenomenon.

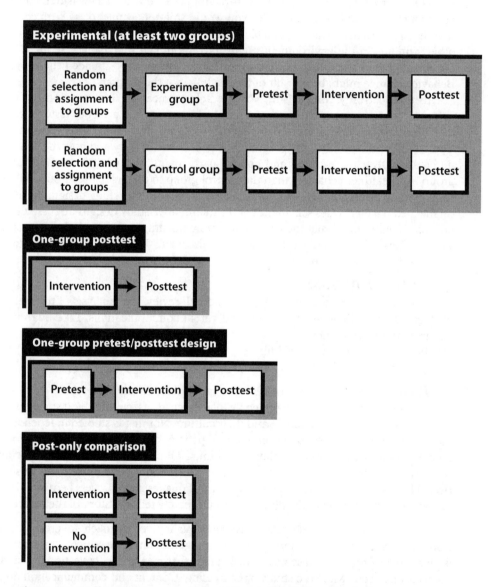

Figure 9.1   Pictorial representation of quantitative study designs.
Many types of study designs exist and often two or more types of designs will be used in one research project. This figure illustrates four types of designs.

Case study.   A case study involves the in-depth study of one case. Many individuals, settings, documents, and communications regarding the case are reviewed and analyzed. A variety of data-collection strategies might be used, such as interviews, content analyses, and observations.

Community-Based Participatory Research

Whether you select qualitative or quantitative designs, **community-based participatory research (CBPR)** provides a framework in which community members and researchers act as equal partners in the process. It begins with a health topic of interest, progresses to gathering information to increase knowledge, and ultimately applies that knowledge to improve the health of a community. The purpose of CBPR, also termed "action research," is to reach community-driven goals while collecting valuable information through research (Minkler, Blackwell, Thompson, & Tamir, 2003). The CBPR process provides an invaluable collaborative research forum, but could also play a role in improving the work of health related agencies. Nonprofit organizations and community health agencies often struggle with reaching their goals because of inadequate strategies, lack of resources, unrealistic expectations from stakeholders, and difficult timelines. CBPR may improve outcomes. Unfortunately, it's not always easy to find community members who have the requisite skills and interest in potential projects. These challenges may create a need for more time and money for the research process than might be needed for other designs. However, devoting the time and resources to this process has the potential to provide dramatic improvements in the success of programs.

According to Metzler and colleagues (2003), the activities important to developing effective community research partners include shared decision making, defining collaboration, establishing research priorities that are meaningful to the community, and securing funding. Minkler (2004) created a framework to help develop community partners. The framework incorporates Kelly's ideas on community-based research (1986) and Jones's thoughts on understanding racism (2004). Minkler's framework helps researchers address "(a) achieving a true 'community-driven' agenda; (b) insider-outsider tensions; (c) real and perceived racism; (d) the limitations of participation; and (e) issues involving the sharing, ownership, and use of findings for action" (p. 684). We strongly encourage you to learn more about the CBPR process and to apply it when you develop a research project.

Establishing a Budget and Creating a Timeline

Each research project must have a unique budget. The steps for developing this budget are the same as those used in a program budget: selecting the categories, determining the implementation phases, estimating costs, documenting in-kind contributions, allowing for contingencies, and calculating the total funding needed. The categories for your budget will be very similar to those in the program budget. See Table 9.1 for a sample budget specific to a research project.

An exclusive timeline for the research project will be helpful as well. See Figure 9.2 (on p. 217) for a Gantt chart specific to a research project.

Table 9.1   Sample Research Budget

Budget Item	Description	Total Cost
Personnel		
Health researcher	960 hours $35/hr	$33,600
Secretary	800 hours $17/hr	13,600
Subtotal		47,200
Personnel benefits	20% of wages	8,000
Total personnel		**$55,200**
Supplies		
Printing	100,000 × .08	$ 8,000
Postage	20,000 × .50	10,000
Office supplies		1,500
Total supplies		**$19,500**
Services		
Telephone	$150/month	$ 1,800
Total services		**$ 1,800**
Consultants		
Data processing	25 hours $18/hr	$ 450
Graphic artist	16 hours $40/hr	640
Total consultants		**$ 1,090**
Contingencies		$ 500
Total contingencies		**$ 500**
Indirect costs	15% of total	**$ 645**
Total costs		**$78,735**

Selecting Measurement Instruments

Qualitative and quantitative research designs may seem to include similar data-collection strategies like surveys, interviews, or observation, but the instruments used are not the same. Quantitative instruments will collect information that is quantifiable while qualitative instruments will collect words, phrases, and observations that can be studied for meaning. Quantitative data-collection instruments include but are not limited to surveys, questionnaires, tests, medical equipment, and checklists. Qualitative data-collection instruments include but are not limited to focus groups, the Delphi technique, interviews, and observations.

The instruments used in data collection must be selected, adjusted, and sometimes written. Instrument selection or development should be viewed as an integral part of the research process. If the instrument is medical equipment, for example, it must have protocols (specific procedures) for clinical measurements. The instrument might also be a paper-and-pencil questionnaire or survey.

Developing a quantitative instrument is a time-consuming and difficult process. As a result, you might tend to develop research objectives and hypotheses based on

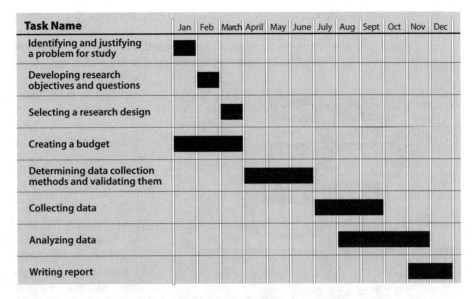

Figure 9.2   Gantt chart for a research project.
Projecting the timeline for the whole scope of a research project will help you focus on each of the very important steps.

available instruments rather than the other way around. We agree that every attempt should be made to find an existing instrument that is appropriate, but, if it is not possible we encourage you to use appropriate development techniques. Let's discuss instrument development as we discuss estimating validity and reliability. Figure 9.3 on the following page illustrates a six-step process for instrument development.

ESTABLISHING THE FRAMEWORK

Establishing a framework for an instrument is like building a foundation for a house. You need to decide on the best material and style for the foundation. In the case of instrument development, you might choose a theoretical base. If so, a health behavior or learning theory will guide the development process. For example, if social cognitive theory is your foundation, your intervention and the entire research project will evolve from the theory. One construct in the theory is self-efficacy. One of your intervention activities might focus on this construct. You might also choose criteria for your foundation. Perhaps study participants must achieve a standard set of behaviors (criteria). If so, the instrument would be guided by these criteria. The good news for you as a researcher is that you will keep the same framework used during intervention development. If theory guided the intervention development, then it will also guide the measurement instrument.

DEVELOPING A SKELETON

You begin by developing a first draft of your instrument. You might start by using an open-ended type of questionnaire that elicits participants' beliefs (Ajzen & Fishbein, 1977); you can talk with individuals who are expert in the measurement of your behavior of interest; and you can review existing literature for suggested forms and formats.

Special attention must be given to both the format and wording of each item during initial drafting. The difficulty lies in creating items that accurately represent the psychosocial variables of interest (such as attitudes, perceptions, and beliefs) and are appropriate for the target populations' culture and local dialect. You will want to search the literature for scale items previously used and adapt those items, if necessary, to the proposed study. Keep in mind that you will need to get the original developer's permission to use or adjust any part of a previously existing instrument. Be sure to consider the cultural appropriateness of both the items and the instrument as a whole.

Imagine that you are asked to study a teen pregnancy program that was based on the theory of planned behavior. The purpose of the program might have been to increase the intention of the teen mothers to select safe ways to discipline their children. You might measure their perceptions of the consequences if they do so and whether those consequences are good or bad (attitudes about the behavior). You might also measure the teen mother's perceptions about who wants them to select safe disciplinary behaviors and if they value the opinions of those individuals (subjective norms). Also, you might measure the control beliefs of the teen mothers. It will take effort on your part to select the best vocabulary for measuring components of the

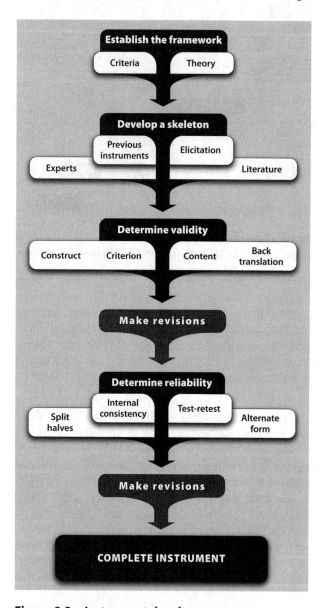

Figure 9.3   Instrument development.
Instrument development is a complex task that requires many steps. This illustration provides a model for instrument development.

theory of planned behavior. You will have to search the literature for an existing instrument. If there is no existing instrument, you will need to find one that was used in a similar situation and adjust it. Once you have developed the skeleton format, estimating the validity of the data collected is the next step.

INSTRUMENT VALIDITY

Determining the degree to which the data collected by an instrument is valid begins with attention to the brevity and clarity of the instrument. Establishing instrument brevity and clarity is particularly complicated when cultural sensitivity of the instrument is a priority. Brislin's guidelines for writing and modifying instrument items have been used widely and adapted for cross cultural instruments (Wang, Lee, & Fetzer, 2006). These guidelines suggest using short, simple sentences of less than 16 words (Brislin, 1986). This is no easy task when you should also repeat nouns instead of using pronouns, avoid metaphors and colloquialisms that could shorten the wording, and add sentences and phrases where needed to provide cultural context for key ideas. Only through collaborative community involvement in instrument development can you be sure that the instrument is sufficiently brief and effectively clear.

Once brevity and clarity have been examined, you will want to consider four major types of validity. These include criterion-related, content, construct, and back translation. Keep in mind that instrument validity is not the same thing as the internal and external validity of a research study.

CRITERION-RELATED VALIDITY

When the scoring of an instrument yields results similar to actual observation of the behavior of interest, the data collected by that instrument is said to have **criterion-related validity.** For example, imagine that a parental discipline survey was developed as an easy way to measure the quality of a teen mother's discipline behaviors. The data would have criterion-related validity if it gave the same estimate of discipline quality as did an actual observation of a teen mother disciplining her children. The observed behavior is the criterion. The process requires a statistical procedure called a *correlation* to determine if a relationship exists between a score received on the instrument and a score on the actual performance of the behavior. The resulting number is called a *validity coefficient.* The validity coefficient can range from -1 to +1. For most instruments, you should look for a moderate to high correlation (ranging between .65 and 1) before you use it.

CONTENT VALIDITY

If the data collected by an instrument accurately reflects an area or domain of knowledge, it has **content validity**. For example, the data from the perceptions-of-discipline survey would have content validity if the instrument used the word *discipline* and other concepts appropriately. In most cases, no specific, well-defined criteria exist from which to determine content validity. Most evaluators rely on experts in the field to assess it. You would ask a panel of experts in parental discipline choices to review the instrument and suggest changes that would make the content stronger. This practice has merit as long as the people you choose truly have expertise in the content.

CONSTRUCT VALIDITY

The extent to which the data collected from an instrument reflects its theoretical base is a measure of **construct validity** (Smith, 2005). Construct validation is not a matter of rapid assessment. Much research in using the instrument and follow-up analysis are required. *Factor analysis* (a statistical procedure) may provide you or your statistician with useful information about your theoretically based instrument. This statistical procedure should be used only in combination with expert knowledge of the constructs to be measured to prevent misconceptualization. Individuals with expertise in the theoretical construct being measured are normally asked to assist in establishing the construct validity of the data collected by an instrument. Experts will have the knowledge to suggest changes that would help it better reflect the theory. It is important to note that professionals evaluating the construct validity of an instrument may not be familiar with the cultural norms and local dialect of the partner population. Thus, an instrument thought to be construct-valid could be virtually ineffective if a particular word distorted meaning within the targeted cultural context.

Plan to involve members of the partner culture in your instrument development. The ideal is to enlist the help of health professionals who are familiar with the construct to be measured and who understand the culture and local dialect. When this isn't possible, a combined group effort should include both construct and cultural experts.

BACK TRANSLATION

An instrument designed for one cultural setting and used in a slightly different culture may cause the researcher to miss aspects of the second culture that are important to the overall picture. The resulting conclusions might then be based on concepts that are nonexistent within the targeted culture or at least partially incorrect. Thus, existing instruments should be used only after modifications are made to fit the specific culture and research situation (Brislin, 1986).

A popular method for validating a translated instrument is **back translation** (Jones, Lee, Phillips, Zhang, & Jaceldo, 2001). If you choose to have your instrument translated into another language, one bilingual individual translates from the source language to the target language. Another bilingual person then translates the resulting target-language version back to the source language. This process may be repeated several times and the first and last source-language versions compared. If the major concept survives the activity, it is regarded as *etic* (that is, readily available words and phrases exist in the two languages that facilitate concept translation). If the concept doesn't survive, it is *emic*, or expressible in only the source language.

In addition to its use when two languages are involved, the back-translation process can be used to modify an instrument to the popular jargon of a community. In this instance you would ask "bilingual" translators who understand both the local jargon and the terminology used in the original instrument to be involved in the process.

Selection of bilingual translators is a critical first step in the back-translation process. The ideal is to choose translators who are members of the partner culture and are keenly familiar with the cultural norms and local dialect of the targeted group. They must also clearly understand the original instrument language and the constructs it is intended to measure. Translators must have an ability to focus on the clear communication of concepts rather than the literal translation of words and phrases. The degree to which they understand both the original instrument and the partnered culture will affect their ability to find target-language equivalents without having to use unfamiliar terms (Jones et al., 2001).

Finding translators who meet the necessary criteria is seldom easy and the ideal is rarely achieved. Translators with differing levels and types of expertise can work as a team. Potential sources are trained professional translators identified by community gatekeepers, health professionals, or university researchers experienced in working with the population as well as members of the cultural group who are studying in a university health program. Because few bilingual individuals are trained translators, a team approach may be more effective.

The results of the back-translation process may seem inconsistent with the original instrument. The critical questions to ask in this situation are (a) whether the original instrument concepts survived the process while words and phrases changed or (b) whether the original concepts were lost in the process. Bringing the translators together with the evaluator to discuss this issue is critical. If the group concedes that the concepts remained intact, the translated instrument is now ready to be subjected to further validation procedures for readability and understandability within the partner culture. However, if the targeted concept was lost in the process, the evaluator should return to the original instrument. It may be helpful to reword the original following Brislin's guidelines and present the altered version to a new set of translators. Another alternative would be to work with the original translators to create items in the targeted language that do reflect the targeted construct. The resulting instrument can then be further validated.

The rigorous process of back translation cannot fully guarantee that resulting scales will be culturally appropriate. Further work is necessary to validate its utility within the partner culture. This work includes testing the instrument for readability and understandability with a subsample of the targeted population.

INSTRUMENT RELIABILITY

It is also important to determine if the data collected by a survey or questionnaire is reliable. Reliability is the degree to which the instrument (survey or questionnaire) will provide consistent results over time. To understand better, think about your bathroom scale. If the scale gives you wildly varying results every time you weigh in, the scale is not reliable. While it's true that your weight will change depending on what you eat or do in the hours before you weigh in, it won't change more than a few pounds in normal circumstances. The most common ways to estimate the reliability of data produced by a questionnaire or survey include test-retest, split-half, and internal consistency strategies.

Test-retest reliability.   The test-retest strategy can be used effectively on surveys or questionnaires with scales; that is group(s) of question(s) about a specific topic or topics. For example, a group of questions on the survey might be about knowledge of healthy nutrition and another might be about healthy physical activity. These groups of questions make up two scales. In test-retest reliability, an instrument is given to the same group of people on two different occasions. A correlation (discussed in chapter 3), is computed on the scale scores from the two test administrations. Results of the correlation will range from negative one (the scores on the first test administration are opposite from the scores on the second administration; one set of scores is high and the other low) to positive one (the scores on the first test administration are similar to those of the second administration). Of course, you will want to see a highly positive correlation (close to positive one). One difficulty with test-retest is determining the amount of time between test administrations. Two weeks to a month is the general amount of time. The idea is to time the second administration so that test takers won't remember what they answered before but also have not learned more about the topic.

Split-half reliability and internal consistency.   These strategies require only one test administration. The split-half strategy can work well when the survey or questionnaire has numerous questions about one topic. The responses on even numbered questions are compared to those on the odd numbered questions. Again, a correlation is computed and the data collected by the instrument will be considered reliable if the correlation is close to one.

Internal consistency demonstrates whether the responses on a survey "hang together," that is if responses are consistent among questions for each person. One common statistical test used to calculate the consistency of responses is Chronbach's Alpha. Interpreting the results of this test is similar to that of interpreting a correlation. The desired result is close to one.

DATA-COLLECTION STRATEGIES

Data are collected in many ways, ranging from observation to complex medical tests. If you will remember, we indicated that there is a difference between research design and data-collection strategies. When you have selected your research design, the data-collection strategy and sampling methods (methods for selecting participants) can then be determined. You will most likely be involved in collecting data through survey instruments, communication groups, or observations. As we have said, these types of strategies can be either qualitative or quantitative but the instruments themselves are designed to reflect the type of data needed. If responses from a specific strategy can be counted, the instrument is likely to be quantitative. If an open-ended response can be expected, the instrument is likely to be qualitative. We'd like to review a few common strategies in the next few paragraphs.

FOCUS GROUPS

As you know from chapter 6, a focus group consists of a small number of people who are asked to participate in a discussion that provides qualitative data. Questions are developed prior to the discussion; during the session, a trained facilitator presents the questions and keeps the discussion moving. This individual does not give opinions or participate in the discussion, other than to clarify what others have said or encourage discussion in greater depth. The participant comments are recorded in some fashion. A second person serves as the recorder so the facilitator can focus on the process of the discussion. Any number of focus groups can be conducted as long as different people participate in each group.

A difficult issue in a focus-group design is determining who will participate. Will you try to get everyone in the partner population to be in a focus group? If the group is too large, will you randomly select a few to participate or will you simply ask for volunteers? If you ask for volunteers, the sampling method is called *convenience sampling.* Your decisions will be based on the research objectives and design, timeline, and budget. Keep in mind that if you want a representative sample, you should include all participants or randomly select some of them.

DELPHI TECHNIQUE

The Delphi technique, described briefly in chapter 6, collects both qualitative and quantitative data. It is another group design, but participants do not meet face-to-face. It is generally used for decision making or consensus building (Raskin, 1994), which can be important evaluation processes if you are trying to determine the value of a health education program.

If you decide to use the Delphi technique, you will need to identify criteria for selecting participants in the study. Your respondents are usually experts in the type of intervention you are delivering. They will need to commit some time to the study because they will take part in several rounds of surveys.

Round 1 is used for collecting baseline data. Participants will be asked to respond to one or more open-ended questions that reflect the research questions. When the surveys are returned, you take the responses and put them in a Likert format (items that require a rating). In round 2 participants are asked to respond to the Likert scale. When those surveys are returned, you place the items that have the highest levels of agreement in a list. During round 3 participants rank the items. You then identify the items that are most frequently ranked the highest. Your objective is to discern consensus among the group members. A fourth round may be necessary to complete the process.

INTERVIEWS

As you are probably aware by now, interviews may be formal or informal, simple or complex. A trained interviewer asks the participant at least one question and facilitates the remainder of the interview in a way that matches the data-collection protocol. If you select this strategy, you might use the same set of questions and same interview protocol for all interviewees (structured), or you might simply ask people to tell you what they think about the topic of study. If the research design is quantitative and formal, the interview questions, setting, and time will be carefully determined before data collection. Participants will be asked to stick to the questions and will be prompted in the same way. As with other data-collection strategies, you will have to make decisions about who will be interviewed. Some qualitative interview protocols use a sampling method called *snowball sampling*. In this method, a few volunteers are interviewed and they are asked to suggest others who could also be interviewed. The number of interviews thereby "snowballs." Use your research plan as your guide.

OBSERVATION

Like an interview, observations might be formal or informal, simple or complex. An observer might have specific things to look for or might note anything and everything seen. If you select this strategy, you will have to decide whether the individuals whom you are observing will be told. People who know they are being observed might change their behavior without even thinking about it. This is called **observer effect**. You will also need to be aware of your own biases. Unless you are careful, your beliefs and attitudes will be reflected in your observation (**observer bias**).

SURVEYS

Surveys can be used in both quantitative and qualitative designs. The type of item or question will determine the kind of data collected. Open-ended items elicit qualitative data, while multiple-choice questions and Likert scales, for example, elicit responses that can be quantified. Surveys are very versatile; they can be used with large or small samples, and they can be conducted over the telephone, through the postal system, in a face-to-face setting, or electronically.

As with other strategies, you will have to make decisions about who will participate. One of the most difficult issues with surveys, however, is determining their appropriateness for your project. For example, surveys that collect information about behaviors, beliefs, and attitudes often use self-report responses. In other words, you are measuring the participants' perceptions, which might not match up with reality. If self-report isn't appropriate for your project, you will want to use another technique, such as an actual observation of behaviors.

Implementation

The research plan must include the implementation phase, during which the measurements (whether surveys, interviews, medical assessments, or observations) are made. The environment plays an important role in this data-collection phase. For example, if a survey is planned but there is no place to sit and write, participants may not focus well on their responses. If a medical assessment of some type is planned without a place for privacy, participants might choose not to take part. Time, place, temperature, noise level, and lighting are among the many issues that must be considered.

Coding and analysis (usually with the aid of a computer) should take place after data are collected. Coding is a way of preparing data for analysis. A simple example of coding would be assigning a 1 to the data if the participant is male and a 2 if female.

Data Analysis

Many social science researchers enjoy the data-collection process because whether the study design is qualitative or quantitative in nature, the process involves working with people. When data collection is complete, the sheer size of the results can be overwhelming even in a small study. However, data analysis provides the basis from which the researcher draws conclusions.

QUANTITATIVE ANALYSIS

Sometimes the word *statistics* is used to mean a numerical description of an event. The frequency of accident-related deaths or incidents of violence in schools are examples of events that can be described with statistics. At other times, the word indicates mathematical procedures that are used to test hypotheses or determine reliability and validity of your instruments.

These two uses of the word *statistics* actually describe two broad categories: descriptive and inferential. **Descriptive statistics** use numbers to organize data. They lend themselves to being displayed through many types of tables, charts, and graphs. Figure 9.4 presents some commonly used formats for illustrating descriptive statistics.

Inferential statistics are used to make comparisons, identify relationships, and draw conclusions about data. Space prevents us from discussing these tests in sufficient detail in this chapter; but if you have not done so already, we encourage you to take a full course in basic statistics so that you are equipped to select the best ways to organize and analyze your quantitative data.

Pie Chart

Immunization status of children age 1–4 in central cities (pop. ≥ 250,000) by financial status, United States, sample year

Poverty

17%
29%
55%

Nonpoverty

10%
27%
63%

◼ Adequately immunized: 3+ doses inactivated vaccine and/or 3 doses oral vaccine

◼ Inadequately immunized: Some vaccine but <3 doses IPV and/or <3 OPV

◻ Not immunized: No vaccine

Pictograph

Figure 9.4   Displaying descriptive statistics.
Descriptive statistics can be illustrated for your participants or in your reports in a number of ways. The illustrations on pages 225–227 provide some examples. These examples have relatively generic titles; in your own reports, you should include specific information regarding the scope of the data illustrated, the location where the data was collected, and the dates it was collected. Careful thought should be given to the types of charts or graphs you select so that your results can be clearly understood.

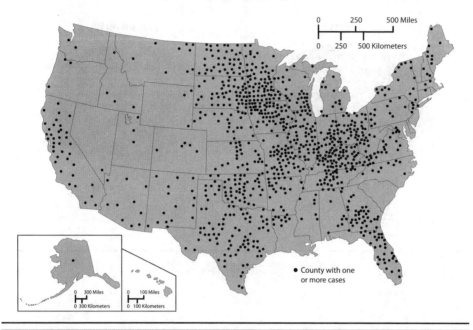

Scatter Plot

Counties reporting one or more cases, United States, sample year

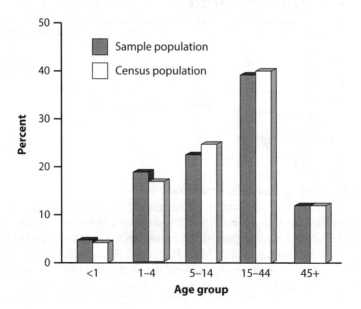

Bar Chart

Percent of age distribution of sample population compared to census population immunization survey, sample city, sample year

Line Graph

Reported case rates by 13 four-week periods, United States, sample year

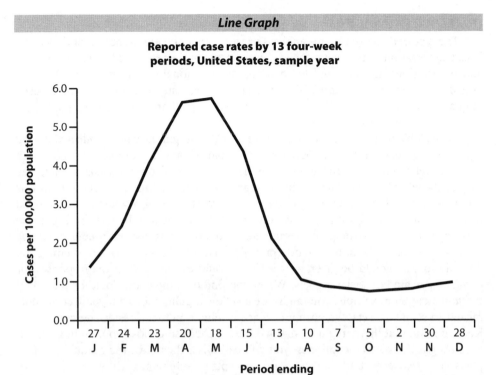

Block Chart

Cases of illness, elementary school sample city, sample year

QUALITATIVE ANALYSIS

The type of data used in this analysis process cannot be represented well with numbers. Conversations, interviews, focus-group discussions, open-ended survey responses, and observations are analyzed for patterns or commonalities in meaning. As mentioned earlier, numerical coding is used in quantitative data analysis but it can be used in qualitative analysis as well. The difference is that qualitative data coding could also use colors, symbols, words, or phrases.

Let us look at an example of qualitative data that might have been collected during a program for teen mothers. Suppose we asked participants to complete a survey with questions related to their satisfaction with the program. One question asks participants to describe what they liked about the program. One person wrote, "This program was fun because people I knew were in it with me." Another person wrote, "I really liked this program because I got to go with my friends." Do you see the relationship in the two responses? Both participants commented about the social aspect (friends or people I know) as a reason for liking the program. Because it looks like a pattern is emerging, "social aspects" would be given a code. You would examine all of the responses for comments related to social aspects. When you find one, the code would be placed by the statement. For example, you might use a yellow highlighter to designate comments related to social aspects or you might place a unique number beside the comments. Keep in mind that there might be many different codes so choose your coding system accordingly. If a pattern continues, you will call this a theme for the group of participants. You may even find that there are concepts or subthemes within the theme. In the end, you will report the major themes and concepts and support your findings with examples of actual statements made by the participants.

The Research Report

The reporting phase of a research project may give the appearance of being the easiest part, but it can be difficult and time consuming. Be sure to allow plenty of time. In this phase, the project must be summarized and the "results" must be articulated.

The report, which is generally prepared at the end of the project, is substantial and formal. According to the National Science Foundation (1997), the report author must consider what the readers of the report need to know, how to best organize the document, how to present conclusions that are very clear as well as those that are not as definitive, and how to protect the confidentiality of the participants in the presentation of the results.

In determining the needs of your audience, you might decide that the individuals reading the report will need sufficient detail to repeat the program in exactly the same way. If this is the case, each phase of the project must be clearly delineated and thoughtful conclusions prepared. On the other hand, perhaps the audience for the report will be the press. They may be interested primarily in a summary of results and conclusions. This type of report might be shorter but no less thought-out. Of course, when you have multiple audiences, you might be called on to do both types of report. Just be patient, collect your thoughts, and prepare the needed documents.

In general, most reports include some background information, the research objectives or questions, the data-collection strategies, a description of data analysis, a listing of the results, and a discussion of conclusions. The report should be well written and interesting to read. If you have used mixed methods (a combination of several research designs), you will want to include participant comments and observations as well as statistics. Be sure to proofread, revise, and proofread again. Small errors can detract from the importance of your message. Remember, form your conclusions carefully. If your audience is in a hurry, the conclusions will be the focus of their reading. Don't forget to provide your participants with the results of the study.

≡ Evaluation: A Type of Research

Health professionals frequently assume that the health of their patients, clients, or participants automatically improves as a result of the programs designed for such purposes. However, you should be aware that some health education programs don't work, or that the hoped-for changes occur as a result of something other than the program. Evaluation must be a part of the program plan. It is also a type of research.

Definition

Green and Kreuter's 1999 definition of evaluation still remains appropriate today. They define evaluation as "the comparison of an object of interest against a standard of acceptability" (p. 220). This is more easily understood when you consider that both the *object of interest* and *standards of acceptability* are identified by your program objectives. The object of interest is the behavior and the standard of acceptability is the "how much" and "when" components of the objectives. Let's look at an example from your program for teen mothers. One of your objectives regarding second pregnancies might have been, "By the end of the year-long program offered by the public health educator, participants will list at least five benefits of remaining abstinent." In the subsequent evaluation, the object of interest is "list benefits of remaining abstinent" and the standard of acceptability is "at least five."

Many individuals believe that the definitions for evaluation will change according to the purpose of conducting it. For example, if cost analysis is the major purpose of the evaluation, you might be defining evaluation in terms of **cost-effectiveness** (an assessment of the program costs and how they relate to the success of the program) or **cost-benefit** (an analysis of the financial gain from the program). On the other hand, if you want to know whether program participants are satisfied with the program, you will probably define evaluation in terms of process (the way in which the program runs).

Purposes

Some common purposes of evaluation include the following:

1. To determine if program objectives have been met.
2. To see if the appropriate participants are involved in the program.
3. To make certain that the interventions match design specifications.
4. To find out what works and what does not.
5. To determine fiscal efficiency.
6. To fulfill grant or contract requirements.

7. To provide marketing material.

8. To determine if the program will work for other people beyond program participants.

9. To contribute to scientific knowledge about health education programming.

≡ Types of Evaluation

Regardless of the purpose, all forms of evaluation fit into two major categories: formative and summative. **Formative evaluations** occur during program development and implementation. These evaluations determine the efficacy of program development and the utility of program implementation for the purpose of program improvement (McDermott & Sarvela, 1999). **Summative evaluations** occur after program completion: immediately, after a specified waiting period, or both. As you know, many health programs use the terms *process*, *impact*, and *outcome* to label their objectives; but keep in mind, some agencies and foundations use only the term *outcomes* for objectives and then divide outcomes into short- and long-term. Don't be concerned, there are just different ways to label objectives. We encourage you to understand the concepts behind the terms. Hopefully, you remember that process objectives are those that provide guidance in program functioning. No matter which term is used for the concept, the types of evaluation used are determined by the types of objectives written during program development.

Process Evaluation

In chapter 7 we defined process as "a series of actions or behaviors resulting in an end." In a health education program, processes of interest might include, but are not limited to, the effectiveness of program implementation, the adequacy of the number of people attending, the suitability of the program schedule, the acceptability of program location, and the satisfaction of program participants with the program. It's important not to confuse processes with impacts or outcomes, which are the results of the program, i.e., whether participants gained knowledge or changed behaviors. Process evaluation measures how well the program fulfills the process objectives. A sample evaluation question written from a process objective might read, "Did program participants feel that the content of the program met their personal needs?"

Can you see how important it is to write clear and measurable program objectives? Your evaluation will be directly related to those objectives.

Impact Evaluation

Impact refers to aspects of health that have changed by the end of the program. Health impacts generally occur more rapidly than health outcomes. Some examples include knowledge level (in almost any health education program), weight loss (in a weight-loss program), and number of cigarettes smoked per day (in a smoking-cessation program). Sometimes health determinants or behaviors are both impacts (short-term) and outcomes (long-term) of health programs. If you choose to conduct an impact evaluation, the short-term program effects will be measured immediately after the end of the program and analyzed.

Outcome Evaluation

A health outcome provides a broader, long-term picture of health. It might refer to determinants of health such as the social and economic environment, the physical environment, and the person's individual characteristics and behaviors (World Health Organization, 2008g) but it might also include the presence or absence of a disease. Health determinants, behaviors, and even the presence of disease can be measured. If you choose an outcome evaluation, the long-term program effects will be measured and analyzed. The major difference between impact and outcome evaluations is the length of time since the program or intervention. Impacts are short-term program results while outcomes are long-term program results.

Regardless of the type of evaluation, you will need to consider the issues that create barriers to effective evaluations. According to Schneider, Milat, and Moore (2016) who interviewed evaluation researchers, issues of time such as starting the evaluation planning too late, limited framework for the evaluation, use of process evaluation only, and busy schedules are the biggest barriers to effective evaluations. Some of the other barriers reported by the interviewees included politics, inadequate resources, and concerns about the consequences of the evaluation (Schneider et al., 2016). We encourage you to understand these barriers and plan ahead so they will not diminish the value of your evaluations.

The Evaluation Plan

The evaluation plan will have its own objectives. If you think of objectives as road maps, it is easier to understand why you might want to develop them to be specific to the type of evaluation. Your evaluation objectives will be directly related to the program objectives. Imagine that your program objective stated, "The infant safety knowledge level of Rising Star participants will increase by 25% after the four classes presented by the health educator." Can you identify the objective type? It is not a process objective; it does not describe a function or process of the program. If you said impact, you are absolutely correct. The objective describes a short-term result of the program.

The evaluation objective linked to this particular program objective might state, "Measure the percentage change in infant safety knowledge between pretest and posttest for program participants." You will have evaluation objectives that link to each of your program objectives and perhaps a few more. For example, you may want to evaluate participant perceptions of whether the program was effective because if participants didn't like it, the word will probably spread and attendance at future programs might be influenced.

The types of evaluation must be clarified (process, impact, or outcome), and the research design must be determined. From this point forward, the evaluation plan will match a research plan.

☰ Ethics in Research

The most basic ethical consideration in research is the protection of your participants. One of the first things to do is to ask them to consent to being part of the research project. Of course, you will want them to feel free to say no. They will feel less hesitant if they understand the research process and how the information will be reported, so be sure to explain the process well. Table 9.2 summarizes risk issues that must be considered in an ethical research process.

Table 9.2   Ethics and Research

Honesty	Strive for honesty in all scientific communications. Honestly report data, results, methods and procedures, and publication status. Do not fabricate, falsify, or misrepresent data. Do not deceive colleagues, granting agencies, or the public.
Objectivity	Strive to avoid bias in experimental design, data analysis, data interpretation, peer review, personnel decisions, grant writing, expert testimony, and other aspects of research where objectivity is expected or required. Avoid or minimize bias or self-deception. Disclose personal or financial interests that may affect research.
Integrity	Keep your promises and agreements; act with sincerity; strive for consistency of thought and action.
Carefulness	Avoid careless errors and negligence; carefully and critically examine your own work and the work of your peers. Keep good records of research activities, such as data collection, research design, and correspondence with agencies or journals.
Openness	Share data, results, ideas, tools, resources. Be open to criticism and new ideas.
Respect for Intellectual Property	Honor patents, copyrights, and other forms of intellectual property. Do not use unpublished data, methods, or results without permission. Give credit where credit is due. Give proper acknowledgement or credit for all contributions to research. Never plagiarize.
Confidentiality	Protect confidential communications, such as papers or grants submitted for publication, personnel records, trade or military secrets, and patient records.
Responsible Publication	Publish in order to advance research and scholarship, not to advance just your own career. Avoid wasteful and duplicative publication.
Responsible Mentoring	Help to educate, mentor, and advise students. Promote their welfare and allow them to make their own decisions.
Respect for Colleagues	Respect your colleagues and treat them fairly.
Social Responsibility	Strive to promote social good and prevent or mitigate social harms through research, public education, and advocacy.
Non-Discrimination	Avoid discrimination against colleagues or students on the basis of sex, race, ethnicity, or other factors that are not related to their scientific competence and integrity.
Competence	Maintain and improve your own professional competence and expertise through lifelong education and learning; take steps to promote competence in science as a whole.
Legality	Know and obey relevant laws and institutional and governmental policies.
Animal Care	Show proper respect and care for animals when using them in research. Do not conduct unnecessary or poorly designed animal experiments.
Human Subjects Protection	When conducting research on human subjects, minimize harms and risks and maximize benefits; respect human dignity, privacy, and autonomy; take special precautions with vulnerable populations; and strive to distribute the benefits and burdens of research fairly.

From *What Is Ethics in Research & Why Is It Important?* by D. B. Resnik, 2007, National Institutes of Environmental Health Sciences—National Institutes of Health. Retrieved from http://www.niehs.nih.gov/research/resources/bioethics/whatis.cfm

It will be important for you to minimize risks that your participants will face. Risks include those that are physical in nature as well as psychological. For example, if you are asking questions that your participants find embarrassing, you are putting them at psychological risk. If you ask them to do something that could cause injury, this puts them at physical risk. It is up to you to protect them.

When you write your report, present data for a group rather than results specific to individuals. If you are presenting specific comments or observations, do not use identifying information if you can avoid doing so. If a participant can be identified, get permission first. Just remember to be honest, respect your participants, and act with integrity.

≡ In Conclusion

Research is the cornerstone for improving health; it provides the documentation and confirmation that interventions work, that patterns created by healthy behaviors exist, for understanding why people behave the way they do, and for choosing new directions in prevention. The best health education programs are developed with evaluation research in mind. We hope you will develop an understanding of rigorousness in research, which calls for appropriate designs and data-collection strategies. When you write your research plan, pay special attention to writing objectives. They should be directly linked to the problem being addressed or, in the case of evaluation, the program objectives. As part of that plan, you will also need to create a feasible timeline and a budget. Devote as much attention to the final research report as to the rest of the research process; the report will document your work. Most importantly, let ethics be your guiding light. Every decision should be informed by both an understanding of and appreciation for ethics in research.

REVIEW QUESTIONS

1. Describe and justify the steps involved in writing a research plan.
2. Discuss the importance of the categories that might be used in a research budget.
3. Select one qualitative design and discuss its strengths and weaknesses.
4. Analyze the benefits of using an experimental design.
5. Give examples of process, impact, and outcome evaluations.

FOR YOUR APPLICATION

This activity has two parts. First, develop an evaluation plan for the program you are developing in your project. If you aren't participating in a project, select or create a simple health education program and develop an evaluation plan for it. Second, write an instrument with just a few items for your evaluation. If it is a quantitative instrument, consider how you might determine reliability and validity. Ask a few friends to take the survey and analyze the results. When your evaluation plan and instrument have been graded, revise them and put them in your portfolio if you are creating one.

PART III

COMMUNICATING NEEDS
AND
MANAGING RESOURCES

10

Community Health
Administration

"But I thought you were going to make those phone calls!" You try to keep the exasperation out of your voice, but this is just one of many similar conversations you've had lately. It seems as though no one involved in this health program knows what anyone else is doing. What was once a good program idea, both wanted and needed by the community, is becoming an organizational nightmare. You hang up the phone and say out loud, "Where did I go wrong?" In desperation, you take out an old textbook that you never thought you'd use again. You look up the terms *management, leadership, administration,* and *coordination.*

Chapter Objectives

1. Detail the difference between leadership and management.
2. Identify techniques for conflict resolution.
3. Define policy and name three components.
4. Describe the difference between procedural policy and public health policy.
5. Name four federal agencies that monitor public health policy.
6. Summarize the purpose and components of the Patients' Bill of Rights.
7. Create ideas for making certain that all people have access to health care.
8. Practice writing policies.

Leadership, Management, and Administration

The magnitude of health disparities in U.S. communities, the interwoven web of causation of our most devastating diseases, and the inability of our health care system to adequately care for all of our sick underscore the importance of inspirational leadership and competent administration. John Holland of the Santa Fe Institute states that health and the health care system are "multi-layered systems largely driven by rapidly changing technology and information." He further states, "Knowing the building blocks of the organizational system and its core processes is critical. Studying the interfaces of the building blocks allows system leaders to ask questions based on the flows or patterns among the processes, identify the feedback loops, explore the interfaces, and ultimately identify an efficient system" (Holland, 2003 p. 3).

What is administration? Are leadership, administration, management, and coordination of services different terms for the same activity? Can anyone be a leader? There are a lot of questions to be answered in this chapter, and we'd like to first discuss the concept of leadership. Leaders get things started, so it's a good place for us to begin.

Leadership

Leadership research conducted in the 20th century generally focused on the leaders themselves; the traits and behaviors observed in successful leaders (Bryman, 1996). Initially, it was thought that leadership qualities were genetic. Later research seemed to indicate that leadership consisted of a set of behaviors that could be learned. Typically such behaviors focused on the transactional interaction between leaders and followers. Toward the end of the century, leadership approaches seemed to combine a number of different traits, styles, concepts, and behaviors; one of which was transformational leadership, which may also be viewed as democratic leadership (Cunningham, Salomone, & Wielfus, 2015).

Transformational leadership differs from previous leadership concepts in that it focuses on the *relationship* between the leader and follower, not merely the transaction. There is an increased moral and ethical focus. Such leaders are interested in the well-being of the people being led, not just getting the job done. The transformational leader begins by determining a vision based on an understanding of the core values of the organization. Next, the leader sells the vision by developing trust with the people involved. This step may take a great deal of time, effort, and charisma. In the end, the transformational leader takes a visible role in the actual move toward the goal (Synique, 2008).

Service leadership became popular early in the 21st century and is similar in many respects to transformational leadership (Cunningham, Salomone, & Wielfus, 2015). This approach utilizes a service-oriented framework in which personnel in an organization and their leaders use service activities to reach mutually determined goals. Every contact with a customer or client is seen as an opportunity to increase loyalty through providing service. Such leadership recognizes that clients are both internal and external (Gronfeldt & Strother, 2006).

In 2008, Burman and Evans published a "charter" for aviation leaders that we feel makes sense for health administrators as well. Much like health care, aviation is a field that is driven by the need for quality and excellence. According to Burman and Evans, leaders must perform the following behaviors:

- Lead by example in accordance with the company's core values.
- Build the trust and confidence of the people with whom you work.
- Continually seek improvement in methods and effectiveness.
- Keep people informed.
- Be accountable for personal actions and hold others accountable for theirs.
- Involve people, seek their views, listen actively to what they have to say and represent these views honestly.
- Be clear on what is expected, and provide feedback on progress.
- Accept people's differences and deal with their issues fairly.
- Acknowledge and recognize people for their contributions and performance.
- Weigh alternatives, consider both short- and long-term effects, and then be resolute in the decisions you make (2008, p. 10).

Strategic Leadership also has similarities to transformational and service leadership styles but adds an important characteristic: preparedness for change. "The Strategic leader has the ability to stay ahead of the curve by anticipating change and motivates an entire company to adapt to it" (Cunningham, Salomone, and Wielfus, 2015 p. 32).

We believe that leadership is a fluid concept that differs by person and situation. Great leaders can be quiet and unassuming or vibrant and vocal. The two overriding traits of successful leaders are the ability to (a) envision the future and (b) motivate people into belief and action. One distressful fact is that there are still many barriers for women with strong leadership characteristics from becoming high-level leaders. According to Haile, Emmanuel, and Dzathor, some of the barriers include organizational cultures, gender stereotypes, lack of willingness to capitalize on women's skills, structural procedures, male chauvinism, and differences in pay. We challenge you to work toward overcoming barriers like these so that the most talented and inspirational people, regardless of gender or skin color, are in leadership positions (2013).

Once a leader has been selected, a path has been selected, and people are ready to move, the actual navigation is often provided by managers. Managers direct people and control schedules and budgets. Leaders are not always good managers and good managers are not always good leaders. Most organizations, however, need both to function effectively.

Management

Table 10.1 compares leadership and management tasks and traits. As you can see from the table, managers are highly involved in the day-to-day operation of an organization. They are charged with maintaining budgets, keeping schedules, maintaining optimum output, and reaching objectives. Managers are those who are responsible for the bottom line. The manager's job may be the most difficult because he or she maintains balance and flow.

Table 10.1   Leadership versus Management

Leadership	Management
Establishes vision	Controls resources
Holds a future orientation	Has a real-time orientation
Maintains a broad perspective	Focuses on details
Deals with change	Organizes activities to maintain status quo
Encourages growth	Schedules daily operations
Supports people	Directs personnel
Takes risks	Minimizes risks

Most people believe that management skills can be learned because they are task oriented. If we were to create a charter for managers, we would include the following behaviors. We hope you agree that these are skills you should have when you enter the workforce, even if you don't start as a manager.

- Manage time proficiently.
- Track activities carefully.
- Evaluate performances professionally.
- Provide clear instruction.

- Resolve disputes appropriately.
- Organize well.
- Listen actively.
- Know policies, guidelines, and rules.
- Write objectives that match organizational goals.
- Use resources efficiently.

Administration

Administration involves both leading and managing as well as coordinating support systems and activities that facilitate the effective running of an organization, institution, or program. Some of the major roles might include quality assurance, finance, human resources, facilities management, and other tasks that further the goals of the organization.

Upon graduation, most of you will work in formal organizations. These include government agencies, schools, nonprofit organizations, private practices, and health care institutions. A formal organization is one that has been established to meet a specified mission. It may consist of a small office with a few positions or numerous sites with a wide variety of departments and personnel. An organizational flow chart describes the structure of an organization, whether small or large. Figure 10.1 illustrates an organizational flow chart for a small organization.

Viewing organizational charts and the titles of personnel can be confusing. The words division, department, area, and section may be used by different organizations to mean the same thing. On the other hand, an organization may use these terms to differentiate the size of various units or types of activities within their structure. Administrative titles are equally confusing and humorous, at times. A mid-level administrator (perhaps the administrator of a division or department) might be called

Figure 10.1   Sample organizational chart.

coordinator, director, manager, chair, or even *head.* Each organization has definitions for each title. Your goal will be to understand the levels. Before you interview for a position, familiarize yourself with the organizational structure of your potential employer.

Most formal organizations exist within a bureaucratic structure in which one or more persons have been given authority to make decisions and take action. The administration of any organization may have several levels that have varying degrees of responsibility and authority. Having the authority to make decisions and take action provides power. So, power is a good thing, right? As usual, the answer is not simple. While power must be present for action to take place, power placed in the hands of an ineffective leader or manager can destroy the organization.

As you all know, there are informal organizations that exist within formal organizations. These informal groups generally represent social networks within a formal organization, and although they may not have recognized authority, they may have a great deal of power. Informal leaders may hold the key to your success as an administrator. It will be important for you to recognize and communicate with the informal leaders.

Promoting cooperation, building collaborative networks, and writing policy are important skills for administrators. We will discuss these next. Administrators also must be effective communicators. We will cover verbal and written communication in chapter 11.

Cooperation and Conflict Resolution

Promoting cooperation, enhancing collaboration, and writing policy are fundamental activities for those who administer health programming. *Cooperation* is a word most of us have heard since our early childhood, along with other phrases such as *play nicely, share, give in,* and *get along.* Most of us can probably remember a time when we were asked to cooperate, but felt that what we were really being asked was to give up some level of control and let some other person have her or his way. Because of those kinds of experiences, the idea of cooperation doesn't always excite people. Giving up control over something about which we feel strongly can be a real challenge. However, most of us can also recall a time when we received help from someone who was willing to cooperate. It's a good feeling when you experience a partnership effort that truly benefits everyone involved. It usually happens in an atmosphere of cooperation.

Promoting Cooperation

So what is cooperation? Is it really giving control to another person and following his or her lead? According to Merriam-Webster's Online (2008), **cooperation** is "to act or work with another or others: act together" or "to associate with another or others for mutual benefit." To explore the meaning of cooperation more fully, consider for a moment two important phrases in these definitions: "to act or work together/to associate" and "for mutual benefit."

If a group of people came together to build a small house, no thinking person would expect all members of the group to have the same types of house-building skills and experience. After all, an electrician who could ably wire the house would not necessarily be well-versed in plumbing. Skilled plumbers aren't always good carpenters, and carpenters may know little about applying stucco, aluminum siding, or brick to the outside walls. But each set of knowledge and skills is needed for successful house building.

These differing skills are needed at different points in the building process. One wouldn't expect the electricians to show up, for instance, until the foundation had been laid and the walls framed. If the roofers insisted on doing their job on the day the foundation was poured, we'd likely begin to worry about their competence. And though each job is important to the overall goal, each differs from the others in the length of time and amount of effort needed.

With so much diversity of effort and focus, how is the group able to achieve any common goal—much less build an entire house? In most house-building efforts, a project foreperson or contractor coordinates the project. This person usually has a blueprint of the house that illustrates how all parts are to be constructed. The contractor uses the blueprint to coordinate individual efforts, constantly checking progress in light of the master house plan. And, because the contractor is the person most aware of the contribution of each group, a full understanding and appreciation of the abilities and efforts of each is paramount to project success.

What can we learn from this illustration of cooperation in action? The concepts are very basic. First, we know that cooperation happens when everyone contributes to the project. However, oftentimes different people must do different jobs at different times, paces, and levels of effort to achieve the common goal. Misperceptions among group members about what others are contributing can lead to jealousy and resentment. A mutual understanding of group-member expectations, from the outset, is very important for achieving and maintaining cooperation.

Second, we know that it helps to have a blueprint and a designated person (or group of people) responsible for coordinating the effort. This person may not necessarily complete individual tasks in the project. Nor does this person need extensive skills in all project task areas. However, the project coordinator should be someone who

- can maintain sight of the big picture and how each individual task fits
- is willing and able to maintain close contact with the project from start to finish
- has strong organization, communication, and negotiation skills
- can respectfully interact with each project contributor in a positive way and, when necessary, resolve conflicts

Conflict Resolution

Most of us tend to interpret the words and actions of others through the lenses of our personal values and experiences (Seelye & Seelye-James, 1996). When values and interpretations differ among individuals, misunderstandings can develop. Consider two highly qualified professionals who are collaborating on a project but have different perceptions about time and commitment. Ann tends to be task-oriented and believes that a committed professional always arrives on time. Ben highly values a cooperative approach and is less concerned about time constraints. Ann interprets Ben's late arrivals to meetings as a sign of low commitment. She decides to take a strong lead to ensure project success. Ben interprets Ann's independent decision making as controlling and aggressive. He stops attending meetings. Mistaken assumptions lead to conflict and the project flounders.

A difference in time orientation is one of the **silent value factors** that are seldom discussed but often contribute to conflict in collaborative efforts (Seelye & Seelye-James, 1996). Though such differences are often expected in cross-cultural situations, they can also influence interaction when no cultural differences are apparent. For example, using formal titles rather than first names may seem cold and distant to some people, whereas using first names can be insulting to others. Avoiding direct eye contact with a member of the other gender may seem respectful to some and devaluing to others. A lecture-based meeting presentation may appear to be the most efficient and logical approach but could cause some of your participants to suspect that you feel superior to the group and wish to control it. Understanding these potential differences is the first step to preventing **conflict**. Because time-orientation differences are a common conflict factor, we invite you to complete the checklists in FYI 10.1 as a starting point.

10.1 Assess Your Time Orientation

Differences in time orientation (monochronic versus polychronic) are a common conflict factor. Understanding those differences can be a first step toward conflict resolution.

How monochronic are you?

- I like to do one thing at a time.
- I concentrate on the job at hand.
- I take time commitments (deadlines, schedules) seriously.
- I am committed to the job.
- I adhere closely to plans.
- I am concerned about not disturbing others (follow rules of privacy).
- I show great respect for private property (seldom borrow or lend).
- I emphasize promptness in meetings.
- I am comfortable with short-term relationships.

How polychronic are you?

- I like to do many things at once.
- I am highly distractible and frequently interrupt what I am doing.
- I consider time commitments more of an objective to be achieved, if possible, than a quasi-legal contract.
- I am committed to people and human relationships.
- I change plans often and easily.
- I put obligations to family and friends before work concerns.
- I consider intimacy with family and friends more important than respecting their privacy.
- I borrow and lend things often and easily.
- I base the level of promptness on the particular relationship.
- I have a strong tendency to build lifetime relationships.

From *Culture Clash: Managing in a Multicultural World*, by H. N. Seelye and A. Seelye-James, 1996, pp. 25–26. © 1996. Used with permission of the McGraw-Hill Companies.

Resolving Differences

How can you avoid conflict that is based on value differences and misinterpretations? Communicate. Communicate clearly by using a variety of written and oral formats. Communicate often by establishing ongoing channels through which information and perceptions are exchanged. Communicate unselfishly by listening as often, or perhaps more often, than you speak. Communicate to understand. Communicate to problem-solve. Communicate to collaborate.

Communicate. But also keep in mind that, regardless of how hard you work as project coordinator to minimize the potential for conflict, it can still occur. In fact, conflict is normal. Members of your coalition, task force, or advisory board may agree with the overall goals of the collaborative effort, but strongly differ when it comes to decisions about how to approach a task, the time frame in which it will happen, the location of task events, or who will be involved. What do you do when the cause of the conflict isn't miscommunication but rather disagreement about the process or expected outcomes? The first step is to gain an understanding of the cause of the conflict, what motivates each person involved to disagree.

People often become involved in conflict because they are stakeholders in relation to the argument issue. A **stakeholder** is a person or organization who will likely gain or lose something as a result of efforts made to reduce the targeted health problem. In decision-making situations, most stakeholders are motivated at least in part by what they and the people they represent stand to gain or lose through the decision. That isn't necessarily a bad thing. A diverse representation of community stakeholders can serve as a healthy set of checks and balances in the decision-making process. The protected welfare of various community groups often depends on advocates who look out for their interests. It is likely, however, that some members of such a diverse decision-making group will disagree from time to time. When that happens, your goal as project administration, manager, or leader will be to facilitate appropriate discussions and negotiations so that the project progresses and, to the extent possible, all groups benefit.

How strong are your negotiation skills? Have you ever attempted to resolve differences between people you care about? If so, you may have concluded that at least one person seemed more interested in personal well-being than the good of all involved. Getting someone like that person to cooperate can be an intellectually and emotionally draining task and you may be tempted to use some choice adjectives such as *stubborn, selfish,* and *impossible* in the process.

If you've had a similar experience, you can probably relate to the dilemma some project coordinators face. The ideal is to resolve the conflict in a way that allows all parties involved to reach a mutually satisfying solution. FYI 10.2 contains tips for conflict resolution (Espinoza, personal communication, August 2008). One step refers to a technique known as **active listening**, or **reflective listening**. In this technique, each person involved in the discussion is required to orally paraphrase or repeat back what was just said by the other person. The purpose of this exercise is for each person to focus on the thoughts and feelings of others rather than on his or her own personal reactions or interpretations. The person whose statements have been paraphrased is then given the opportunity to correct mistaken interpretations and elaborate for deeper understanding.

FYI

10.2   Tips for Dispute Resolution

DO	DON'T
• Know that conflict is normal and healthy.	• Think that everyone responds to conflict in the same way.
• Realize that differences may not be as great as perceived.	• Respond purely on emotion.
• Try on the other hat—listen.	• Suppose that you know everything.
• Be creative in considering resolutions.	• Deem that your truth is the only truth.
• Watch for potential conflict and understand it before it escalates.	• Believe that conflict resolution is simple.

In our example, Ann and Ben could use active listening to discuss their frustrations and seek conflict resolution. For instance, Ann might say, "Ben, I don't think you are really committed to this project and it frustrates me." Ben's reflective response could be, "You don't think I care about the project? What makes you think that?" Ann might then launch into a description of how Ben is always late for meetings and doesn't seem to care about deadlines. At this point, Ben could respond in at least two different ways. He could abandon the active listening technique, become defensive, and react. On the other hand, he could take a deep breath and attempt to focus on Ann's reasoning and feelings rather than his own. In doing so, his response could be more reflective. "Ann, until now, I didn't realize that my 'late arrivals' irritated you. It isn't because I don't care. It's just that traffic holds me up. Besides, I've been thinking that you don't really want my input on this."

It would then be Ann's turn to paraphrase rather than react. A reflective response would be, "Why do you think I don't want your input?" This would allow Ben to explain how hurt he felt when Ann moved ahead on decisions without him, and two mature professionals would have the opportunity to view the situation through the eyes of the other.

Their new appreciation for each other's perspective could then be applied in the next resolution step, finding mutual ground for agreement. In our example, both individuals agree on the importance of the project, which implies that they share mutual goals. A return to common goals reminds individuals that they are partners rather than adversaries. Competition can then give way to flexible collaboration.

Because Ben and Ann share a common goal, they can collaborate in order to reach it. They might, for example, alter meeting schedules and locations to reduce Ben's traffic barriers. Ben could commit to leaving his home earlier and Ann could agree to be more flexible and work on other projects should Ben be late. The two could agree to identify and work toward important deadlines, but adopt a more flexible approach to less time-dependent tasks.

The individual strengths of each person could also be applied more effectively to different aspects of the project. Ben's strengths might be in interacting with other people who are important to project success, while Ann might prefer to take on greater responsibility for needed organizational aspects. The two could learn to trust each other more in these responsibilities, respect and appreciate the asset inherent in their differences, and communicate more freely to prevent future misunderstandings. The approach would not guarantee consistently smooth interaction, but effective collaboration could hardly occur without it. The same concepts of individual collaboration and conflict resolution can be applied to group and community settings. Although the processes become more complex in broader interactive settings, some of the same principles apply.

Community Development

Think back for a moment to other chapters in which we've discussed the definitions and roles of communities in health education. By now you have had the opportunity to explore concepts of how individuals within a community form bonds driven by values, interests, needs, and capacities. We hope you appreciate how important it is to partner with the community from the earliest stages of the needs assessment and to maintain community connections throughout program planning, implementation, and evaluation. If so, you may have reached the same conclusion that many in our profession hold: A community that has the power to create its own solutions is the most likely to have success in improving the quality of life of its members.

If community building and empowerment are so important, can they be fostered? The health professionals involved must hold the philosophy that community connectedness serves as a foundation. The strategies selected must be geared toward building community, not just isolating a problem or two in the community as targets for health programs. And, significantly, the community must possess the capacity to become involved in the process. One of your first goals may be to help the community become aware of its existing competencies so that it can capitalize on strengths and rectify gaps. Community-based participatory research or action research, discussed in chapter 9, may be an effective method for identifying community strengths. Other practical community building and organization suggestions are listed in FYI 10.3.

But, wait a minute! Didn't we tell you in an earlier chapter that the health problems you are hired to address will likely be dictated by agency missions and available grant money? How can you reconcile the need to target pre-designated goals with what we've said here about beginning with community concerns? It is possible that the agency decision makers who set those targets are quite aware of the need for community ownership and, before you were hired, set the wheels in motion for effective community partnerships. You should be able to learn a lot by talking to your superiors and coworkers, along with community members, to understand how decisions were made.

If you find that the community was not involved in the decision-making process, the concepts and methods of community organization and building should still be applied. You can begin talking about the targeted health problem with various community groups and gatekeepers, along with representatives of other agencies and community health organizations. Ask for their perceptions about the extent of the problem and potential community-based solutions. If awareness of the problem is lacking, awareness-building messages can be disseminated through the media, town hall meetings, pamphlets, health fairs, presentations to organizations, and focus groups. The

10.3   Community Building and Organization Suggestions

Following these community building and organization suggestions can help a community identify its own health problems and potential solutions.

Support community issues	Start where the community is, and let community members make the decisions. Be a catalyst or facilitator of those decisions, not a decision maker.
Foster issue awareness	Talk with various groups of community members to raise awareness levels. Offer ideas for how community members might convert concerns into action.
Expedite information collection	Provide information about where to access resources. If needed, be willing to research information and pass it on to community members.
Develop community competence	Identify natural leaders and helpers within the community. Help them identify and tap into their own networks of support. Encourage and support collective problem solving and resource development. Emphasize capacity building and assets mapping.
Advocate for the community	In staff meetings or other settings in which community members are not present, speak on their behalf in a supportive, respectful manner.
Mediate when negotiation is needed	When needed, help resolve differences between community stakeholders by emphasizing the mutual benefits of cooperation and negotiating mutually acceptable compromise to reach common goals.

Sources: *Community Health Education: Settings, Tools, and Skills for the 21st Century*, by D. J. Breckon, J. R. Harvey, and R. B. Lancaster, 1998, Gaithersburg, MD: Aspen; and "Improving Health Through Community Organization and Community Building," by M. Winkler and N. Wallerstein, 1997, in K. Glanz, F. M. Lewis, and B. K. Rimer, *Health Behavior and Health Education: Theory, Research, and Practice*, pp. 241–269, San Francisco: Jossey-Bass.

time and effort you invest to gain community support will be well worth it in the long run. Without it, your programs may be viewed in the community as just another come-and-go event that is best ignored.

Coalitions

Once community support is in place, there are other steps you can take to further develop community organization and foster community building. The asset-mapping and capacity-building efforts should help identify community agencies and organizations other than the one in which you work that could contribute to and benefit from collaborating on community health projects. Shared ideas and resources can streamline costs, reduce duplication, and improve the quality of resulting programs (Payne, 1999). For these reasons, we encourage you to consider forming a coalition.

A health **coalition** is a "group of individuals and/or organizations with a common interest who agree to work together toward a common goal" (KU Work Group, 2018a). Coalitions are often formally structured with written goals and designated responsibilities (Parker et al., 1998). They can be useful throughout all aspects of a community health effort, offering guidelines and resources for everything from needs assessment to program evaluation (KU Work Group, 2018a). It is important, however, that specific coalition tasks remain consistent with designated goals.

One way of using a coalition in an effective manner is to ask its members to brainstorm a list of immediate and long-range objectives and tasks that, if accomplished, can help the coalition meet its goals. For example, consider a fictitious coalition whose primary goal is to reduce the incidence of HIV infection among adolescents in the community. There are several different tasks or projects a coalition could initiate to help accomplish this goal. Among them could be a needs assessment to identify HIV/AIDS-related attitudes, knowledge, and risk behaviors among local adolescents; an HIV/AIDS awareness campaign through local newspapers and radio and television stations; a telephone AIDS hotline that adolescents could call to ask questions; and an HIV testing and referral program that adolescents could readily access. Each of these activities would match the coalition goal of reducing the incidence of HIV infection. Each could be carried out over time and, in some cases, simultaneously if varying clusters of coalition members served as leaders and members of subgroup task forces.

A coalition of this breadth would require careful coordination and consistent communication among coalition members. Each task force would need clearly communicated directives, specific objectives, and designated deadlines by which a particular task objective should be met. Consistent periodic coalition meetings, with task-force reports requested at each meeting, provide the accountability check needed to encourage progress. The person asked to coordinate this effort could be you. As you can see, both managerial and leadership characteristics would be useful.

Keep in mind that coalitions aren't always a good choice. Coalitions can help you accomplish more than you could within the capacity of your single agency and community contacts. However, coordinating a coalition usurps a large amount of time, energy, and resources. And barriers to progress can arise within coalitions if individual members push personal agendas or continue to react negatively to earlier problems with other coalition members. So, before you form one, carefully consider its usefulness and cost in light of your community's intended objectives. Invest the time needed to learn all you can about potential coalition members and how they are viewed by the community before inviting them to the table.

Partnerships

In some instances, a coalition may be deemed less desirable than a simpler partnership established between your agency and a single community group or organization. The political lines and historical perspectives are often less complicated in these types of relationships. Thus, progress on designated tasks can, in some ways, advance more quickly. However, the simpler partnership approach can also reduce the scope of what you are able to accomplish because you will have fewer resources and contacts.

A partnership with a community organization is a good place to start when the goal can be adequately accomplished through the partnership capacities. You and your partner organization can establish clearly stated objectives and initiate important tasks. Then, as the work progresses and the need for broader involvement arises, other groups can be invited to join in your well-established efforts. The guidelines in Figure 10.2 can help you establish a strong partnership from the beginning.

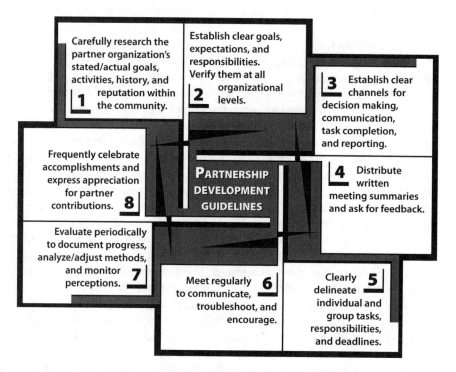

Figure 10.2   Guidelines for establishing effective partnerships.
These guidelines can facilitate mutually beneficial outcomes.

≡ The Role of Policy in Administration and Coordination

When was the last time you heard someone mention the word *policy* in a conversation? You might have been in a department store attempting to return some merchandise. Or you could have been in your supervisor's office asking why changes couldn't be made. If you've ever been told you couldn't do something because it would violate a policy, you may be tempted to think the purpose of any policy is to make life difficult. Yet, despite occasional frustrations, most of us recognize that, when needed, a carefully developed and applied policy has its merits.

Policy Defined

Westerinen (2003) defines **policy** as "a definite goal, course, or method of action to guide and determine present and future directions" (p. 3). This definition is relatively easy to use because it touches on two important characteristics of a policy: goals and guidance. Policies provide the guidance or direction for reaching goals.

PROCEDURAL POLICY

An organization's **procedural policy** is the set of rules and regulations by which an institution or organization operates. Procedural policy serves as a guideline for *how* things are accomplished. For example, suppose you worked in a hospital patient education program and had a great idea for a health education program you'd like to develop for the hospital's employees. How would you go about gaining permission to develop it? And, if permission were granted, would there be rules about using hospital time versus your own time to work on it? Where would you go to gain access to supplies and other resources? Who would need to see memos about its development and who would sign off on important papers and contracts? The answers to such questions would depend on organizational regulations and the procedural policies that guide such things as how decisions are made, resources are requisitioned, tasks are accomplished, and reports are disseminated.

Procedural policies often focus only on how tasks are to be accomplished. They don't always explain *why* the task should be initiated in the first place. Examining the reason for the task or health program takes us back to Westerinen's policy definition, which included goals as part of a policy's driving force. Adding an objective component to the definition creates a more complete perspective on policies and policy development. Objectives that are clearly stated in an organization's written policies help justify the health services and promotion programs provided by that organization. They help organizational decision makers stay on track as they make choices about how they will use precious resources to improve health and quality of life in their communities.

PUBLIC HEALTH POLICY

Developing policy to help decision makers stay on track also works at the national level. Many national initiatives to enhance the well-being of U.S. citizens begin as national policies. National policies do not have to be health-specific to have an impact on our nation's health. Policies that affect housing, education, and crime control, for example, influence the health and well-being of U.S. citizens.

FEDERAL POLICY MAKERS

Specific components of the federal government direct and monitor health-specific policy development. As we have stated in previous chapters, the Department of Health and Human Services holds primary responsibility for national health services and initiatives in the United States. The department's programs are administered by eleven operating divisions, including eight agencies in the U.S. Public Health Service and three human services agencies. National health policies are largely generated and maintained within this organization through its agencies. One of those, the Health Resources and Services Administration (HRSA), directs health policy initiatives and service programs to underserved and special-needs populations through five bureaus and ten offices.

"HRSA is the primary federal agency for improving health care to people who are geographically isolated [and] economically or medically vulnerable" (HRSA, 2018).

The Centers for Disease Control and Prevention promote health policy as it relates to prevention initiatives for specific health issues, such as chronic disease prevention, environmental health, and injury prevention. The CDC works directly with health departments and other partners to research public health concerns that could impact health policy issues. They respond to federal policy makers with the following services:

> rapid and reliable response to congressional requests for information; congressional briefings on broad public health issues and specific CDC programs; technical assistance on public health policy and legislative initiatives; CDC materials, services, and tours of facilities, including new state-of-the-art labs; discussions with scientific experts on programs of interest; participation by agency leadership and scientific experts in local public health-related events; and e-mail updates on key CDC topics. (CDC, 2006b)

The Agency for Healthcare Research and Quality (AHRQ) supports research and subsequent policy development that improves the quality of health care, reduces health care costs, and broadens health service access. It also provides evidence-based information on health care outcomes and quality of care. AHRQ's User Liaison Program helps state and local health policy makers by providing research results through various formats such as workshops, electronic courses, and teleconferences.

The United States Food and Drug Administration (FDA) works to keep foods, drugs, medical instruments, and other products safe. The Center for Food Safety and Applied Nutrition (CFSAN), part of the FDA, oversees a research program that provides information for regulatory decisions and the development of policies (FDA, n.d.).

POLICIES AND THE LEGISLATURE

Public policies are often put into effect as a law, ordinance, or resolution (Breckon, 1997). Ideas for legislated health policy initiatives can originate from a variety of sources, including members of Congress, the executive branch, committees, government health agencies, voluntary health agencies, special interest groups, and many other sources.

Once introduced as a bill, a health-related policy initiative will be submitted to a legislative committee that will likely conduct hearings on the proposed bill and, subsequently, rewrite, amend, approve, or reject the bill. A bill that has been approved by a committee is then placed before the Senate or House of Representatives for consideration. A number of health agencies and organizations are actively involved in efforts to influence health policy legislation. In chapter 12 we will explore this advocacy process in more detail.

PATIENTS' BILL OF RIGHTS

A health policy concern that received national attention was the concept of protecting patients' rights in relation to health care (Reardon, 1999). In 1998, President Clinton directed the Department of Health and Human Services and other federal agencies to comply with the Consumer or Patients' Bill of Rights (USDHHS, 1998). As can be noted in FYI 10.4, these rights focus on accessibility to quality health care. Late in the 20th century there appeared to be a growing sentiment that current man-

10.4   Patients' Bill of Rights

The Patients' Bill of Rights focuses on accessibility to quality health care among health care consumers.

1. Consumers have the right to receive accurate, easily understood information and some require assistance in making informed health care decisions about their health plans, professionals, and facilities.

2. Consumers have the right to a choice of health care providers that is sufficient to ensure access to appropriate high-quality health care.

3. Consumers have the right to access emergency health services when and where the need arises.

4. Consumers have the right and responsibility to fully participate in all decisions related to their health care.

5. Consumers have the right to considerate, respectful care from all members of the health care system at all times and under all circumstances.

6. Consumers must not be discriminated against in the delivery of health care services consistent with the benefits covered in their policy or as required by law based on race, ethnicity, national origin, religion, sex, age, mental or physical disability, sexual orientation, genetic information, or source of payment.

7. Consumers who are eligible for coverage . . . must not be discriminated against in marketing and enrollment practices based on race, ethnicity, national origin, religion, sex, age, mental or physical disability, sexual orientation, genetic information, or source of payment.

8. Consumers have the right to communicate with health care providers in confidence and to have the confidentiality of their individually identifiable health care information protected.

9. Consumers have the right to a fair and efficient process for resolving differences with their health plans, health care providers, and the institutions that serve them, including a rigorous system of internal review and an independent system of external review.

From *Report to the Vice President of the United States: Status of Implementation of the Consumer Bill of Rights and Responsibilities in the Department of Health and Human Services*, U.S. Dept. of Health and Human Services, 1998, Nov. 2. Retrieved from http://aspe.os.dhhs./gov/health/vpreport.htm

aged health care initiatives were not working and that drastic measures were needed to return the power of health care decision making to the doctor and patient rather than health maintenance organizations (HMOs) (Online NewsHour, 1999; Reardon, 1999). Congress passed a law in 1999 to allow patients to sue their HMOs if they were refused needed health care. In the wake of that legislation, some HMOs voluntarily relinquished the health care decision-making power back to physicians (Online NewsHour, 1999).

THE UNINSURED

At one time a concern for policy makers was the number of employers who were dropping or decreasing health insurance benefits. According to the Henry J. Kaiser Family Foundation (2018),

In the past, gaps in the public insurance system and lack of access to affordable private coverage left millions without health insurance, and the number of uninsured Americans grew over time, particularly during periods of economic downturns. By 2013, more than 44 million people lacked coverage. Many people do not have access to coverage through a job, and some people, particularly poor adults in states that did not expand Medicaid, remain ineligible for financial assistance for coverage. (para. 7 & 8)

Unfortunately, uninsured individuals are the most likely to be in poor health (Henry J. Kaiser Family Foundation, 2004). This concern has since been lessened because

on March 23, 2010, President Obama signed comprehensive health reform, the Patient Protection and Affordable Care Act, into law. The changes made to the law by subsequent legislation focused on provisions to expand coverage, control health care costs, and improve [our] health care delivery system. (Henry J. Kaiser Family Foundation, 2018 para. 1)

Lack of insurance promotes delays in seeking medical attention, a lower likelihood of filling prescriptions or taking medications as frequently as prescribed, and fewer expenditures on preventive strategies. Lack of legislation providing guidelines for health insurance companies promotes actions such as non-coverage for previous health conditions, or higher expenses for some people. Lack of legislation regarding health insurance for all impacts when and how people access care. As was demonstrated in 2010, a change in leadership at the national level can have dramatic impacts on the health of the nation due to policy changes. In 2018, due to another federal leadership change, confusion about health care policies presented many problems for U.S. citizens. Lack of agreement among federal legislators and between the legislators and the President caused state and federal actions to be taken that decreased the effectiveness of the Affordable Care Act. Health professionals and political leaders alike MUST create policies that will consistently produce tangible health benefits for all citizens.

The Process of Policy Development

National public health policies serve as guidelines for establishing health program priorities in the United States. For instance, a law that provides health insurance for uninsured American children (State Children's Health Insurance Program administered by the Centers for Medicare and Medicaid Services), is a direct outcome of public health policies. But why do those specific policies exist and how were they developed?

DECISION MAKING

The *Healthy People 2000, 2010, and 2020* goals, described in chapter 1, are products of national health policies. But why did the policy developers target the specific health problems described in those documents? Health policies have historically been driven by economic, social, and political concerns (Ibrahim, 1985). Epidemiological statistics such as mortality and morbidity rates are often categorized by demographic characteristics (such as age, gender, ethnicity, and socioeconomic status) to identify groups at risk. The impact of existing health services and programs on the health status of these groups is also considered. And, in some instances, a politically influential figure can be instrumental in swaying policy decisions (Ibrahim, 1985). These three components (existing needs, current program impact, and available support) are important considerations in any effort to develop health policies.

Most new policies are developed because someone perceived a need for change. Perhaps you have recently benefited from a new university policy that expanded library operation hours. Why would university officials put such a policy in effect when they know it will cost more money? It is because they have considered your needs. But how did they know you needed those changes? We hope they didn't guess. The appropriate approach would have been to survey a representative sample of students to find out about library access needs and interests, consult with library administrators to assess their perceptions of need and feasibility, and test the newly designed service to observe the degree to which the change would make a difference. These actions would be taken before the proposed policy was officially enacted to ensure a *cost-effective* approach.

In the same manner, health policy development should be based on sound needs-assessment efforts and careful interpretation of the results. A scientific investigation into existing health status and needs in a population is the first critical component of policy development. Perceived needs among population members and the professionals who deliver health programs should be identified in this step.

Second, the availability of resources and the feasibility of being able to maintain the proposed policies must also be considered. The overwhelming list of needs within some communities can confuse policy developers. The goal is to develop policies that reflect a balanced perspective, one that considers actual and perceived needs in light of service feasibility.

This balanced perspective can then help you move to the third component of policy development, that of soliciting support from those who have the resources and political influence to assist with policy adoption. We will discuss this issue more fully in chapter 12 when we address advocacy concepts. For now, it is sufficient to know that political power is a critical component of policy development and adoption.

WRITING POLICY

Green and Kreuter (1999) state that a well-written policy has three components: "(a) the clear statement of a problem (or potential problems) that needs attention, (b) a goal to mitigate or prevent that problem, and (c) a set of strategic actions to accomplish that goal" (p. 386). With those three requirements in mind, where would you begin in the process of policy development? Assume, for a moment, that you work for a large manufacturing company where many of the employees smoke cigarettes. The company decision makers have already identified the problem, which is that employees are smoking on the job. You've been asked to write a policy that addresses the problem.

Your statement of the problem could be written in a number of ways, as long as it identifies the problem of smoking employees. The second part of the policy, a goal to mitigate or reduce the problem, would likely include a statement about reducing the frequency of smoking on the job or creating a smoke-free environment. The third part, the set of strategic actions needed to accomplish that goal, would likely be difficult to put into effect, especially if you realized that any policy you created could upset some of the employees.

The nature of the policy you would develop and strategies used to implement it would greatly depend on your philosophy and goal. If your ultimate goal is to have no smokers on the payroll, your strategic approach could embrace quick, drastic action, such as posting no-smoking signs throughout the building and automatically firing any employee caught violating the rule. If, on the other hand, you desire to keep smokers in your employ but still maintain a smoke-free environment, you might take a more gradual approach that provides advance notice to employees, designated smoking areas, and smoking cessation classes for employees who smoke. Your goal would dictate your policy and how you applied it.

≡ In Conclusion

Whether or not your title is that of manager, we encourage you to continually build skills in the areas of time management, project tracking, dispute resolution, organizing, listening, interpreting policy, and allocating resources. These are skills that will help you succeed in any job. When it comes time for you to assume a leadership role, we hope you will lead by example, build trust, accept differences, communicate effectively, recognize accomplishments, assure quality, and make resolute decisions.

The concept of synergism illustrates how we view the connection between leadership, cooperation, and policy development; that is, the combined partnership efforts of collaborating parties produces a greater result than the sum of efforts independently exerted by each party. Effective coordination of health programs and services is dependent on a collaborative effort toward policy development and goal attainment. Your efforts toward these goals may not always produce the desired effect and, even when they do, the results sometimes emerge very slowly. However, even in small, gradual increments, collaboration can be effective.

REVIEW QUESTIONS

1. Write an essay that compares and contrasts leadership and management and explains why they are both important.
2. Describe the process of cooperation and how to promote it.
3. Identify techniques for conflict resolution.
4. List ways in which coalitions and partnerships can be developed.
5. Define policy and name its three components.
6. Describe the difference between procedural and public health policy.
7. Name four federal agencies that monitor public health policy.
8. Summarize the purpose and components of the Patients' Bill of Rights.
9. Write a procedural or public health policy for your community.

FOR YOUR APPLICATION

Creating a Community Coalition

Select a local age- or ethnicity-specific community and a health problem it faces. Use your project community if applicable. Create a proposal for a coalition whose primary goal would be to address the health problem in the community you selected. Your proposal should include:

- A coalition mission statement and goals. Each goal should represent a specific project or task needed to accomplish the stated mission.
- A list of potential strategies needed to accomplish each goal.
- A list of national and/or state organizations or agencies that could provide support.
- A list of local organizations, agencies, institutions, and other community groups that could provide support.
- A timeline for the coalition to follow in completing designated tasks.

When your coalition assignment has been graded and revised, place it in your portfolio if you are preparing a portfolio.

11

Communicating Health Information

The young woman shifts her baby to the other hip and opens the pamphlet you just handed to her. She's in need of health information that will help her make critical decisions for her baby's health, but will a pamphlet be enough to convince her to get her baby immunized? Did the explanation you gave make sense to her? She's a new mother, there are other needs in her life that impact the decisions she makes about the health of her child. The few minutes you have to convince her to come back next week are fading, and it appears that it is the information you can share verbally that will truly make an impact. You feel that every word counts. So, what do you say and how do you say it effectively?

Chapter Objectives

1. Describe the skills necessary for effective communication.
2. Explain each component of the health communication model.
3. Generate an example of each of the four stages of health communication.
4. Discuss the role media advocacy plays in health education.
5. Explore reasons why health literacy is so important.
6. Practice effective communication skills.
7. Critique examples of health education print and digital materials.
8. Apply the SMOG technique to determine the reading level of text-based health education materials.
9. Create a plan for health communication that includes social media.

≡ Effective Communication

"A tip from a former smoker: Be careful not to cut your stoma." This jarring command from the CDC's Tips From Former Smokers health communication campaign is placed atop a photo of a shirtless man shaving, his neck craned back to reveal his gaping stoma (see FYI 11.1). A caption identifies him as "Shawn, Age 50, Diagnosed at 46. Washington State." At the bottom of the page, smaller text reads, "Smoking causes immediate damage to your body. For Shawn, it caused throat cancer. You can quit. For free help, call 1-800-QUIT-NOW."

The CDC launched Tips From Former Smokers in 2012 as a cross–media platform campaign, communicating its message through billboards and posters; online video; podcasts; social media; the CDC mobile app; public service announcements; and print, television, theater, and radio ads. The campaign features real smokers who have quit or people whose health has been affected by secondhand smoke. Each gives the audience an example of how tobacco can destroy individuals both physically and emotionally. After its 2012 launch, the CDC reported that the campaign had increased weekly calls to its quit-line by 75% and had drawn 38 times more visitors to the Tips website every week. The Twitter hashtag #CDCTips has been used many

FYI

11.1 Shawn's Tip

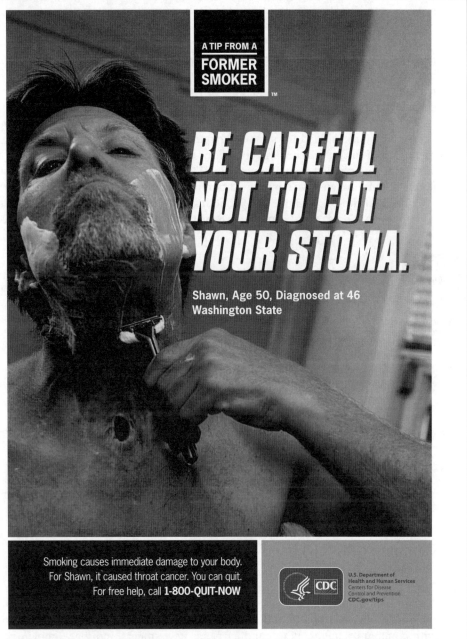

Courtesy of the Centers for Disease Control and Prevention (CDC) *Tips From Former Smokers*® campaign. Retrieved from http://www.cdc.gov/tobacco/campaign/tips/resources/ads/tips-ad-shawn-full-v1a.pdf.

thousands of times by both individuals and organizations, creating a public conversation about the dangers of smoking and institutional responses to it. Some would argue that fear tactics were driving this campaign. Others might counter that the campaign and its "shock value" caught people's attention and woke them to the physical and even emotional realities of nicotine addiction.

No matter how one chooses to look at it, it was evident that with a series of short, straightforward messages that involved its target audience, the creators of the Tips campaign were able to heighten awareness of the physical and psychological impacts of smoking. This example demonstrates the power of communication and how clear, concise, and relevant health messages can "mobilize communities and individuals to adopt healthy behaviors, direct policy makers' attention to important health issues, and frame those issues for public debate and resolution" (Harvard School of Public Health, n.d., para. 1).

As we've mentioned in previous chapters, effective communication plays a vital role in the diffusion of a health behavior or innovation. Moreover, it is pivotal in collaboration and conflict-resolution efforts. We've also discussed the usefulness of careful and culturally sensitive communication in a variety of health education efforts (see FYI 11.2). However, we have not yet addressed the issue of what communication *is* and how you can use it to be an effective health educator.

FYI

11.2   Health Communication: Related Topics in This Text

Chapter	Health Communication Topic
2, 4	Communication styles (and culture)
6	Community participation and capacity building
8	Social marketing, health literacy, multiple intelligences, and theory of the diffusion of innovation
9	Research reports
10	Collaboration and conflict resolution
11	Communication models, communication strategies and principles, cultural communication, and health literacy
12	Advocating for health
13	Obtaining accurate information from resources

Communication Defined

Communication is "the process of transmitting ideas and information" (KU Work Group, 2018b, Chapter 6, section 1, para. 2). Communication is a vital component of community health, especially as it relates to health education. It permeates every area of responsibility and can become your most valuable tool as you interact with community members to conduct needs assessments and plan, implement, and evaluate programs. It is particularly important in the process of **community capacity building**, which we described in chapters 2 and 6, because you may need it to help community members raise community awareness about an existing health problem; influence public opinion about the need to address the problem; and mobilize support from institutional, political, and community leaders and stakeholders (Harvard School of Public Health, n.d., para. 1).

Accurate Communication

"I communicated to him that I was going to finish the job. He just didn't listen!" You can probably imagine the tone of frustration that accompanied this statement. Few things are more irritating than to believe you have successfully communicated with another person, only to later discover that the person didn't understand at all. Do you think whomever our speaker is referring to simply didn't listen? It's possible. Picture two people, Vanessa and Cruz, who are busily putting away groceries. Vanessa talks as she works. Cruz interjects a few "um-hums" here and there as he places cans on a shelf. What Vanessa doesn't realize is that, for some reason, Cruz isn't hearing what she thinks he hears. Days later, Vanessa discovers through a friend that Cruz did not believe she had told him about her plans and reacted negatively when she carried them out. Miscommunication led to misunderstanding, and problems resulted.

There could be a number of reasons for this miscommunication, including the actions, thoughts, and cultural norms of both people involved. True communication depends on both the giver and the receiver of a message. The absence of clear communication can quickly lead you astray when you are attempting to serve as a resource person or program coordinator (Seelye & Seelye-James, 1996). Miscommunication can foster frustration and resentment and destroy important working relationships. It can result in wasted time and resources when you have to backtrack and reconstruct project components. It can also affect your credibility in the community and reduce community members' motivation to become involved.

Accurate, effective communication is also important within the context of the basic philosophies of community health that we discussed in earlier chapters. If the primary goal of community health was to force people to do what we believe is best for them, the communication process would be simple. We would merely need to clearly state what we expect from people and graphically describe the consequences for those who do not comply. We would not need an entire chapter focused on communication because most people are already familiar with how direct orders are communicated.

We do need this chapter, however, because community health is not primarily about enforcing directives. It is, instead, about helping people to help themselves. From this perspective, the focus isn't on you, the health professional, and your expectations. *The decision-making power lies in the hands of the people you serve.* Their beliefs, expectations, values, desires, and concerns will ultimately dictate their health-related behavior. Your role is to facilitate healthy decisions by providing information, resource access, and guidance as needed. And, in some instances, you may also discover a need to persuade, motivate, and encourage healthy choices.

That's why community health professionals rely on effective communication. Designing something intended to communicate—like the immunization pamphlet given to the young mother in our opening scenario—can be a challenge. How do you persuade a young woman whose life views are different from yours that the temporary discomfort of an injection is a good thing if it protects her baby from disease? You already know the answer. It begins with effective communication. Effective communication depends not only on the people involved, but also on the nature and quality of the message itself and the channel through which the message is delivered. The process is a bit more complex than it first appears. To understand it more clearly, we introduce you to a useful model.

Health Communication Model

Jerrold Greenberg (2003), a professor emeritus and well-known health educator, contributed much to what is known in the field about the process of health communication. His **health communication model** illustrates how communication works (Figure 11.1). On the surface, the communication process seems simple. The *sender* (Vanessa in our illustration) attempts to convey a *message* (that she plans to do something) through a communication *medium,* or channel of message delivery (orally, as she puts away groceries), to the *receiver* (Cruz). That sounds straightforward enough, doesn't it? However, if the process is so simple, why does miscommunication occur? Let's explore the possibilities as they relate to each of the four model components.

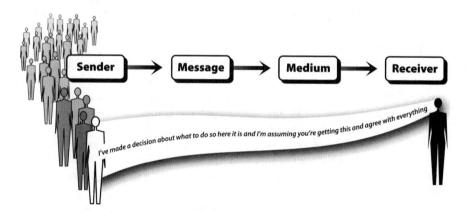

Figure 11.1   Health communication model.
This model shows a linear flow of health communication that reminds us to consider factors that influence each component and shape the degree to which clear, effective communication occurs.

SENDER

Have you ever been totally certain that you said something in a particular way only to discover later that what you said and what you thought you said were two different things? Perhaps you made a statement in conversation and immediately realized that your wording conveyed something other than what you intended. Such situations can be embarrassing, but they are a useful example of how the sender plays an important role in the communication process.

How the sender processes information, decides upon the message to be conveyed, and formulates the message to be expressed are critical to message development. Possible contributing factors to the miscommunication in our illustration may have included inconsistencies between what Vanessa intended to say or believed she said and what she actually stated. A clearly communicated message begins with careful decision making and message construction on the part of the sender.

Before we move on to the second component of the model, let's discuss who the sender is in most health situations. Greenberg (2003) points out that most community health educators think of themselves as the message senders. After all, we are the ones hired to communicate health education messages. But isn't the sender also considered the originator of the message? The sender in our illustration certainly originated her message about her plans. But are community health professionals truly the originators of health education messages about, for example, the effect of physical activity and diet on one's health? Or are we simply the messenger, the deliverer, the medium through which the message is sent? Greenberg (2003) maintains that society is the true health education message sender and that we, as health professionals, are the message conduit. Understanding that difference serves as a reminder that we must carefully consider the accuracy and quality of the message we are sending before we send it.

MESSAGE

In our example involving the two grocery-bearing friends, we know little about the message itself. We know only that it was about some decision Vanessa had made about something she planned to do. Whether that decision was a good idea and how it would affect others seems irrelevant to our discussion about how it was miscommunicated. However, as a health professional, the nature of the messages you will be asked to convey is a critical issue. It's important to consider message accuracy and message appropriateness.

Many confusing health-related messages are transmitted to our society through the news media, infomercials, books, magazines, and the Internet. Many of them are products of sensationalized half-truths, money-making schemes, or misguided individuals who mean well but mistakenly believe and spread inaccurate health information. As a health professional, you are responsible for the accuracy of the health messages you deliver. That is why it is important for you to understand research methodology and the difference between evidence-based fact and opinion. In chapter 13, we will discuss the importance of knowing where to go for accurate information as a resource person. For each message you send, you will need to first consider who originated that message and on what research evidence it was based.

Message appropriateness is another important aspect to be considered. For example, the message that regular physical activity can positively contribute to one's health may be accurate. But the term *regular physical activity* can mean different things to different people. What is considered an appropriate physical activity type, frequency, and intensity for one person might place another at risk of injury. We need only compare the needs of an Olympic athlete to those of a sedentary 80-year-old adult to understand the importance of adapted messages. Another example relates to pregnancy prevention. It would be necessary to understand the cultural values and religious beliefs of your audience before you demonstrate how to unroll a condom on an anatomical model of a penis or before even using the word *condom*. In fact, the word *contraception* could be offensive to some groups who do not endorse contraceptive use. The phrase *family planning* may be a more appropriate choice. Both examples underscore how health messages should be presented in a way that is appropriately tailored to match the needs, cultural values, and abilities of the message receivers.

As we stated in chapter 8 when we discussed social marketing and the diffusion of innovation theory, presenting the message in a way that appropriately appeals to individual values, culture, and readiness for change increases the chance that the message will be accepted. Some individuals in our society suffer from what is referred to as **iatrogenic health education disease (IHED)** (Greenberg, 2003). Though IHED isn't truly a diagnosable disease, the phrase is used to describe a state of mind in which a person feels overwhelmed by the onslaught of health-risk messages. As a result, the person believes that trying to live a healthy lifestyle is futile and gives up on trying to maintain healthy behaviors (Greenberg, 2003). If you have ever heard someone say, "We all have to die of *something!*" or "Oh, *everything* causes cancer!" you may have been listening to a person suffering from IHED. To guard against this, your messages should be appropriately tailored to the receiver's sense of what is reasonable and worthwhile.

MEDIUM

As we stated earlier, Greenberg (2003) would likely contend that you, the health professional, are the message medium, the channel through which the health message is delivered. From a different perspective, pamphlets, Web pages, oral presentations, newspaper articles, blogs/vlogs, social media pages, mobile apps, and PSAs could also be considered examples of message mediums. Whether you consider yourself or these message delivery channels as the medium, it is important that you pay close attention to how health messages are delivered.

You may have noted in our miscommunication illustration that both parties were busily putting away groceries as the message was delivered. Can you imagine Vanessa bending down to put something on a bottom shelf just as she began her message about her plans? While her back was turned Cruz could have momentarily stepped into a closet pantry and never even heard her statement. Or, through the noise and shuffle of activity, he may have heard only part of what she said. In either event, one could conclude that the chosen message channel left a lot to be desired.

This is why the selected message medium or channel is so important. Your message can be accurate and appropriately adapted to your intended audience. It may be worded in a way that effectively appeals to audience needs, values, and levels of readiness for acceptance. Yet, with all those important components in place, the communication process still may break down due to a faulty message medium. That medium must be a consistently reliable channel to the audience, one that can be depended upon to deliver the message to the right place at the right time.

RECEIVER

Finally, we arrive at the place where blame was placed in the beginning. Vanessa's comment that "He just didn't listen!" placed all the blame at Cruz's feet. We've already considered the possibility that it wasn't Cruz's fault—that the problem could lie with the sender, message, or medium. But let's reconsider. After all, Cruz was providing some indication that he was listening with each "um-hum" he offered. It is possible that Vanessa clearly stated her plans in an audible format, and Cruz was there all along to receive every word, but didn't. He may not have been really listening at all. Or he may have been listening but didn't really place importance on what she said and, thus, quickly forgot it. Or he may have listened carefully but, because he and Vanessa process information differently, may have placed an entirely different interpretation on what she said.

The receiver obviously plays a vital role in the message communication process. In health education settings, the receiver could be the person whose health needs you are attempting to assess and address with health programs. It could also be the community gatekeeper or stakeholder whose support you need for your assessment and programming efforts. The receiver could be someone whose resources you hope to attain for use in your efforts through grants, donations, or volunteered services. In each of these situations, knowing your communication goal is important.

The Communication Effect

Before developing a specific message and choosing an audience-appropriate medium or message channel, the message sender should carefully consider the desired communication effect, or outcome. For instance, is the purpose of a message to simply provide information, or is it intended to persuade the message receiver to adopt a particular health attitude or behavior? The difference between these two goals could drastically alter your communication approach.

There was a time when public health educators believed that we needed only to impart health-related knowledge to bring about positive changes in health behavior. If we simply told people, for example, that smoking causes cancer and regular physical activity can help prevent heart disease, then people would automatically stop smoking and become active—or so it was believed. Thus, we needed only to bridge knowledge gaps with informative health messages, and all people everywhere would live healthier lives. Right? Wrong!

You may recall our discussions in previous chapters about the multitude of factors that influence health attitudes and behaviors. You may also remember that knowledge about health is only one factor, which, in the face of all those other influences (such as values, habits, peer pressure), carries very little weight on its own in health-related decisions. That is why developing effective health communication messages is such a challenge. In addition to providing needed health information in a format that is easily understood, the messages you send must also appeal to the message receiver's value system. They must motivate your receivers to overcome any perceived barriers that might prevent them from adopting healthy attitudes and behaviors.

Persuasive Communication

If health communication focused only on developing clearly stated health information, health educators might not be needed. After all, many professional disciplines train their members to clearly present information. However, there is a real art to knowing how to assess and adapt health-related messages to the needs and values of a variety of audiences and to package those messages in ways that can persuade receivers to change attitudes and behaviors.

This art is known as **persuasive communication**. A return to our discussion in chapter 8 about the theory of diffusion of innovation could be helpful in understanding this art within the context of mass communication. We encourage you to develop persuasive communication skills and seek opportunities to practice applying them through a variety of media (see "For Your Application" at the end of this chapter). Never forget, however, that persuasive communication is not the same thing as **coercion**, which means manipulating or even forcing people to do what you want. The decision to adopt or reject a health-related attitude or behavior is not yours. Your job is to provide needed information, training, and resources for positive health behavior change and to attempt to respectfully persuade and encourage the adoption of attitudes and behaviors that are clearly in the best interests of your audience. However, the decision belongs to the message receiver, not you. Adopt a respectful approach in your health communication efforts and you will likely avoid crossing the line between the professionally appropriate tone of persuasive communication and inappropriate coercion.

Regardless of whether your message is intended to inform or persuade, the receiver is the pivotal component in the communication process. The receiver is the component over which you have the least amount of control. For that reason, it is critical that you learn all you can about the receiver's thought processes, needs, values, and preferred communication channels.

Learning Styles and Information Processing

People think in different ways, and that's why communication can sometimes be a challenge. The ideas formulated by the message sender do not always match the thought processes of the receiver. What may seem to you to be a perfectly clear pamphlet about the need for immunizations may not make any sense at all to another person. Or perhaps your pamphlet helps clarify the issue for one mother, but she would achieve full understanding more readily by listening to oral testimony from another teenage mother who provides the same information but in story form.

Differences in learning and information-processing (cognitive) styles have been researched for years (Anderson & Adams, 1992; Bean, 1996; Evans & Cools, 2011; Gardner 1993), and much of this information is reflected in the multiple intelligences model we described in chapter 8. Here we wish to add only that understanding the differences in individual information processing represented in the model will greatly enhance your communication efforts.

Some controversy exists in the literature about whether learning and communication-style differences can be detected across cultures. Numerous studies have been cited to provide evidence that distinct *cultural* differences exist in relation to these styles (Anderson & Adams, 1992; Cushner, 1994; Ginsberg & Vlodkowski, 2009; Renzuli & Yun, 2001). Others argue that such studies do not provide conclusive evidence (Kitano, 1997). As with other cultural differences, these distinctions appear to emerge among groups of individuals who closely adhere to their cultural roots. In fact, some scholars suggest that culture shapes not only *what* one thinks, but also *how* one thinks and learns (Cushner, 1994; Evans & Cools, 2011; Renzuli & Dai, 2001). However, when we ask how culture may impact learning and communication, we broach a controversial and sensitive area. There is evidence to support that culture and learning are connected in important ways. Early life experiences and the values of a person's culture affect both the expectations and the processes of learning and communication. If this relationship is true, could we then assume that students who share cultural characteristics have common learning or communication style patterns? The word *assume* is a call out here. One should not assume anything. Therefore, working across cultures to communicate requires continual reexamination of one's assumptions, expectations, and biases which is what it means to exercise **cultural humility**.

We call this to your attention to make two points. First, the U.S. is rich in diversity; therefore, developing tailored messages and offering them in multiple formats and channels is important to reaching your intended audience. Second, we caution you to carefully consider both sides of the cultural distinction argument so that you don't make the mistake of either ignoring culture-specific differences or of stereotyping those who share certain cultural characteristics. Whenever time and resources allow, a balanced, multiple-strategy approach is a good idea. In order to work effectively as a community health professional, you will need to not only communicate effectively, but be able to deliver your message cross-culturally. This takes time and effort on your part to learn a different perspective, as well as practice skills that can help you deliver your message to a variety of audiences. You may wish to further your knowledge of effective cross-cultural communication by enrolling in a course at your local university or participating in online training through a local agency in your community. FYI 11.3 contains a comparison of cultural values, while strategies for effective cross-cultural communication are included in FYI 11.4. We encourage you to practice these strategies as well as seek out additional opportunities to strive for cultural competency in your everyday life.

FYI

11.3 Comparing Cultural Values

Values Typical of Some Cultures	Common "Western" or U.S. Values
Fate	Personal control over the environment
Tradition	Change
Human interaction dominates	Time dominates
Hierarchy/Rank/Status	Human equity
Group welfare	Individualism
Birthright inheritance	Self-help
Cooperation	Competition
Past orientation	Future orientation
"Being" orientation	Action/Goal/Work orientation
Formality	Informality
Indirectness/Ritual/Privacy	Directness/Flexibility/Openness
Spiritualism/Detachment	Materialism

Adapted from *Community Health Education and Promotion: A Guide to Program Design and Evaluation*, by N. Di Lima and C. Schust, 1997, Gaithersburg, MD: Aspen Publishers.

11.4 Enhancing Cross-Cultural Communication

Messages are conveyed both verbally and nonverbally. A tilt of the head or a certain inflection can give a message a whole new meaning. You should be aware of variations in nonverbal and verbal communication to avoid misunderstandings or unintentional insults when working with individuals and families.

Nonverbal Communication	Interpretations
Silence	You may find silence is awkward, intimidating, or a waste of time. However, many cultures value silence and view it as a normal part of a conversation. Conversely, some cultures find it socially appropriate to talk over another person or begin talking before the other person has finished. Being aware of the other person's natural pauses and interruptions will enhance the communication process and help foster respect.
Distance	The appropriate physical distance between people in a social setting varies from culture to culture. Provide people with options for space preference, such as saying, "Please have a seat wherever you feel comfortable."
Eye Contact	The amount of eye contact that is comfortable also varies from culture to culture. Do not be offended if some individuals do not hold your gaze; this could actually be a cultural sign of respect, not disinterest.
Emotional Expression	Expression of emotion may also be influenced by culture. Some cultures value stoicism, while other cultures are more accepting of displays of emotion. Varying beliefs about the origins and treatment of pain may also influence emotional expression from culture to culture.
Body Language	Gestures, motions, and positioning of the body can be interpreted differently depending on the culture. A hand signal commonly used as a funny expression in one culture can be an offensive insult in others. Conservative use of body language is prudent when you are uncertain of cultural norms relating to body language.
Oral Communication	
Greetings and Formality	In some cultures, it may be okay to greet your new female client with "Hey, Mary," while in others, a "Señora Hernandez" would be most appropriate. Do not assume that a first-name basis is appropriate for all client relationships. It could be inferred as disrespect, and you will lose credibility with your client. Avoid terms of endearment such as "dear" or "honey," and do not refer to adults as "boy" or "girl." If you're unsure how to address your client, simply ask what they would prefer.

Rapport	It's important to establish some form of trust with your client, even if you've just met. You can use small talk to demonstrate that you're open and friendly, and then transition into more pointed, open-ended questions such as, "How are you?" and "How may I help you?" If the client is not very responsive, you can always offer some suggestions and options. Be sensitive to personal boundaries; some questions could be viewed as invasive. Be sure not to interpret a client's non-response or silence as disrespect. Patience will go a long way toward building relationships in a short amount of time.
Subject Matter	Do not ever assume that because you are a health professional that people will be willing to discuss their health behaviors with you. Certain subject matter may simply not be culturally appropriate to discuss. For example, asking about family, sexual orientation, spouses, or religious beliefs may be taboo depending on one's culture and gender. Consider phrasing questions so they are less pointed; or, you can simply reassure clients that they "do not have to answer if they do not feel comfortable."
Translating	Language is a common barrier for health professionals trying to work with diverse populations. Working with a translator will help you deliver the health message in the most direct way. The translator could be a bilingual colleague, or it could be your client's family member. However, children are not always the most appropriate translators because the subject matter or ideas may be beyond their understanding or maturity. While working with the translator, avoid slang terms, lengthy sentences, or complex ideas. Instruct interpreters to use the client's own words instead of paraphrasing and ask for further clarification if a word or phrase is unclear. Allow sufficient time for the client to hear and formulate answers to questions.

≡ Communication Strategies and Principles

Now that you have a firm understanding of the communication process and your role and purposes in health communication, we can begin to explore methods that have been proven to enhance the likelihood of successful communication. We first present some general strategies for the development and implementation of health communication. We follow that with some broad communication principles and strategies that can be adapted to most media. In subsequent sections, we also provide basic guidelines for selected media.

Stages of Health Communication

The circle in Figure 11.2 illustrates four stages of health communication (NCI, 2008) that can help you develop effective messages. Note that the first two stages are steps you should take before the communication is implemented. After reading the ear-

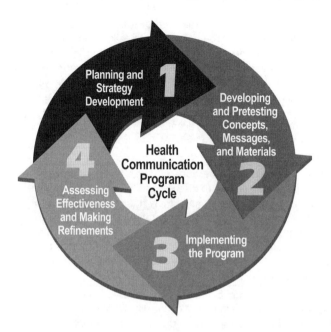

Figure 11.2   Stages of health communication.

Adapted from *Making Health Communication Programs Work: A Planner's Guide,* National Cancer Institute at the National Institutes of Health, U.S. Dept. of Health and Human Services, 2008. Accessed from http://www.cancer.gov/cancertopics/cancerlibrary/pinkbook.

lier chapters in this book, you should be able to anticipate that a thorough needs assessment and detailed plan are recommended before any health education effort begins. This includes efforts toward effective health communication.

Let's suppose for a moment that you work in the community education division of a nonprofit refugee assistance program for Sudanese immigrants in your city. You've been asked to enhance awareness in the local refugee community about the need for annual well-woman checkups and the availability of free cervical screenings at the grant-funded refugee clinic nearby. You begin with stage 1, planning and strategy development, which entails a preliminary needs assessment. As with any needs assessment, you first study existing data and then collect new data to fill in any information gaps. The goal is to identify specific beliefs and norms within the Sudanese refugee community that may serve as either barriers to or promoters of the likelihood that Sudanese women will obtain screenings and routine follow-ups. (Return to chapter 6 for a reminder of needs-assessment components and strategies.) Stage 1 would end with clearly defined communication goals and objectives that are designed to address influencing factors.

You would then be ready to move on to stage 2, to develop communication channels and materials that best match your selected audience's needs and preferred information sources (such as social media sites, blogs/vlogs, mobile apps, specific radio stations, local eating establishments, newspapers, and organizational newsletters). We encourage you to solicit as much input as possible from community members; in doing so, expect to receive a variety of suggestions about channels and formats. Individuals who share similarities or group titles do not necessarily access the same communication channels. Find out about communication channels that have been used in the past to reach members of the community, and analyze existing communication materials to determine strengths and weaknesses of past and current efforts.

Communication channels for refugees or asylees can be very complex due to within-group diversity and the fact that acculturation may impact individuals in different ways. For example, Sudanese women who have lived in the U.S. for more than five years may still live in the same area of town, but may think very differently than those who have just arrived. The definition of the "Sudanese refugee community" follows the same distinctions and limitations we discussed in earlier chapters when attempting to identify other recognized community groups. You may, for instance, be able to access some Sudanese refugee women through other organizations whose specific purpose is to provide service to and support for the community. However, some Sudanese refugee women, especially those who have lived in the U.S. longer, may not choose to access information through these organizations any longer. They may have developed a sense of distrust or no longer feel they need assistance. They may, however, receive your message about the need for annual checkups via their friends who do participate in those organizations. Or you may more readily reach these women through churches, grocery stores, the local health department, or through respected community leaders.

It is a good idea at this stage to draft and test several different message channels (such as brochures, videos, or public service announcements on radio). Ask community gatekeepers and health experts with knowledge about local Sudanese culture to critique each and provide suggestions. Then do a **pilot test** of the revised message formats and channels and obtain feedback from representatives of the intended audience. Ask those representatives to give you their honest impressions of the message and its format, the degree to which the message could be understood, recalled, and accepted as important and culturally appropriate. Make revisions based on their feedback.

In our example, let us assume that the outcome of the first two stages was the development of a flyer in the Zaghawa language and Arabic to distribute in the Sudanese refugee community. The flyer encourages women to seek well-woman checkups offered at the nearby free clinic and attempts to overcome barriers that often prevent these women from obtaining the checkups. Your flyer also contains the contact information of the free clinic as well as the names and phone numbers of contact individuals there. You also train volunteers from the community to present this information at local organizational meetings and worship centers that specifically serve the Sudanese refugee community. In addition, you decide to develop a public service announcement for the small radio station that is run by, and serves, Sudanese refugees. In the message, a woman identifies herself as a Sudanese woman who arrived in the U.S. two years ago. She describes how the free well-woman exam her sister received detected an early form of cervical cancer and saved her sister's life. She describes the care and respect her sister was given at the clinic and from the local refugee agency that helped her find the financial means to cover her treatment. The woman encourages women to join her as she, too, will seek the screening. The last few seconds of the PSA provide a heartfelt appeal to the listener to break through the barriers and schedule a checkup. Listeners are then given the clinic's phone number, which is also provided on the flyer.

You now have implemented three different communication channels (stage 3). The radio PSA serves as one. The volunteer presenters who distribute the pamphlet serve as a second channel. If the presenters' audiences respond to the appeal, the flyer alone may serve as a third channel as it finds its way into the hands of other Sudanese refugee women who never hear the presentation. How will you know whether any of the three channels is working and whether you should continue to invest time and money into some, none, or all three? That's where stage 4 comes in. You won't know unless you track the messages.

You can choose from several tracking strategies. You could ask the volunteer presenters to keep records of the frequency, location, and date of each presentation; the number of people who attend them; and the number of pamphlets distributed at the end of each meeting. You could also record the number of times the PSA was aired with dates and times of day noted. But those counts would only tell you how often you presented the message. They would tell you nothing about whether you achieved the intended communication outcome and if so, which channel was responsible. That is, did the communication increase the frequency of annual well-woman checkups among targeted members of the Sudanese refugee community?

Measuring the communication effect would require a different kind of tracking, one that would allow you to survey those who received the message to learn how they perceived the message and whether it motivated them to complete an annual checkup. After your campaign begins, you could also survey those who visited the clinic to determine whether any were motivated to make an appointment by one of the communication channels and, if so, which one. A review of chapter 9 will help you generate other evaluation possibilities. For our purposes here, note that evaluation and revision are important components of health communication.

General Communication Principles

The National Cancer Institute (NCI, 2008), part of the National Institute of Health (NIH), provided an overview of how the public commonly perceives health messages (FYI 11.5). Understanding these perceptions can help you shape your health messages so that they are more likely to be accepted. First, the NCI points out that few people understand the concept of *health risk*. That is why the public is more likely to react strongly to such low-risk possibilities as homicides and accidental deaths that are often sensationalized by the news media, yet may ignore information about chronic diseases (such as heart disease, stroke, diabetes) that represent a greater health risk (are a more likely possibility) for most Americans.

To counter this imbalance, it might seem logical to focus our communication efforts on risk-awareness messages. However, messages that frighten the audience can backfire by producing feelings of helplessness and denial. When someone says, "Everything causes cancer," it underscores the dangers of using fear tactics in your communications. A well-balanced message can include an explanation of related health risks, but should not target fear as the intended outcome.

In the same sense that few people understand the concept of health risk, the general public has little confidence in or understanding of scientific research (Losh, 2012; National Science Board, 2004; NCI, 2008). People tend to embrace easy solutions and absolute answers and expect to find them in scientific research results; they have little patience with discussions about the need to replicate studies over time to test for consistency. Few understand how variability in study participant numbers and characteristics, methods used, and research settings can bias results. Even fewer know the difference between an association that only proves two factors coexist and a well-designed cause-and-effect study. For this reason, oversimplified news media coverage of a man who drank throughout his life and lived to be 100 years old, for instance, can quickly become accepted as conclusive evidence that alcohol intake increases longevity.

11.5   Public Perceptions about Health Messages and Suggested Communication Strategies

These suggested communication strategies (right column) are based on what is known about common public perceptions (left column) and how they affect people's acceptance of health messages.

Common Public Perceptions	Suggested Communication Strategies
• Few people understand the concept of health risk.	• Personalize new information.
• Fear tactics sometimes backfire.	• Focus on positive outcomes of positive behaviors. (Avoid fear tactics.)
• The public may not believe or understand science.	• Minimize use of scientific jargon.
• People respond to easy solutions and absolute answers.	• Keep messages simple.
• People tend to live for today, not tomorrow.	• Accentuate immediate health and non-health benefits.
• Health may not be a priority.	• Personalize messages.
• Individuals do not feel personally susceptible.	• Suggest "do-able" first-step solutions.
• The public holds contradictory beliefs.	

Adapted from *Making Health Communication Programs Work*, National Cancer Institute at the National Institutes of Health, U.S. Dept. of Health and Human Services, 2008. Retrieved from http://www.cancer.gov/cancertopics/cancerlibrary/pinkbook/.

The irony in this is that few people dwell on the future; long-range health risks and related information are seldom a priority (NCI, 2008). These tendencies apply especially to the younger members of our society and to those at lower socioeconomic levels. But no matter who your audience is, your health messages should emphasize immediate health and non-health benefits to adopting healthy lifestyles. An example would be to explain how regular physical activity results in immediate stress reduction and weight management benefits, to show that people who are active report more positive perceptions about life and are more productive. These short-range, non-health benefits may create a greater message appeal and have greater impact than would a discussion about how physical activity can reduce risk of long-range heart disease.

Our perceptions about personal susceptibility to a particular health problem are usually lower than our actual risk rates (NCI, 2008). Yet individuals can also hold contradictory beliefs about how people, in the abstract, are susceptible to a multitude of health dangers. To return to an earlier example, picture a smoker who doesn't believe he or she is at personal risk of developing lung cancer but insists that all things cause cancer. The smoker may believe that we will all eventually die of cancer anyway and that quitting smoking will do little to change that. To counter low levels of perceived susceptibility and contradictory beliefs, design your messages in a way that personalizes the issue and provides clear, simple suggestions that won't overwhelm your message receiver.

Mediums for Communicating Health Information

There are various mediums used to communicate health messages. Public service announcements (PSAs) and brochures were mentioned earlier. Radio ads, press releases, blogs, social media, news features, flyers, billboards, and interviews are other ways to deliver your message (see FYIs 11.6 and 11.7). An exhaustive discussion of all of these mediums would fill an entire book. Therefore, let us recommend a very helpful website sponsored by the University of Kansas called the *Community Toolbox* (https://ctb.ku.edu/en). This website is a "living document" developed by a number of professional community groups, organizations, and foundations whose members are interested in promoting community health and community development (KU Work Group, 2018b). From it, you can download skill-building information on more than 150 community health topics. Among those topics are a variety of practical "how to" articles that relate to the development and use of professional presentations, fact sheets, pamphlets, PSAs, and grant proposals. The website provides a much broader array of resources than what we have mentioned here. We invite you to visit this site for more detailed information about how to effectively apply health communication theory, principles, and skills when selecting and using such mediums. Tips for writing an effective press release are covered in FYI 11.8 (on p. 278), with an example in FYI 11.9 (on p. 279).

FYI

11.6 Tips for Creating Appealing Posters and Flyers

Posters and flyers are common channels for health communication. They rely on words and images to get their main point across. When creating your poster or flyer, consider the following:

- Simplicity is key—try not to have too many different elements vying for the reader or the viewer's attention.
- Large, colorful images will grab your reader's attention. Lots of contrast helps, too.
- A novel image is another good way to catch your audience's eye.
- Make sure that your images are culturally appropriate and do not lead to stereotyping.
- Your poster should be easy to read from a distance.
- Colors can have different effects: greens, blues, and purples tend to be soothing while red, orange, and yellow tend to excite and attract attention.

Mistakes to Avoid

- Visual clutter—too much of "a good thing" is not necessarily good. Keep it simple.
- Unclear and misunderstood wording can confuse (or even anger) the reader.
- Typos or spelling errors—can discredit the source and look unprofessional.
- Poor quality photo or artwork is bad for your organization's public image.

Adapted from KU Work Group for Community Health and Development, 2018b, Chap. 6, Sect. 11: *Creating Posters and Flyers*. Lawrence: University of Kansas. Retrieved from http://ctb.ku.edu/en/table-of-contents/participation/promoting-interest/posters-flyers/main. Copyright © 2018 by the University of Kansas for all materials provided via the World Wide Web in the ctb.ku.edu domain.

11.7 Arranging and Developing News Stories

There are many good reasons for publicizing your organization or event on television or in the newspaper. Benefits may include gaining increased publicity, heightening community awareness and support, and attracting not only attention but possible funding.
Consider the following when arranging for a news story:

- Timing: schedule your news story to appear around the time of your event and take advantage of national dates and awareness campaigns (e.g. National Health Education Week).

- Contact a local health professional or feature reporter. Keep in good contact with this individual as he or she may serve as a continual contact for future events.

- Take a human angle. People love human interest stories.

- Prepare a press release (FYI 11.8).

- Include pictures in your news story.

- Provide contact information for your organization.

Adapted from KU Work Group for Community Health and Development, 2018b, Chap. 6, Sect. 4: *Arranging News and Feature Stories*. Lawrence: University of Kansas. Retrieved from http://ctb.ku.edu/en/table-of-contents/participation/promoting-interest/news-feature-stories/main. Copyright © 2018 by the University of Kansas for all materials provided via the World Wide Web in the ctb.ku.edu domain.

Writing for Success

An important first step in good writing is knowing *why* you are writing and for *whom* the message is intended. Then create an outline or cognitive map of your intended message so that you have a clear vision of the major points you wish to communicate. A number of different types of writing styles and formats could be appropriate, depending on your writing purpose and audience. These can range in complexity and length from single-statement public service announcements to brief informational brochures and flyers to full articles intended for a general audience or a professional community. Across these formats, however, there are some general rules of thumb you can follow for effective writing (FYI 11.10 on p. 280).

In many cases, the most powerful, thought-provoking statements are those that are clear and concise. Marketers have known for years that people tend to respond to short slogans they can easily remember. We need only to watch an evening of television or observe the ads on various websites to find examples of that concept. Good writers follow the same guideline by deleting unnecessary words or phrases and simplifying sentence structure. Imagine if the concise slogan from the Tips From Former Smokers anti-tobacco campaign, "Be careful not to cut your stoma," were transformed into something like, "If you have a stoma, it is important to be careful not to cut it while shaving." Do you see how the addition of just a few words changes the overall effect of this message?

Three additional tips for concise writing are to avoid excessive use of prepositional phrases, delete unnecessary words, and use verbs in an active voice. Consider the statement, "The attitudes of the community are so powerfully strong that the program offered by our agency will need to focus on them." The phrases "the attitudes of the community" and "the program offered by our agency" could be shortened to "community attitudes" and "agency program." The word "powerfully" in the phrase "so powerfully strong" could be deleted without losing meaning. Sentences should always be in the *active voice*; make the organization or person who will do the action (the agency) the subject of the sentence and use a verb in the active voice. Thus, a shorter statement could be, "The agency program should focus on the strong community attitudes." The "For Your Application" at the end of the chapter contains an editing exercise that will allow you to practice this simplification process.

11.8   Writing a Press Release

Headline Is in Title Case Meaning You Capitalize Every Word Except for Prepositions and Articles of Three Letters or Less and Short; Ideally It Is Not More Than 170 Characters and Does Not Take a Period

The summary paragraph is a synopsis of the press release in regular sentence form. It doesn't merely repeat the headline or opening paragraph. It just tells the story in a different way. The summary paragraph is mandatory at FPRC.

City, State (FPRC) Month 1, 2005—The first paragraph, known as the "lead," contains the most important information. You need to grab your reader's attention here. And you can't assume that they have read the headline or summary paragraph; the lead should stand on its own.

A press release, like a news story, keeps sentences and paragraphs short, about three or four lines per paragraph. The first couple of paragraphs should cover the who, what, when, where, why, and how questions. A press release is usually no more than 250 words.

The rest of the news release expounds on the information provided in the lead paragraph. It includes quotes from key staff, customers, or subject matter experts. It contains more details about the news you have to tell, which can be about something unique or controversial or about a prominent person, place, or thing.

"You should include a quote for that human touch," said Gary Sims, CEO of the Free Press Release Center. "And you should use the last paragraph to restate and summarize the key points."

This is the example press release template for use at the Free Press Release Center. The last paragraph can also include details on product availability, trademark acknowledgment, etc.

About ABC Company:

Include a short corporate backgrounder about the company or the person who is newsworthy before you list the contact person's name and phone number. Do not include an e-mail address in the body of the release. Your e-mail address goes only in the "Contact E-mail" box when you submit your press release. To stop spam, your address will not appear on the site, but rather people will be able to contact you via a special contact link displayed with your press release.

Contact:

David Brown, Director of Public Relations

ABC Inc.

555-555-5555

http://www.YourWebAddress.com

From *Sample Press Release*, Free Press Release Center, n.d. Retrieved from http://www.free-press-release-center.info/sample-press-release.html

The **SMOG formula** presented in Figure 11.3 (on p. 281) can be used to adapt your written materials to specific audience reading levels. More specific guidelines for its application can be accessed through the Community Toolbox Web page. Your word processing program probably has a feature that can help you assess readability. The back translation process described in chapter 9 can help you adapt your message to a culturally appropriate format. Because you will likely have spent a great deal of time working with the material at this point, you will need to submit the final draft to people who can read it with a fresh eye and suggest further changes. Don't skip this step! A final edit by other health experts and community leaders, followed by a pilot test among community members, can save you the cost and embarrassment of distrib-

11.9   Sample Press Release

A Broken Engagement Could Bring Relief for Orphans in Sierra Leone

Spanaway, WA (PRWeb) November 16, 2006—International charity, All As One, is hopeful that the upcoming Warner Bros. film, *Blood Diamond*, will raise awareness about the decade-long war in Sierra Leone and the children who are still suffering its effects. One supporter of the cause will be auctioning his diamond ring from a broken engagement and donating the proceeds to All As One, in an effort to shine a light on the continuing issue of "conflict" diamonds, while benefiting the children of Sierra Leone in the process.

The civil war in Sierra Leone, funded by corruption and the "blood" diamond trade, was devastating to the people and economy of the country. Though the conflict ended in 2002, it is the children who are still suffering the most. Operating by donations from individuals across the world, All As One's Children's Center in Freetown provides shelter, food, clothes, education, and medical care for orphaned and destitute children, who would otherwise be living on the streets.

Deanna Wallace, a resident of Washington and founder of All As One, is a mother of twelve—ten of whom came to her through adoption, both internationally and domestically. She says, "In Sierra Leone's past, orphans were raised by their extended families. But the war has ravaged the country, destroyed villages, and left Sierra Leone's citizens in poverty. The government simply does not have the resources to begin implementing child welfare programs or orphanages." Complicated adoption procedures and restrictions, many imposed by the U.S. government, make the need for organizations like All As One even greater. "For many of these children, this is the first, and possibly the only, home they will have" Wallace says. "But they are thriving at the Children's Center—here, they have a chance to learn, play, and just be kids."

The eBay auction will run from December 5–15, to coincide with the December release of the film. Wallace hopes the film and the auction will bring needed attention and support to a country much of the world has forgotten.

For additional information about All As One or the upcoming auction, contact:

Jen Brauer, Public Relations/Media Contact, US
jen@allasone.org
511-923-3632
or visit http://www.allasone.org

Photos are available upon request.

From All As One (allasone.org). Used with permission.

11.10   **Rules for Good Writing**
Practicing these rules will enhance the efficacy of your health education messages. **To prepare for writing:** • Identify why you are writing. • Identify your audience. • Create a message outline or cognitive map. **To write concisely:** • Use active voice. • Delete unnecessary words. • Avoid strings of prepositional phrases. **To adapt materials to the intended audience:** • Use SMOG or your word-processing program to determine reading levels. • Use back translation to determine cultural appropriateness. **To correct mistakes and evaluate finished products:** • Edit more than once. • Have a "fresh" pair of eyes review the final draft. • Pilot test materials.

uting materials that contain misspelled words, incomplete sentences, or confusing text. The Community Toolbox website also contains specific guidelines for materials development and pretesting.

INFORMATIONAL PIECES FOR LAY NEWSLETTERS

We encourage you to consider regular newsletter mailings to keep community members apprised of agency or program activities and related national and local news. A number of word-processing programs contain newsletter templates that are simple to use, and there are also digital templates that you can download online and disseminate through e-mail. Access to the Internet for late-breaking health news and graphics makes newsletter production a straightforward task. Before you develop your own, study newsletter content and layouts from a variety of sources and apply the tips for good writing provided in FYI 11.10. Advice from a graphic artist or journalist can improve the quality of your product.

BROCHURES AND PAMPHLETS

An effective brochure or pamphlet should have a single theme. You cannot cover all aspects of a particular health topic in one brochure. As stated earlier, use an outline and keep the message simple. For example, if the purpose of your brochure or pamphlet is to convince a teenage mother to obtain immunizations for her baby, limit your message to reasons why she should get them and where she can get them. Don't get bogged down in related but unnecessary details about, for example, the human immune system or symptoms of childhood diseases. Apply the rules of thumb listed in FYI 11.10 and use bulleted lists where appropriate. With digital design tools so accessible now, it has become easier to create print and electronic materials. However, it is

The SMOG readability formula is commonly used to determine the reading level of written materials. To calculate the SMOG reading grade level, begin with the entire written work that is being assessed and follow these four steps:

1

Pick 30 sentences,* 10 each from near the beginning, in the middle, and near the end of the text.

2

From the sample of 30 sentences, circle all of the words containing three or more syllables (polysyllabic words), including repetitions of the same words, and total the number of words circled.

3

Estimate the square root of the total number of polysyllabic words counted. This is done by finding the nearest perfect square and taking its square root.

4

Finally, add a constant of 3 to the square root. This number gives the SMOG grade, or the reading grade level that a person must have reached if he or she is to fully understand the text being assessed.

SMOG Conversion Table**

Total Polysyllabic Word Counts	Approximate Grade Level
0–2	4
3–6	5
7–12	6
11–20	7
21–30	8
31–42	9
43–56	10
57–72	11
73–90	12
91–110	13
111–112	14
113–157	15
157–192	16
193–210	17
211–240	18

* Visit the NIH Web site for details about pamphlets and fact sheets. http://rex.nci/nih.gov

** Developed by Harold C. McGraw, Office of Educational Research, Baltimore County Schools, Towson, MD.

From *Making Health Communication Programs Work: A Planner's Guide*, National Institutes of Health, U.S. Dept. of Health and Human Services, 2002, NIH Pub. 92-1493.

Figure 11.3   The SMOG readability formula.

worth the expense to enlist the help of an experienced graphic artist or photographer for advice about layout, graphics/visuals, typefaces, and paper. We live in a fast-paced, visually stimulated society, so visual appeal is extremely important.

In preparing your work, talk to people from the intended audience to understand some of their perceptions and attitudes about the topic. This will help you better understand your intended audience and focus on presenting what is most relevant. When you're finished designing your materials, pretest them with members of your intended audience to make sure that the wording, images, and content are appropriate. **Pretesting** allows you to gain initial feedback from your audience before the final version is created. This preview allows your intended audience to offer you suggestions for refining your work so that it creates the impact you had hoped.

PUBLIC SERVICE ANNOUNCEMENTS

Public service announcements are short video or audio messages provided to radio and television stations. Generally, PSAs are sent as ready-to-air audio or videotapes, although radio stations (especially community or public stations, such as campus radio, PBS, and National Public Radio) sometimes prefer a script that their announcers can read live on the air. PSAs are usually 30 seconds or less and can be as simple as a person talking into the TV camera, urging someone to not drink and drive, or they can be elaborate productions that are scripted with actors, music, and story lines.

Broadcast media—radio and television—are required by the Federal Communications Commission (FCC) to serve "in the public interest." Most stations use PSAs as one way to meet this requirement. While they aren't required to donate a fixed percentage of air time per day to PSAs, stations do have to state in their licensing and renewal applications how much air time they plan to devote to PSAs. Most stations donate about a third of their commercial spots to noncommercial causes; in other words, if a station has 18 minutes of commercials in a given hour, six minutes of that will probably be devoted to PSAs (KU Work Group, 2018b).

PSAs require a bit of work on your part, and they tend to be ineffective at influencing policy. Some also criticize PSAs for being fear based and oversimplified. Consider using them when you have a specific action you want the viewer or listener to take, or when they can be coordinated with other activities designed to influence people's behavior. FYI 11.11 provides some suggestions for creating an effective PSA.

SOCIAL MEDIA

Social media are applications that use the Internet to connect people in virtual communities, allowing them to create, share, use, and modify content such as text, images, audio, and video (Kaplan & Haenlein, 2010). People now spend more time on social media sites than on any other kind of website, making it a key platform for health communication (Nielsen, 2012). Social media is most effective if integrated with other media as part of a cohesive campaign with a consistent message. The CDC's Tips From Former Smokers campaign, discussed at the beginning of this chapter, is a good example of such cross-platform communication.

While hundreds of social media platforms exist, Facebook and Twitter are two of the most used. Facebook is a social networking website that lets users create profiles and exchange messages and media, both publicly and privately. Organizations can also create Facebook profiles where they are able to post information and interact

11.11 Creating a Public Service Announcement

Here are some key points to remember when writing a PSA:

- Keep the language simple and vivid since you will often have 30 seconds or less to get your message across.
- Use "hooks," words or phrases that grab attention, to attract and sustain your audience.
- The PSA should request a specific action, such as calling a number to get more information.
- Choose points to focus on—don't overload the viewer or listener with too many different messages.
- Avoid scare tactics.
- Brainstorm: Get together with your colleagues and toss around ideas about ways to illustrate your points. You may want to look at other PSAs for ideas.
- Check your facts. It's very important your PSA is accurate.
- For 10-second spots, keep word length to 20–25; for 15 seconds, 30–35, and for 30 seconds, 60–75 words.

Adapted from KU Work Group for Community Health and Development, 2018b, Chap. 6, Sect. 7: *Preparing Public Service Announcements*. Lawrence: University of Kansas. Retrieved from http://ctb.ku.edu/en/table-of-contents/participation/promoting-interest/public-service-announcements/main. Copyright © 2018 by the University of Kansas for all materials provided via the World Wide Web in the ctb.ku.edu domain.

with other users. Twitter is an interface that lets users post short messages, or "tweets," of up to 140 characters. Users choose a name, called their "handle," and can add "hashtags" to connect their tweets to others on the same topic. For instance, the CDC uses the handle @CDCTobaccoFree and the hashtag #CDCTips for its tweets related to the Tips From Former Smokers campaign. Other Twitter users can reference that handle or hashtag to comment on the campaign.

As with traditional media, use the rules for good writing listed in FYI 11.10 when writing for social media, always keeping your objectives for writing and your target audience at the forefront of your mind. FYI 11.12 suggests additional tips for communicating through social media.

BLOGS AND VLOGS

Blogs and vlogs, short for "weblogs" and "video weblogs," allow creators to post entries regularly, using text, video, or both. Major health organizations maintain blogs on a wide range of topics for various audiences. Blogger and YouTube are the most popular tools for creating a blog or vlog, but you can choose from many other interfaces or host one on your own website.

The general rules of writing (FYI 11.10) apply to blog posts and vlog scripts, as do many of the tips for social media (FYI 11.12): keep your audience and purpose in mind, post new content regularly and frequently, promote your blog or vlog across multiple media, develop a strategy for allowing and responding to user comments, and use metrics to evaluate what impact your content is having. In each post, try to

11.12   Writing for Social Media

Keep content short and simple

People have short attention spans when they're using social media, on the order of a few seconds per post—if that. To increase the chances that other users will read and click on your posts, keep them bite-sized.

Facebook

- Keep posts under 250 characters, including spaces, to let them appear on other users' news feeds.
- See Figure 11.4 for an example from the CDC.
- Keep comments on other users' content under 1,000 characters. Include a website link for additional information.

Twitter

- Try to keep tweets under 120 characters to make them easier to share.
- For instance, @CDCTobaccoFree tweeted on February 5, 2014, "#CDCTips ads are back to encourage smokers to #quitnow & quit for good. Learn more: http://1.usa.gov/1hY04rH."
- Use hashtags (like #CDCTips and #quitnow) to allow users to click through to related content.
- Include a website link for more information (the one above leads to a news story on the CDC website about the Tips From Former Smokers campaign).

Determine how often to post and stick to a schedule

Once your content gains other users' attention, keep them engaged by providing more content regularly. The CDC recommends posting on Twitter and Facebook at least once a week. Whatever interval you choose, keep it regular to encourage your audience to start expecting and using the information you provide.

Include an action item to engage users

The most effective and memorable uses of social media involve a call to action, whether implicit or explicit. On Facebook, for instance, organizations can encourage readers to act by posting questions that lend themselves to conversation in the comments, hosting contests, creating quizzes, posting videos, and providing infographics, photos, badges, and widgets that are easy to share.

Develop a strategy for responding and interacting

When you post content, other users will respond to it. You may also want to respond to other users' posts. Consider in advance how your organization will approach both activities. For example, responding to negative comments with additional information rather than simply removing them can build credibility among other users.

Evaluate effectiveness

Most social media platforms have statistics available to track metrics such as clicks and time spent on the Web page. Facebook Insights and Twitter Analytics offer this information to users. Set quantitative goals for your organization's social media use, make a plan for determining whether they've been met, and decide how you're going to respond if they haven't been. For example, will you retire a Twitter feed if you don't have a certain number of followers by a given date?

Source: "CDC Social Media Tools, Guidelines, and Best Practices," Centers for Disease Control and Prevention, 2014. Retrieved from www.cdc.gov/socialmedia/tools/guidelines/index.html

Figure 11.4   CDC Tobacco Free Facebook post.
The CDC Tobacco Free Facebook page included this photo with the following caption:
"A slip doesn't mean you can't quit for good. Stick to your smokefree goals, find support
from loved ones, and get back to quitting the right way."

Image courtesy of the Centers for Disease Control and Prevention (CDC) *Tips From Former Smokers*® campaign;
photo credit: iStock. Retrieved from https://www.facebook.com/cdctobaccofree.

include a call to action, whether you're asking readers to use specific resources, attend
an event, or just think about your topic in a new way.

A few particular communication strategies apply to blog and vlog content. First,
in both text and video formats, favor stories over abstract content. For instance, the
CDC's Tips From Former Smokers campaign includes a series of videos, and each
features one former smoker relating how smoking damaged his or her health and happiness. These anecdotes represent people's experiences on a large scale, but hearing,
"I quit smoking the day my leg was amputated" is more powerful and memorable
than hearing, "Smoking increases the chances of having type 2 diabetes, which can
lead to amputation" (CDC, 2013a). To tell stories, use plain language rather than jargon, technical information, and detailed charts and graphs (CDC, 2014b). If your
audience would find those resources useful, provide information about where to find
them, including links to online content.

Within a blog or vlog, take a consistent approach to the content. Keep blog posts and videos about the same length every time so that your audience knows what to expect. The CDC (2014b) recommends creating videos less than three minutes long to encourage viewers to watch the whole thing. Use the same formatting from post to post to further build audience identification. For instance, you might begin each video with a title in the same format and conclude the video with your website address.

MOBILE APPLICATIONS

Mobile applications—small software programs for mobile phones and tablet computers—can provide people with regular, reliable, useful health information that's easy for them to share with others. With increasing frequency, people are using their phones to access the Internet, and they tend to use mobile applications, or apps, to connect far more than they use their phone's Web browsers (Nielsen, 2012). Like any software, apps take expertise and time to develop and maintain, so consider whether your organization has the resources to invest in an app.

One unique property of a mobile app is that people can use it anywhere they can bring their smart phone. The best app designs incorporate the mobile environment creatively. Many mobile devices are GPS enabled, for instance, allowing apps to tailor content to real-time user location. Interactive features allow users to easily share content and access resources. For example, if you provide a phone number, e-mail address, or website, you can design it to link to the mobile device's phone, e-mail application, or browser apps, and consider allowing users to log in through Facebook. Since mobile devices are often small and navigated with a finger instead of a mouse, designs should also be light on text and favor a vertical layout to minimize horizontal scrolling.

LETTERS AND MEMOS

Frequent letters and memos sent through the postal service or e-mail can be an effective tool for keeping a variety of team members apprised of your progress and plans. As with other written materials, brevity is important. Try to limit letters to one page and memos to one or two paragraphs. When appropriate, use a business-style heading that lists "Date," "To," "From," and "Re" so that readers can quickly identify the purpose and content of the letter or memo.

PROFESSIONAL ARTICLES

Most professional journal articles follow a thesis-based structure, meaning that they begin by introducing the reader to a specific question, problem, or issue. The introduction explains why the question or issue is significant by reviewing and citing professional literature on the subject. If the paper is a *scientific article,* meaning that it describes and reports the results of an experiment or applied program, a description of the methods or program implemented should follow the introduction section. Next comes the description of the results or outcomes, a discussion of the strengths and weaknesses of the study or program, and the author's interpretations and conclusions (Garrard, 1999). The article must also include a bibliographical format that allows you to cite each source used. Each journal has its own author guidelines, usually printed in every issue, that describe how to format a manuscript you plan to submit. Pay careful attention to these guidelines and study several past volumes of your target journal to note commonly published topics and writing styles.

Manuscripts submitted for publication in professional journals are usually subjected to a rigorous review process before they are placed in print. The journal editor who receives your manuscript will first read it to determine whether your manuscript topic matches journal goals and readership interest. If the editor believes so, he or she will then send out copies of your manuscript to journal reviewers who have knowledge about your manuscript topic. Each reviewer will submit a recommendation about whether the manuscript should be rejected, accepted for publication as written, or accepted if certain revisions are made. In the case of the last recommendation, the reviewer will also provide directions for suggested manuscript changes. The editor will then synthesize responses from all reviewers and make a decision about rejection or acceptance of your manuscript for publication in the journal. If "accepted with revisions," you may ask the editor to clarify suggestions before submitting a revised manuscript. It sometimes takes as long as a year or two for a manuscript to progress from your seed of an idea through manuscript development and submission to a printed journal article. Writing for publication takes lots of practice, patience, and persistence. We recommend that you begin by looking for opportunities to be a co-author with professors who have publication experience.

PUBLIC SPEAKING

Think back to the last time you heard a good speaker deliver a message. What made you think the speaker was so effective? It probably had something to do with your degree of interest in the speech topic. However, an interesting topic isn't the only characteristic of a good speech. A skilled speaker can make almost any topic sound interesting. However, public-speaking skills do not come naturally to most people; if you've ever attended a banquet or wedding reception you can attest to this. Rather, accomplished speakers have honed their skills over time. FYI 11.13 on the next page lists some qualities of a good speaker, many of which you can develop with practice. What other qualities are missing from this list?

TELEPHONE VOICE

The tone of voice you use in a telephone survey or business conversation can make a difference in how well your words are accepted. In most cases, using a slightly lower and deeper tone than you usually use in common conversation can convey warmth and confidence. Practice speaking in a calm, carefully concise manner and enunciate your words distinctly. Adopt a cheerful telephone demeanor, even when talking to a difficult person, and you will be surprised with the results.

PRESENTING FOR LAY AUDIENCES

Three key elements to a successful community presentation are the right background conditions, the right preparation, and the right delivery (KU Work Group, 2018b). You can gain understanding and some control over the background conditions by studying your prospective audience. Ask questions about their demographics (for example, age, socioeconomic status, ethnicity), knowledge about and attitudes toward the presentation topic, and their expectations of you and your presentation. Consider recruiting key stakeholders and community gatekeepers to attend the presentation to help them recognize the need for community action. Whenever possible, study the presentation setting ahead of time to check room size, temperature, acous-

11.13   Qualities of an Effective Speaker

The qualities of an effective speaker go beyond good preparation and include skills related to verbal and nonverbal communication.

An effective speaker:

• begins the speech with an attention-catching statement or story.

• tells the audience what to expect in the speech.

• limits the speech to 3 or 4 main points.

• includes the whole audience through frequent eye contact.

• uses stories and illustrations where appropriate.

• uses pleasant and appropriately animated facial expressions.

• uses an outline to enhance flow.

• never reads notes to the audience.

• projects the voice to the back of the room.

• uses differing voice inflections and appropriate nonverbal body language.

• speaks slowly, clearly, and concisely.

• uses visuals to illustrate major points.

• involves the audience as much as possible.

• summarizes the speech by reiterating its major points.

• limits the speech to the designated time frame.

tics, seating arrangements, and audiovisual equipment. Find out in advance who will be present to help you with last-minute adjustments if needed.

Good preparation begins with a clear presentation objective. Let's return to our earlier example in which you were asked to address the need for well-woman check-ups among members of the Sudanese immigrant community. Suppose that you are preparing to make one of the community presentations we described, and let's work through some basic preparation steps (FYI 11.14).

Your presentation objective might state that you wish to convince members of the audience to get an annual well-woman checkup and encourage others in the community to do the same. Your main presentation outline should contain information designed to persuade your audience (that is, reach your presentation objective). For example, your points could include a brief description of the risks involved in bypassing annual well-woman checkups, an acknowledgment of past barriers to checkups for members of the Sudanese immigrant community, a summary of how some women's health clinics have begun to address the problem and are accessible, a list of the benefits of participating, and directions for calling to set up an appointment. You could then create bulleted lists under each of your main points that would contain key subpoints. From there, you could expand your outline into a full presentation.

11.14   Preparing for a Presentation

Following these simple presentation preparation steps can strengthen message delivery and acceptance:

• Write a clear, brief presentation objective.

• Develop a presentation outline.

• Select supporting materials.

• Create visual aids.

• Practice.

Adapted from KU Work Group for Community Health and Development, 2018, Chap. 4, Sect. 5: *Making Community Presentations*. Lawrence: University of Kansas. Retrieved from http://ctb.ku.edu/en/table-of-contents/assessment/getting-issues-on-the-public-agenda/community-presentations/main. Copyright © 2018 by the University of Kansas for all materials provided via the World Wide Web in the ctb.ku.edu domain.

We recommend that you use a software program for slide presentations (such as PowerPoint, Prezi, or Keynote) to develop your outline. Most programs will allow you to add detailed notes beneath each slide created, and you can then convert the results to a variety of visual formats, including computerized slides projected onto a screen with a data projector, a video or mixed media presentations (with programs like Adobe Spark or iMovie), or even paper printouts for poster displays. FYI 11.15 on the following page contains valuable design tips for any visual format used (and you can use multiple formats in the same presentation).

Don't forget to practice your presentation and delivery! What looks good on paper doesn't always sound good in an oral format, and the length of time needed for the presentation will likely be important. Begin with an opening sentence that will grab your audience's attention. At the end, summarize the main points you just delivered and appeal to your audience's values and concerns as they relate to your presentation topic. Memorize the key points of the presentation so you can concentrate on a professional delivery, but plan to use your presentation notes to help you stay focused.

As you practice your presentation, visualize speaking to your audience or stand in front of a mirror. Concentrate on projecting your voice to the back of the room, but in a relaxed, expressive tone that exudes appropriate levels of enthusiasm and confidence. Work on including all members of the audience through frequent eye contact and avoid turning your back to the audience when referring to visual aids. Instead, stand to the side of the visual and face the audience as you describe the visual.

PRESENTING FOR PROFESSIONAL AUDIENCES

Much of what we recommend for community presentations also holds true when presenting to professional audiences. However, whereas professional and technical terminology is considered jargon and should be avoided in community presentations, it is more likely to be understood and expected among professional audiences. We suggest that you use professional terminology among your professional peers to

11.15 Tips for Creating Effective Visual Aids

These tips for creating effective visual aids improve the appearance and acceptance of the health message:

- Limit each visual to one main idea.
- Use no more than 6–8 lines of text per graphic or slide.
- Use bulleted lists and key phrases rather than sentences.
- Use plain language; avoid jargon.
- Double-space between text lines.
- Use large, bold, crisp fonts.
- Check for visibility from the back of the room.
- Only show information you plan to discuss.
- Plan to quote and clarify each graphic or slide.
- Turn off the projector lights when you have no slides to project.
- Cover the next graphic or slide until you are ready to address it.
- Use chart formats effectively:
  + Horizontal bars: to compare categories
  + Vertical bars: to show change over time
  + Line graphs: to show trends across time periods
  + Pie charts: to show amounts as a percentage of the total

Adapted from KU Work Group for Community Health and Development, 2018, Chap. 4, Sect. 5: *Making Community Presentations*. Lawrence: University of Kansas. Retrieved from http://ctb.ku.edu/en/table-of-contents/assessment/getting-issues-on-the-public-agenda/community-presentations/main. Copyright © 2018 by the University of Kansas for all materials provided via the World Wide Web in the ctb.ku.edu domain.

enhance your credibility as well as audience understanding. This does not mean your language will be obscure or your meaning hard to discern. Your primary goal should still be communication. Professional audiences are also more likely to expect and appreciate your knowledge of the professional literature and how your work relates to other studies and theories. We encourage you to develop a strong research and theory-based understanding of your work so that you can convey to your professional peers how your work contributes to universal understandings. When presenting at professional conferences, it often helps to provide a handout to your audience that contains an abstract of your presentation and a list of references or recommended readings. Expect some audience members to want to contact you later to learn more about your work and explore future collaborative efforts. Maintaining contact with your professional peers through conferences and seminars can be your professional lifeline. We highly encourage you to participate in professional meetings and present your work so that others may learn from and add to your understanding.

Health Literacy

As we mentioned earlier in this text, one of the most pressing community health issues today is health literacy. Factors relating to poor health literacy in the U.S. include the consistent finding that the literacy demands of most printed health materials exceed the reading abilities of many American adults (Center for Health Care Strategies, Inc. [CHCS], 2013; Weiner et al., 2004). With up to 90 million Americans having difficulty with reading basic information, calculating numbers, or communicating with health providers (CHCS, 2013, page 1), there has never been a greater need for you to learn more about how to develop health communication materials that are easily understood by those who have less than a sixth-grade reading ability. This starts with knowing and understanding your intended audience and assessing factors that impact decision making among this group (see chapter 6). In order to create health communication materials like the ones described in this chapter for those with lower literacy skills, you may need to attend a workshop, a professional conference, or visit some websites such as the Center for Health Communication at the Harvard School of Public Health (www.hsph.harvard.edu/chc) to get a better understanding of what works when designing for this special population.

As explained in FYI 11.16, using more pictures and less text, eliminating jargon or slang terms, and curtailing the use of polysyllabic words (3 syllables or more) in your text will help (CHCS, 2013, p. 2). However, learning to effectively communicate information that often is complicated takes practice. We urge you to explore ways to improve your health communication skills as you further your professional development.

11.16   Designing Health Materials for Those with Lower Literacy Skills

1. **Culture is key. Know your audience.** Pay special attention to their preferences, values, language, and dialect. Talk to individuals from your audience, and talk to a variety of people. Ask for feedback from your audience before you publish or distribute your materials. Revise if necessary.

2. **Present the information in a simple manner.** When preparing the written content:
   - Write as if you are speaking to the reader.
   - Present only the most important information.
   - Use headings and subheadings to signal to the reader about upcoming information. Break up large amounts of information into easy-to-read sections.
   - Use short sentences and short paragraphs. Sentences should be no more than 25 words, and paragraphs should be no more than 60 words.
   - With audiences for whom English is a second language, it is preferable to write in their native language. If that is not possible, consider using materials written for lower literacy levels in their second language.
   - Set quotes or phrases off to the side of the main body of text. Use buzzwords to draw the reader in or to notify them of information.
   - Leave an adequate amount of white space along the margins and throughout the publication. This is especially important for low-literacy audiences. Avoid overcrowding each page with words.

(continued)

3. **Use photos and graphics.** Many times, a picture really *is* worth 1000 words! A well-designed graphic can clarify the message being presented or even replace large blocks of text.
   - Avoid stereotyping by carefully selecting images. Again, culture and audience preference play an important role in deciding what is an acceptable image or graphic to include.
   - Seek specific feedback regarding potential images you intend to include in your publication.
   - Show various types of families in your publications. Include pictures of two-parent families, single-parent families, multi-racial families, and families that depict grandparents raising grandchildren, among others.
   - Show images that reflect a variety of different types of residences.
   - Show people in a variety of occupations, including those that are nontraditional. An example might include a male nurse, a female engineer, or a person with a disability in a job most often held by people without visible disabilities.

4. **Keep the reading level below a 6th grade level.**
   - Avoid using polysyllabic words (more than 3 syllables).
   - Do not use slang or jargon.
   - Use SMOG or another readability formula to check the complexity.

Sources: "Tips for Designing Publications for Underrepresented Audiences," by P. D. Ingram, M. H. Dorsey, and S. Smith, 2004, *Journal of Extension,* 42(4). Retrieved from http://www.joe.org/joe/2004august/tt2.php; *Making Health Communication Programs Work: A Planner's Guide,* National Institutes of Health, U.S. Dept. of Health and Human Services, 2008. Retrieved from http://www.cancer.gov/pinkbook

≡ In Conclusion

Communicating effectively is at the crux of community health. Whether you are communicating with people face-to-face in personal conversations or group presentations, through written media, or via public service announcements, the basic concepts remain the same. State your message clearly and concisely. Remember that simple statements and messages are often powerful motivators. Use visuals and illustrations whenever appropriate, and communicate your message in a variety of formats as frequently as possible. Communicate to inform. Communicate to empower. Communicate to progress. We encourage you to begin developing these skills immediately and practice them as often as possible. "For Your Application" provides a suggestion that will help you incorporate several communication formats into one experience and document them in your professional portfolio.

REVIEW QUESTIONS

1. Describe some skills that are necessary for effective communication.
2. Name and describe each component of the health communication model.
3. Explain what is meant by iatrogenic health education disease.
4. Differentiate between persuasive communication and coercion by providing an example of each.
5. Name and give an example of each of the four stages of health communication.

6. Provide at least four strategies for improving cross-cultural communication.

7. Explain how each of the following communication mediums could be used to help deliver a health message to your intended audience: press release, PSA, tweet, and brochure.

8. Name at least six characteristics of a good speaker.

9. Locate a brochure that is intended for a general audience and suggest at least four tips for transforming it so that it is suited for those with lower literacy skills.

10. Analyze why health literacy is a pressing community health issue.

FOR YOUR APPLICATION

Learning to Write Concisely

Convert each of the following sentences into a more concise statement by rewriting to avoid excessive prepositional phrases, delete unnecessary words, and use active voice. Ask a friend to do the same and compare your results.

1. The incredibly high incidence of hypertension among males of African American descent has been reduced by education programs.

2. The common opinion that AIDS is something that happens only to members of the gay community is held by students who attend the local high school.

3. Educational programs that prevent needless accidental injuries have been designed by a large number of the employees of the agency.

4. Preventive health services that are available and affordable were already mandated by the members of the community.

Gaining Communication Experience

Volunteer to deliver a health education presentation to a local community group. Thoroughly research the professional literature and use Internet resources to obtain the information you need and ideas about how to communicate it. Create a slide presentation, poster, and/or informational pamphlet or flyer to be distributed to your audience at the end of the presentation. Ask the audience and, if possible, an experienced presenter to evaluate your presentation and materials.

Observing Health Communication Delivery

Attend at least two health-related events or presentations in your community and take notes on the delivery of each presentation. Design an evaluation form based on the content of this chapter and additional resources you find, evaluate each presentation and presenter, and reflect on the presentations' strengths and weaknesses. How could the delivery of the information be improved? (Note: Instead of attending a presentation, you could find and view a presentation online.)

Developing Health Education Materials for Low Literacy Populations

Obtain a print or electronic health-related brochure or educational resource from a local clinic, grocery store, health department, or nonprofit agency. Assess the reading level of the brochure using the SMOG formula or your word-processing language tool, and revise this brochure to appeal to a group with lower literacy skills. Justify your changes based on what you've read in this chapter as well as other credible sources.

12

Advocating for Community Health Needs

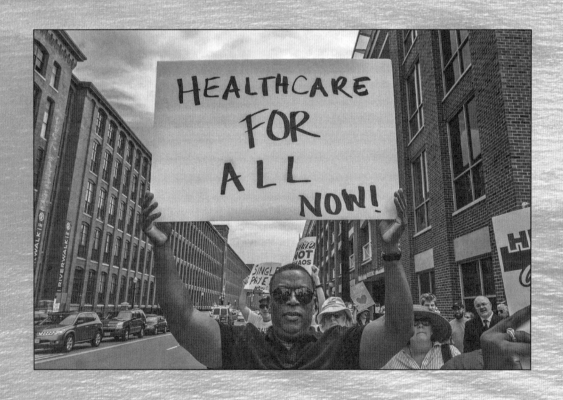

In an effort to collect data for a community needs assessment you are preparing for a local nonprofit, you come across some unsettling information on the county's website. Over 42% of children in your county are overweight or obese yet none of the schools require daily physical education. As a health professional, parent, and resident of the county, you feel the need to advocate for change, but you don't know where to start. How do you convince other parents, policy makers, educators, and other health professionals to support your cause? With little experience in policy making or politics, how do you advocate for legislative action and garner community support? How do you get people to care about the health needs in your community?

Chapter Objectives

1. Define terms and concepts used in health advocacy.
2. Justify the importance of health advocacy.
3. Describe methods of advocating for health issues.
4. List tips for writing advocacy letters, using media, and visiting policy makers.
5. Identify organizations that advocate for health.
6. Review examples of health advocacy activities.
7. Outline advocacy survival skills.
8. Design advocacy materials specific to a particular health issue.
9. Describe the steps involved in creating a social media strategy for an advocacy campaign.

≡ What Is Advocacy?

Have you ever encountered a situation where you thought "That's just not right! There ought to be a law!"? That's how advocacy begins. **Health Advocacy** is defined as "the processes by which the actions of individuals or groups attempt to bring about social and/or organizational change on behalf of a particular health goal, program, interest, or population" (Gold & Miner, 2002, p. 31). Advocacy extends beyond the bounds of this definition, however, and takes many forms. Advocacy can include large-scale efforts such as actively working to create social movements that motivate people to change the social, political, legal, economical, and medical environments. It can also include individual-level efforts such as actively participating in the democratic process and expressing your rights as a citizen of the United States or your country. Advocacy is also standing up for individuals who cannot speak for themselves. When used effectively, advocacy can have a tremendous impact on personal and public health. FYI 12.1 provides a more thorough description of advocacy and what it commonly entails.

12.1   Examples of Advocacy

- Advocacy is active promotion of a cause or principle.
- Advocacy involves actions that lead to a selected goal.
- Advocacy is one of many possible strategies, or ways to approach a problem.
- Advocacy can be used as part of a community initiative, nested in with other components.
- Advocacy is not direct service.
- Advocacy does not necessarily involve confrontation or conflict.
- Some examples may help clarify just what advocacy is:
  + You join a group that helps build houses for the poor—that's wonderful, but it's not advocacy (it's a service).
  + You organize and agitate to get a proportion of apartments in a new development designated as low to moderate income housing—that's advocacy.
  + You spend your Saturday handing out information for the American Lung Association—that's not advocacy (it's a service).
  + You hear that the local recycling center is going to be closed down and you band together with many others to get the city to preserve this site, or find you a new one. Some of you even think about blocking the bulldozers, if necessary. That's advocacy.

Adapted from KU Work Group for Community Health and Development, 2018, Chap. 5, Sect. 4: *Systems Advocacy and Community Organizing*. Lawrence: University of Kansas. Retrieved from http://ctb.ku.edu

Skills for Successful Advocacy

Leaders in the field of community health increasingly recognize that the discipline's mission is to address not just individual health but also the social, political, and economic structures that serve as barriers to community health and well-being. Health educators and community health professionals serve as leaders in addressing conditions that diminish health. However, many community health professionals do not receive any, or receive very limited, training in advocacy in their academic program or workforce training (Radius, Galer-Unti, & Tappe, 2009; Ward & Koontz, 1999). The goals of this chapter are to introduce you to health advocacy as well as to highlight skills and strategies that will help you to bring about change within your own community. There are several key components to effective advocacy that health educators must be aware of in order to achieve the intended goal. These include:

- "rightness" of the cause
- power of the advocates (i.e., more of them is much better than less)
- thoroughness with which the advocates researched the issues, the opposition, and the climate of opinion about the issue in the community
- skill in using the advocacy tools available (including the media)
- selection of effective strategies and tactics (KU Work Group, 2018e)

The process of advocacy is many things to many people. It may be lobbying on Capitol Hill in Washington, DC, with the purpose of educating and influencing policy makers; encouraging insurance companies to cover prevention services; or standing up at a school board meeting to campaign for a comprehensive health education curriculum. Advocacy can be local or national, can be directed toward policy makers of all kinds, and can be used to change many environments. See FYI 12.2 for some terms you may come across while participating in or researching advocacy.

FYI

12.2   Advocacy Terms

Following are some of the common terms used in the advocacy process.

Health Advocacy	The process by which the actions of individuals or groups attempt to bring about social and/or organizational change on behalf of a particular health goal, program, interest, or population.
Lobbying	To conduct activities aimed at influencing public officials and especially members of a legislative body on legislation. Lobbyists are usually paid to do this work.
Grassroots Lobbying	Any attempt to influence the public or segment of the public to take action on specific legislation.
Appropriations	Money that has been set aside by formal action for a specific purpose.
Entitlements	A government program providing benefits to members of a specified group or the funds supporting or distributed by such a program.
Discretion	The power of free decision or latitude of choice within certain legal bounds.
Constituent	One who authorizes another to act as agent.

Sources: Definition for *health advocacy* from the *2000 Joint Committee on Health Education and Promotion Terminology*, 2000. Definition for *lobbying, grassroots lobbying, appropriations, entitlements, discretion*, and *constituents* are from *Merriam-Webster's Collegiate Dictionary*, 11th ed., 2003, Springfield, MA: Merriam-Webster. Cited in "Putting Advocacy into Action" by S. E. Ward and N. Koontz, 1999, *Eta Sigma Gamma Monograph*, 17(2): 36–40.

▤ Basic Tools of Advocacy

Among the basic tools of advocacy are: knowledge, voting, electioneering, coalitions and partnerships, lobbying, grassroots activities, media, personal communication or legislative advocacy, and technology. A brief description of each tool is discussed below, and FYI 12.3 provides a snapshot of advocacy tools and strategies: good, better, and best.

Knowledge

Information, of course, is the basis of knowledge. We have talked about information gathering in several chapters. We have discussed assessing individual and community needs through various methods, and we have discussed libraries, local health departments, voluntary health organizations, the Internet, and many other sources of information. In the case of advocacy, information and knowledge provide you with the power to affect others. We are not suggesting that to be an advocate you have to be an expert. But you do need sufficient knowledge about an issue to be able to provide adequate decision-making information for those to whom you are advocating.

FYI

12.3   Advocacy Tools and Strategies: Good, Better, Best

Strategy	Good	Better	Best
Voting behavior	Register and vote.	Encourage others to register and vote.	Register others to vote.
Electioneering	Contribute to the campaign of a candidate friendly to public health and health education.	Campaign for a candidate friendly to public health and health education.	Run for office or seek a political appointment.
Direct lobbying	Contact a policy maker.	Meet with your policy makers.	Develop ongoing relationships with your policy makers and staff.
Integrate grassroots lobbying into direct lobbying activism	Start a petition drive to advocate for a specific policy in your local community. Use the Internet to access information related to health issues.	Get on the agenda for a meeting of a policy-making body and provide testimony. Build a webpage that calls attention to a specific health issue, policy or legislative proposal.	Teach others to use the Internet for advocacy activities.
Media advocacy: Newspapers, letters to the editor and op-ed articles	Write a letter to the editor.	Write an op-ed piece.	Teach others to write letters and op-ed pieces for media advocacy.
Media advocacy: Acting as a resource person	Respond to requests by members of the media for health-related information.	Issue a news release.	Develop and maintain ongoing relationships with media personnel.

From "Advocacy 101: Getting Started in Health Education Advocacy," by R. A. Galer-Unti, M. K. Tappe, and S. Lachenmayr, 2004, *Health Promotion Practice, 5*(3): 280–288.

Voting

Participating in advocacy is as simple as casting a vote on Election Day (although, depending on the state and the election, the technology used, and the number of voting sites in your area, it may take more time than you had planned). The freedom to participate in representative democracy, to have a say in who will be elected, is a privilege that many people in the world do not get to exercise. You might take your own right a step further and encourage others to register or, better yet, volunteer to help register the people in your community. There has been, and continues to be a great need to help people get registered.

Fortunately, voter participation in the U.S. has improved over the years, especially in the 2016 election. According to the DeSilver (2017), about 55% of those who were of voting age cast a vote on Election Day, and this included 87% of registered voters. This figure was up from previous U.S. elections, but compared to other parts of the world, the U.S. has one of the poorest voter participation rates among modernized countries in the world (see FYI 12.4).

Those who *willingly chose not to vote* as well as those of voting age who *were ineligible to vote* comprised about 45% of the population in 2016 (DeSilver, 2017). People fail to exercise their right to vote for a number of reasons, from "I didn't have time," to "I don't have confidence in the government," to "I was not allowed to vote" (FYI 12.5 on p. 302).

Voting is the most fundamental type of advocacy because voters determine who will serve as elected officials. These elected officials formulate policies that impact our everyday lives, including where and how we vote. **Gerrymandering**, for example, is when lawmakers manipulate the boundaries of (an electoral constituency) so as to favor one party or class (Pew Research Center, 2016). **Electoral fraud**, also known as **voter fraud**, varies from country to country. Generally, it includes illegal voter registration, intimidation at polls, and improper vote counting. Even though technically the term *electoral fraud* covers only illegal acts, the term is also used to describe acts that are unethical, outside the spirit of electoral laws, or in violation of the principles of democracy. For democracy to work, we must not just exercise our own right to vote, but also safeguard the rights of others who may be vulnerable to political and unethical party tactics.

Electioneering

Another basic advocacy tool is to support a candidate's campaign or run for office, which is also termed *electioneering* (Galer-Unti, Tappe, & Lachenmayr, 2004). Though it is illegal and unethical for government and nonprofit organization employees to engage in electioneering as a representative of that organization, as a private citizen, one can support a candidate's run for office.

Coalitions and Partnerships

As mentioned in chapter 10, coalitions involve coordinating individuals or organizations into a team that can work toward a common goal. Good examples include the child protection teams that many cities have formed. Such teams consist of individuals from all of the agencies in the city that are in a position to help abused children. Refer back to chapter 10, where we include some strategies for building coalitions.

12.4 U.S. Voting Behavior Compared to Other Countries (2017)		
Country	**% of voting age population**	**% of registered voters**
Belgium (2014)*	87.21	89.37
Sweden (2014)	82.61	85.81
Denmark (2015)	80.34	85.89
Australia (2016)*	78.96	90.98
South Korea (2017)	77.92	77.23
Netherlands (2017)	77.31	81.93
Israel (2015)	76.10	72.34
New Zealand (2017)	75.65	79.01
Finland (2015)	73.14	66.85
Hungary (2018)	71.65	69.68
Norway (2017)	70.59	78.22
Germany (2017)	69.11	76.15
Austria (2017)	68.79	80.00
France (2017)	67.93	74.56
Mexico (2012)*	65.97	63.08
Italy (2018)	65.28	73.05
Czech Republic (2018)	63.44	66.57
UK (2017)	63.25	69.31
Greece (2015)*	62.14	56.16
Portugal (2015)	61.75	55.84
Spain (2016)	61.17	66.48
Slovakia (2016)	59.43	59.82
Ireland (2016)	58.04	65.09
Estonia (2015)	56.82	64.23
United States (2016)	55.70	86.80
Luxembourg (2013)*	55.12	91.15
Slovenia (2014)	54.09	51.73
Poland (2015)	53.83	55.34
Chile (2017)	52.20	49.02
Latvia (2014)	51.69	58.80
Switzerland (2015)*	38.63	48.40
Iceland (2017)	NA	81.20
Japan (2017)	NA	53.65
Turkey (2017)*	NA	85.43

Note: Voting-age population (VAP) turnout is derived from estimates of each country's VAP by the International Institute for Democracy and Electoral Assistance. Registered-voter (RV) turnout derived from each country's reported registration data. Because of methodology differences, in some countries estimated VAP is lower than reported RV. Current voting-age population estimates for Iceland, Japan, and Turkey unavailable.

*National law makes voting compulsory. In addition, one Swiss canton has compulsory voting.

From *U.S. Trails Most Developed Countries in Voter Turnout*, by D. DeSilver, 2017, May 15, Pew Research Center. Retrieved from http://www.pewresearch.org/fact-tank/2017/05/15/u-s-voter-turnout-trails-most-developed-countries/

12.5   Why Registered Voters Say They Did Not Vote in 2016

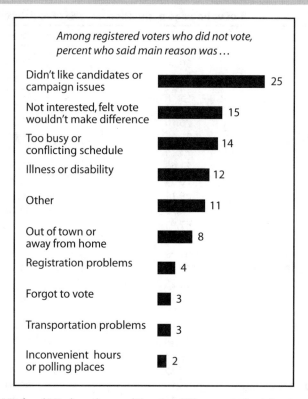

Among registered voters who did not vote, percent who said main reason was …

Reason	Percent
Didn't like candidates or campaign issues	25
Not interested, felt vote wouldn't make difference	15
Too busy or conflicting schedule	14
Illness or disability	12
Other	11
Out of town or away from home	8
Registration problems	4
Forgot to vote	3
Transportation problems	3
Inconvenient hours or polling places	2

Note: "Don't know," "Refused," "Bad weather conditions," and "No response" not shown.
Source: Pew Research Center analysis of the 2016 Current Population Survey, November Supplement.

From *Dislike of Candidates or Campaign Issues Was Most Common Reason for Not Voting in 2016.* Pew Research Center (2017, June 1). Retrieved from http://www.pewresearch.org/fact-tank/2017/06/01/dislike-of-candidates-or-campaign-issues-was-most-common-reason-for-not-voting-in-2016/ft_17-06-01_nonvoters_allreasons/

Lobbying

Lobbying is a form of advocacy. The distinction between the two terms (lobbying and advocacy) is sometimes subtle yet important. Lobbying refers specifically to *paid* advocacy efforts that attempt to influence legislation. On the other hand, when non-profit organizations advocate on their own behalf, they seek to affect some aspect of society, whether they appeal to individuals about their behavior, employers about their rules, or the government about its laws (Connecticut Association of Nonprofits Advocacy, 2003). This distinction is helpful to keep in mind because it means that laws limiting the lobbying done by nonprofit organizations do not govern other advocacy activities. Advocacy can be focused but is generally broader, covering more issues. You need to be aware that if you are employed by a state or federal agency, you cannot represent that organization through lobbying. You may advocate for health issues as an individual, but you cannot serve as a paid lobbyist. The American School Health Association and other professional organizations hire lobbyists to talk with policy makers about health issues.

Grassroots Activities

Grassroots activities are those for which the impetus comes from the people rather than city officials or even local health educators. This "impetus" might even come from a sixteen-year-old high school student. Take for example, Lauren Maunus, who was a sophomore at South Fork High School in Stuart, Florida, when she became a young advocate because of her sister, Rachel. Rachel, like a growing group of Americans, is allergic to peanuts and tree nuts, which can cause anaphylaxis—a reaction to a food or other stimuli that threatens breathing and blood circulation. On average, five Americans die each day from anaphylaxis (Safe Kids Worldwide, 2013), and food allergy prevalence has increased by over 55% in the last decade. Going to school every day and entering the cafeteria was like entering a minefield for Rachel and others like her because the Food Allergy Labeling and Consumer Protection Act (which requires the top eight allergens be identified on all food products) does *not* apply to food sold in public school cafeterias. Therefore, Rachel and other children with similar food allergens are vulnerable to anaphylaxis because the school does not have to disclose ingredients or allergens in the food they serve. That just didn't seem right to Lauren, so she drafted a bill to identify best practices for handling food allergens in the schools. The bill also included education for all food service personnel and required all food items offered in Florida school cafeterias to contain nutrition and allergen information, be posted on school district websites, and be included at the point of sale. Lauren worked hard to garner support from youth, parents, administrators, and policy makers in Florida. The education she proposed became included in guidelines published by the Florida Department of Agriculture and Consumer Services (DACS) and had the force of law. Lauren didn't just stop there, however. She formed a coalition of organizations that are working to protect the estimated 5.9 million American kids with food allergies. These organizations include: the Florida Medical Association, the United Way, the Parent-Teacher Association, and the National Foundation for Celiac Awareness.

Lauren's example demonstrates the power of grassroots advocacy and the will of a young woman to create a safer environment for her sister and for others impacted by food allergens. You, too, can help individuals or groups within your community mobilize to effect change in health-related policies. These grassroots efforts have a profound ripple effect; by engaging people at the local level, you can build consensus, impact social norms and "group think," and make change happen at the legislative level. Mark Pertschuk, director of *Grassroots Public Health: Preemption and Movement Building in Public Health, Phase 2,* a program funded by the Robert Wood Johnson Foundation, further explains:

> Recent research has even uncovered a link between local policy campaigns and
> healthy social norms. In other words, when public health movements build from

the ground up and lead to local policy, the community is more likely to experience a shift in thinking around the issue at hand, whether it's tobacco control or obesity prevention. (2012, par 2)

Media

Daniel Schorr, a commentator for National Public Radio, once stated, "If you don't exist in the media, for all practical purposes, you don't exist" (Bernhardt, 2006). The potential for media to promote awareness of health issues is evident every day as you turn on the TV, listen to the radio, open up a magazine, or surf the Internet. As Smith and Wakefield (2005) note:

> Media shape attitudes and beliefs, act as agents of public education, and play an important role in determining the policy agenda. They serve as a forum for the elucidation of concepts such that they are subject to public consideration and comment, influencing which issues people think about and how people think about the issues. (p. 472)

Media advocacy is "the strategic use of any form of media to help advance an organization's objectives or goals" (U.S. Administration on Aging, 2008, para. 1). Community health organizations and health professionals now recognize the importance of media advocacy in promoting their health issues, missions, and/or agendas. On a daily basis, an average American is bombarded with more than 3,000 commercial messages, most of them counter to healthy living (Baker, 2017). In order to compete with this barrage as a health professional, you will need to know how to effectively package and deliver your message so that it has the biggest impact. Examples of media advocacy include:

- A *press release* highlighting a "no cell phone zone" call to action, sponsored by a local parent organization that seeks to ban the use of cell phones in schools.
- A *letter to the editor* of a newspaper from the director of a women's health organization highlighting a popular misconception or factual errors cited in the previous newspaper report on the HPV vaccine. The letter provides a link to the organization's website, which lists facts, supporting sources, and contact information.
- A *blog* sponsored by the American College Health Association about the need to legislate "smoke-free" campuses across the United States.
- A *radio interview* with a representative from a local breast health organization about the need to change medical coverage of mammography for those under 40 who have a family history of breast cancer.
- A *public service announcement* (PSA) sponsored by Mothers Against Drunk Driving that urges people to vote against lowering the federal legal drinking age.
- A *website* like the Health Education Advocate that educates the public on the need for health care reform in the United States (www.healtheducationadvocate.org).
- A *social networking group*, such as the one hosted by Pioneers for the Cure, that encourages Facebook users interested in breast health to join the group and share the message of breast health with others as well as fund raise for research efforts.
- A short *online video* created to promote an anti-bullying campaign using a *mobile app* called iMovie.

The Internet and Social Media

The Internet is a powerful tool for advocacy; creating and posting a message to educate or motivate your constituent base can be completed in seconds. Taking advocacy online widens your audience and may help you garner support quicker than traditional face-to-face methods alone. Online strategies for advocacy include things such as blast e-mails, sending template letters or online petitions to constituents, creating websites to educate others about the issue or connect people to resources and key contacts, hosting webinars to increase understanding of the issues, and using social media. As mentioned in chapter 11, social media such as Facebook and Twitter, can have tremendous rewards for your local, state, and branch advocacy efforts if you're creative and persistent. Common social media platforms for advocacy (at the time of this text edition) include Facebook, Twitter, Instagram, and Snapchat, but new tools are unveiled every week. Talk to others about what they're doing, and see how your efforts can fit into or shape what's already happening. Social media is about connection and dialogue—it's not a monologue. Furthermore, use of social media should be strategic. Consider components such as your target audience, objectives, social media channels, key messages, and measures for success when planning your social media strategy. A worksheet for planning a social media advocacy strategy is provided in Appendix C. It is best to use both traditional and electronic formats for health advocacy. FYI 12.6 provides CDC's top lessons learned from using social media. For further information and tips, reference *Tips for Using Social Media for Advocacy* by Lori Fresina and Diane Pickles at powerprism.org.

Mobile Health Tools

Mobile health, or *mHealth*, "is a term used to describe the practice of using mobile technologies—mobile phones, text messaging services or applications—to support public health and medicine" (Centers for Disease Control, 2011, p. 21). The use of mobile and wireless technologies to support the achievement of health objectives has the potential to transform the face of health promotion and health care delivery across

12.6   CDC's Top Lessons Learned from Using Social Media

The CDC social media team compiled the following list of lessons learned over the last few years:

1. **Make Strategic Choices and Understand the Level of Effort.** Be strategic and follow demographic and user data to make choices based on audience, communications objectives and key messages. Be sure to assess the level of effort needed to maintain these channels such as time and commitment. Often, the resources needed to start and maintain social media projects are different than traditional communication efforts.

2. **Go Where the People Are.** Social media can help reach people where they are—millions of people use social media and spend a lot of time in these spaces learning, sharing and interacting. The popularity of key social media sites can be assessed by reviewing user statistics and demographics. Additionally, there are several niche social networking sites that target specific groups, like moms, physicians, or racial and ethnic groups; or sites that focus on a particular topic like travel or health.

(continued)

3. **Adopt Low-Risk Tools First.** If you are starting out and finding resistance to using social media among your communication team or stakeholders, it may be helpful to first adopt low-risk solutions and later build on your successes. Products such as podcasts, videos and widgets are easily downloadable, and can be accessed from partner sites and posted on your website.

4. **Make Sure Messages Are Science-Based.** As with any effective health communication, messages developed for dissemination through social media channels should be accurate, consistent and science-based.

5. **Create Portable Content.** Develop portable content—such as mobile applications, widgets and online videos—that can easily extend reach beyond your website to provide credible, timely, and accurate content for partners and others who want to help spread your health messages.

6. **Facilitate Viral Information Sharing.** Make it easy for people to share your messages and become health advocates. This can be accomplished by using social media sites such as Facebook and YouTube that encourage sharing among users, or you can use tools with sharing features, such as widgets or eCards.

7. **Encourage Participation.** Social media allows for the tailoring of messages to help express empathy and acknowledge concern, promote action and listen to what people are saying about health-related topics in your community. Two- way conversations can foster meaningful communication with your audience that can help to facilitate relationships, sharing and interaction.

8. **Leverage Networks.** Social media allows people to easily establish and access networks on a regular basis. For example, Facebook reports that half of all Facebook users have at least 200 friends. By strategically leveraging these established networks, you can facilitate information sharing, and in turn, expand the reach of your health message.

9. **Provide Multiple Formats.** Providing messages in multiple formats increases accessibility, reinforces messages and gives people different ways to interact with your content based on their level of engagement and access to media.

10. **Consider Mobile Technologies.** More than ninety percent of adults in America subscribe to mobile services. Mobile technology is personal, portable and affordable. It allows the sharing of health information through text messaging, mobile websites and mobile applications.

11. **Set Realistic Goals.** Social media can raise awareness, increase a user's knowledge of an issue, change attitudes and prompt behavior change in dynamic, personalized and participatory ways. However, like traditional communication, social media alone may not be able to meet all of your communication goals or address all of the target audiences' needs. Set your goals accordingly.

12. **Learn from Metrics and Evaluate Your Efforts.** Digital communications offer many metrics that you can use to focus and improve your communications efforts. Metrics can help you to report usage, monitor trends and gauge the success of specific promotions or outreach efforts. By analyzing the feedback from these metrics you can adjust your social media strategy, reshape messages, improve processes or shift tactics.

Excerpted from *The Health Communicator's Social Media Toolkit*, Centers for Disease Control and Prevention, 2011. Retrieved from http://www.cdc.gov/socialmedia/tools/guidelines/socialmediatoolkit.html?

the globe. According to the World Health Organization (2011), a combination of factors is driving this change, including: rapidly evolving technologies, the increasing need for portability of information, a continual uptake in mobile and smartphone use, and systems-level integration of mobile health into existing electronic health services.

According to Johnson and Wannemacher, there are three unique characteristics of mobile applications:

- Simplicity—making the application suitable for regularly scheduled tasks using a minimum number of steps/clicks,

- Immediacy—providing the capability to instantly deliver pertinent content to users who carry phones with them literally on a constant basis, and

- Context—delivering services relevant to a customer's location and circumstances (2011, p. 11).

Mobile technologies include the following:

- Mobile websites: A website that has been designed for viewing on mobile phones and other handheld devices such as digital tablets (e.g., iPads). Mobile websites are increasingly responsive in nature, which means that they can adjust to any size device from desktop computers to smartphones.

- Mobile applications: A mobile application, or "app" that runs on smartphones and other mobile devices (like a tablet) that make optimum use of the handset's native functions, such as the camera, offline/data usage, and "push notifications." Types of health-related apps include: calorie counters, running or walking route maps, hospital and clinic waiting room "check ins," eCards (FYI 12.7) related to health that you can send as postcards, healthy restaurant locators, and prescription refill reminders (just to name a few!).

FYI

12.7   Example of an eCard Sent to a Cell Phone

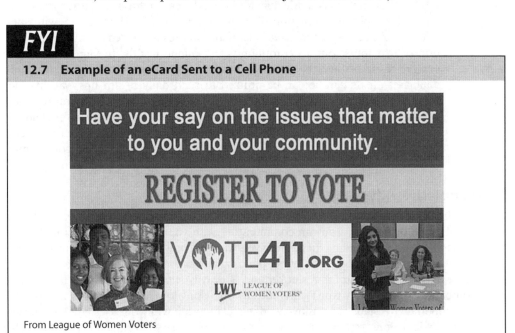

From League of Women Voters

Mobile apps can also be used as powerful educational, tracking and advocacy tools. For example, organizations like Becky's Fund, a national non-profit which seeks to increase awareness and advocacy to reduce interpersonal violence, offers a number of technology safety tips for its audience and for organizations providing interpersonal violence-related services as well as advocacy notifications. One such tool, Guardly, is a mobile app for smartphones used to empower individuals in an emergency situation. It can help students and others faced with dating violence, abusive relationships, or a simple desire to feel safe when walking alone at night (Schaffhauser, 2012). With a click of a button, a person who feels threatened may notify her customized safety network on social media that there is an emergency. Her network can then track her location in real time and mobilize help (including calling 911). Mobile apps can also be used by organizations to educate subscribers about their issues; recruit new members and volunteers; alert subscribers about lobbying events, rallies, and fund-raising efforts; and connect subscribers to other mobile tools such as text messaging. While developing a mobile app is getting easier for the non-techie consumer, it still involves a considerable amount of technical expertise and resources.

- SMS text messaging: SMS text messages are the most common type of mobile data service and are the simplest mobile delivery method. Mobile texting can include up to 160 characters, is more likely to be read than e-mail (Anderson & Jiang, 2018), can be sent quickly from organizations, and target audiences typically have the device readily available—in one's hand or nearby (in the case that they own a smartphone). The CDC reports that "text messaging is quickly becoming a vital tool for the delivery of health information and engaging users to improve their health" (CDC's Health Communicator's Social Media Toolkit, 2011, p. 22). Speed is a critical factor with advocacy efforts, and text messaging allows for rapid dissemination of information to reach "the masses" with specific calls for action. There have been many studies published about the application of text messaging to community and public health. In fact, you should explore some of them by doing a search in your university's online research databases. Texts can be can be utilized to send daily health tips, vaccination reminders, smoking cessation intervention messages, and medication reminders. And in reference to advocacy, text messaging can also be used for sending out voting reminders; generating advocacy alerts; disseminating electronic petitions; raising funds (e.g., "text HOPE to donate $10"); organizing community forums, town hall meetings, and assemblies; and recruiting volunteers.

Legislative Advocacy

Legislative advocacy is actually a form of personal communication with legislators (local, state, or federal). You can communicate with your legislators by writing letters, calling, visiting, or e-mailing. In general, you want to know about the person with whom you will be communicating—his or her philosophies and voting records on health issues. After all, if your legislator is a smoker and is heavily supported financially by tobacco companies, you probably won't gain much by discussing tobacco control with him or her. It is important to establish a positive working relationship with your legislator by contacting the office before you visit and providing some preliminary information. You will probably talk with a staff member during this preliminary call and perhaps even during the visit. Don't be put off by this. Staff members will take your information to the legislator, especially if you provide accurate information succinctly and in a straightforward fashion.

The timing of your visit or letter determines the potential impact. A letter or visit that provides information after a vote has been made is meaningless, even if the information would have changed the vote. On the other hand, a letter or visit immediately before an impending vote might play an important role in changing the vote. In order to time your communication well, you need to learn about the legislative process and keep abreast of the issues that are being addressed. The Internet can help you stay up-to-date.

WRITING YOUR LEGISLATOR

Letters can be effective means of influencing legislation. Your letters can be sent via postal mail, fax, or e-mail. The same guidelines apply to each format. You can

12.8   Meeting with Your Members of Congress

One of the most effective ways to influence the policy-making process and build a relationship is to visit with your senators and representative, or their staff, in person.

Tips for Arranging a Meeting

Call or e-mail to request an appointment. If you want to meet with your legislator in the district, send the request to the district office. Congressional member websites often have online submission appointment requests available.

Follow up by phone. Do not hesitate to call the office if you do not receive a response to your initial request.

Be sure to identify yourself as a constituent. Include information about who you are, the nature of your visit (identify what you want to discuss), when you would like to meet and the names of any friends or colleagues who may accompany you.

Call or e-mail to confirm the appointment.

Sample Request for an Appointment

DATE

The Honorable **XX**

Attention: Scheduler

Dear Senator/ Representative **XX**,

As a constituent and public health professional, I am writing to request an appointment with **[Senator/ Representative XX]** in **[name of town where nearest district office is]** on **[insert date and times available]** to discuss public health funding.

Please contact me to let me know when the **[Senator/Representative]** or the relevant staffer might be available to meet. I will follow up with you in the next week by phone. Thank you for considering my request.

Sincerely,

[Name]

[Contact information]

From *Meeting with your Members of Congress* (n.d.). American Public Health Association (APHA). Retrieved from https://www.apha.org/policies-and-advocacy/advocacy-for-public-health/speak-for-health

also write your members of Congress to request an in-person meeting. See FYI 12.8 for tips for arranging a meeting.

CALLING OR VISITING YOUR LEGISLATOR

Making a personal phone call or visiting your legislator's office can have a powerful impact on policy decisions. Legislators want to know how their constituents feel about the issues being addressed. Your visit will be more impressive if a large group of you contact a number of legislators about the same issue. FYI 12.9 presents tips for making a personal visit to your policy maker.

Survival Skills for Advocacy

The work involved in advocacy is not for the faint of heart! It takes ongoing commitment and energy to drive forward policy and social action. Add to your skills arsenal by adopting some of the "advocacy survival skills" from the Community Toolbox (KU Work Group, 2018e) outlined below.

Accentuate the Positive!

Keep your eyes open for positive events that happen in conjunction with or as the result of your community initiative.

- When you notice something positive happening, even if it's something small, recognize it publicly. Call a local media representative or construct a press release.
- Thank others for their efforts. Pay them public compliments. This will help motivate people to contribute in the future, knowing that you appreciate their involvement!
- Being conscientious about thanking people will help set you apart from other groups that only complain.

Highlight Values and Accomplishments

Always accentuate the positive values and vision relating to your organization's work. For example, you may ultimately be working toward improved community health, safe workplaces and streets, a clean community environment, or quality education. Everybody wants to experience these things, so it's difficult for opponents or skeptics to argue against the kind of values you promote.

- Prevent wasteful arguments or resistance by keeping public attention focused on values and principles that benefit everyone and that help move your initiative along.
- Communicate to others your group's accomplishments: the new programs, policies, and practices it helped bring about.

Measure Success Each Step of the Way

Sometimes people can get discouraged if it seems like months have gone by without any significant gains. If members of your group aren't able to see any progress

12.9 Tips for Making a Visit to your Policy Maker

One of the most effective ways to influence the policy making process and make a lasting connection is to visit with your legislators in person. Most legislators have regular office hours, in their district offices and in the Capitol, during which they and their staff are available to their constituents. To arrange a meeting with your policy maker

- **Send a letter, a fax, or call requesting an appointment.** If you want to meet with your legislator in the district, send the request to the district office. If you will be visiting the Capitol, send the letter to that office.

- **Be sure to identify yourself as a constituent** and address the letter to the legislator and to the attention of the appointment scheduler. Include information about who you are, the nature of your visit (identify what you want to discuss), when you would like to meet, and the names of any friends or colleagues who may accompany you.

- **Follow up by calling the policy maker's office** to which you sent the letter and ask to speak with the scheduler or the staffer who handles appointments. Explain who you are and why you are calling, referring to the letter you sent. If the legislator is unavailable at that time or will not be in the area on the date you would like to meet, the appointment scheduler may offer you another date/time or provide you the opportunity to meet with the legislative staff who handles the issue.

- **Send a letter or make a phone call confirming the appointment.**

During the meeting with your policy maker

- **Arrive on time.** If meeting with a staff member, be sure you have the correct contact name. Do not underestimate the power of the staff person in helping to shape the policy maker's opinions and positions on issues or a particular piece of legislation.

- **Bring two or three colleagues with you.** Prior to the meeting, you should agree on what points will be made and which one each of you will discuss.

- Try to deliver your message in three minutes. Be sure to introduce yourself and your colleagues and explain why you are concerned about the issue and why you have expertise regarding the issue. Be concise, polite, and professional.

- **Be prepared** to answer questions. When asked what you want, clearly explain.

- **Be a resource for the policy maker and his/her staff.** Offer your time and assistance if he/she wants to talk about your areas of interest and expertise in the future.

- **Provide material to support your position.** Leave behind a business card and a one-page fact sheet summarizing your position.

- **Follow up with a thank you letter.** Be sure to include any additional information you may have promised or that may be relevant to the issue.

From *Tips for Making a Visit to your Policymaker* (n.d). American Public Health Association (APHA). Retrieved from https://www.apha.org/-/media/files/pdf/advocacy/policymaker_visit_tips.ashx

after dedicating a lot of time and effort to your mission, their interest and motivation won't last very long. People like to see results, no matter how small. Sometimes, significant progress on a particular community issue is slow to show itself. To break up the time that passes without major breakthroughs occurring, develop a plan of action that has some shorter term or intermediate objectives. For example, let's say that your organization has an outcome objective to provide necessary immunizations to at least 98% of all children ages two or younger within your county within three years. You need those three years to establish the program and get community support; however, you need to measure success throughout this time period as well. To do so, you can plan a number of activities that will allow you to determine whether you are moving toward your goal. Referring to the example above, you may host some educational workshops in the community for mothers with children two years or younger. Measure attendance and change in knowledge and attitudes about immunization at these outreach activities to determine if your program is getting closer to achieving its goals. Do the mothers feel more compelled to have their children immunized? Is the attendance at these events high? Is your marketing working effectively? Celebrations along the way to "the big win" will build the confidence and reputation of your group.

Frame the Issues

If opponents to your program put forth criticisms, don't respond in the terms set forward by your opponents. Instead, shift support away from their perspective by framing the issue in your own voice. Here is a great example provided by the Community Toolbox (KU Work Group, 2018e):

> There is a growing group of individuals who claim that mothers on welfare take advantage of "the system" by having more babies to get "free money" from the government. This sentiment is in direct opposition to your agency, which seeks to help mothers who have uninsured children get the care they need. Rather than attack or take an aggressive stance, responding to their criticism by underscoring that no woman could possibly profit from the small amount of extra money a month per child the state pays, you choose to reframe the issue by focusing on what contributes to mothers being on welfare in the first place: lack of employment opportunities, lack of education or training, inadequate day care, etc. (chap. 30, sect. 2, para. 4)

Develop a Public Identity

If you are too closely linked with a larger and better-known organization, the public may transfer its positive and negative image of the larger organization to your small group. Therefore, it's important to carve out your own identity and let the public know you are unique. For example, there are many breast health organizations in the U.S. that are funded by Susan G. Komen, a breast cancer foundation. In fact, it is possible to see at least two or three breast health organizations in the same community funded by this one foundation. Being affiliated with a big foundation such as this can have benefits, but also can have drawbacks. If your mission and objectives are not uniquely your own, people may have a hard time remembering your agency or assume it offers the same services as the funding source. Not only is it important to carve out your own niche, it will make you more effective in reaching your intended clientele. For example, perhaps your mission is similar to other breast health organizations in the area (i.e., to save lives), but what makes you distinct from others is that you serve primarily Latina women and offer events at local churches. Or, perhaps you are the only agency that provides prosthetics and wigs, while another agency provides mobile mammography. You're all similar enough to be working together toward your mission of saving lives, but unique in the services you offer and strategies you use to achieve this goal.

Know Your Facts

Understand your organization's issues and actions inside and out. This involves being able to quote a source of information or point to reliable statistics for claims you make publicly. Facts should guide your actions and public statements. If you are caught with inaccurate information or documentation, you could seriously damage your organization's reputation, embarrass yourself, and take attention away from important issues.

Keep It Simple

Small successes help build morale and sustain commitment to the issues. They don't always happen as a result of complex, super-involved actions. Offer simpler, short-term solutions that move toward a bigger solution: In other words, gradually build toward a greater complexity. For example, if a goal of your organization or program is to help orphans in Sierra Leone secure a better future, you could become paralyzed by all of the factors that impede this goal. Instead, begin with a needs assessment, identifying areas of priority. For example, what can your organization do in terms of providing some of the most basic needs for these children—such as shelter, food, medical care, or education? Perhaps your program can only focus on one of these based on your resources, or perhaps quite a few. Whether your budget is ample or lean, it is always important to develop simple, realistic, and measurable objectives that will help you chart your course.

Be Passionate and Persistent

As we mentioned earlier, advocacy is not for the faint of heart. However, persistence and passion are two tools that will help you fight the uphill battle. Solutions must be supported by the community, not just a few, and having passion and persistence will help others see the value of your work and become invested in your mission. Creativity, persistence, and passion fuel health advocacy, so it's important that you engage yourself and others in activities that will allow you to experience internal as well as external rewards so you have the momentum to proceed.

Be Prepared to Compromise

Building healthy communities sometimes calls for compromise with groups whose goals may not be identical to your own. Although you want to stay true to your vision, be open to alternative plans of action or compromises that, although not ideal, may get you closer to your goals. Here is another great example provided by the Community Toolbox (KU Work Group, 2018e):

Tobacco control advocates in San Francisco wanted to include bars in a policy to ban smoking in public places. The advocates realized a ban on smoking in bars was considered too extreme by the general public, and including bars in the list of targeted establishments would greatly decrease support for the ban. The advocates decided to drop bars from their list of places to target. This was perceived as a reasonable compromise by the public, and the ordinance passed. (chap. 30, sect. 2, para. 5)

Capitalize on Opportunity

Look for opportunities to promote your goals and seize them when they come along. This may involve lying in wait for an appropriate, "natural" time when you can capitalize on some event related to your objectives. For example, February, a time associated with love for others, may be the perfect time to spread the message of breast health with mothers, aunts, sisters, girlfriends, and other loved ones. Or perhaps a well-known celebrity recently announced she has been diagnosed with breast cancer—now that the media has captured people's attention, perhaps it's a great time to flood your community with messages about mammography, survival, and hope.

Stay the Course

Advocates have successfully gone head-to-head with some pretty powerful people, including politicians, CEOs of well-known businesses, and national lobbying organizations like the National Rifle Association. Facing such influential opponents can be daunting, especially when they have greater name recognition and more resources to oppose you. As an advocate for your community, you will have some credibility with the public—after all, you're fighting for their well-being, whether that means safer streets, decent jobs, cleaner air, or better access to medical care. The public will recognize this! The bottom line is this: If you are intimidated into inaction, your opponents will automatically win and nothing will change.

Look for the Good in Others

When you encounter members from groups that disagree with your goals or viewpoint, don't assume they are "out to get you" or ready to pick a fight. If an opponent criticizes your organization, begin by assuming the person doesn't have the same understanding that you do and is speaking out of a lack of information. Educate the opponent and the public about how they may be misinformed.

Keep Focused on the Goal

Opponents may try to distract you from your advocacy activities by attacking you personally. By responding to their name-calling, you waste precious energy and lessen your chances for future cooperation or compromise with these people. Also, your public image may suffer if the general public sees you involved in mudslinging. Instead of giving in to the temptation to fight back, stay focused on the really important issues at hand. Sometimes it may be necessary to respond to their attacks in order to maintain your credibility in the eyes of the public. When you do, make sure your defense or counter attack is well documented with facts and data to back you up.

Make Issues Local and Relevant

When you bring your issues to the local level, you increase your chances for public support. Issues become relevant to community members when they are close to home. For example, Mothers Against Drunk Driving (MADD) has been successful in many communities because many people know someone who has lost a child to an alcohol-related accident. Some ways to really bring issues home to people in your area include using local statistics for the issue, capitalizing on local role models like business people or volunteers, or presenting the issues in a certain way to help community members understand how they will be affected. The Community Toolbox (KU Work Group, 2018e) offers yet another perfect example:

> Imagine that your organization works to build self-esteem and create life options for local teenage mothers. Invite local business people to speak to your organization on how they are working to create more part-time employment for teens and suggest what kind of skills the employers would like future employees to obtain. Perhaps you can create a mentoring pool where professionals from your community would work with these young mothers to help them develop career goals. (chap. 30, sect. 2, para. 7)

Find Common Ground and Generate a Large Support Base

Sometimes it may seem as if becoming part of an advocacy movement automatically puts you in opposition to state and federal policies, politicians, community leaders, and private organizations. Even though there may be some differences between your group and key segments of the community, you may all be more or less working toward the same broad goals of promoting healthier communities. It's important to include people from "inside the system" in your advocacy efforts. This helps you not only widen your perspective on the issues, but it helps you identify "ins" with key agencies and people who can provide valuable support and clout to your efforts.

Tie Your Advocacy Group's Efforts to Related Events

Watch for events that might be relevant to your group's objectives or tactics. Linking to such events helps publicize your cause and strengthen your position in the community. For example, advocates wanting to increase public assistance to individuals who cannot pay for their electricity bill could link their cause to the recent death of a local man who died of heat exhaustion when he couldn't afford to fix his air conditioner.

≡ In Conclusion

Community health professionals must unite and advocate for important health issues. The power of many voices can make a difference in health outcomes. Advocacy is not a single activity. Knowledge, coalitions and partnerships, lobbying, grassroots activities, traditional and new media, and legislative activism are excellent advocacy tools. Be sure to employ the tips and guidelines for advocacy that other advocates have found to be useful.

REVIEW QUESTIONS

1. Define the advocacy terms presented in this chapter.

2. Compare four advocacy tools.

3. Describe topics you feel are important to cover in a training session for people who wish to visit a policy maker.

4. Select a health issue that you believe warrants advocacy. Research this issue and identify credible sources that represent contrasting viewpoints. Write a few paragraphs highlighting the important facts about your issue.

5. Prepare a phone script related to a health issue of your choice that you would use to contact your legislator's office. Deliver your message and reflect on whether or not your efforts were effective.

6. Identify a health issue that is not presented in the chapter but that you consider an important advocacy topic. Justify your choice.

FOR YOUR APPLICATION

Preparing for Advocacy

Select a health issue that you think warrants further advocacy in your state.

1. Collect some information about the issue.

2. Create a one-page fact sheet that you could give to other health educators who would be willing to join you in advocating for the issue.

3. Ask some of your classmates to comment on or make additions to your fact sheet.

Putting Advocacy into Practice

Select a health issue that warrants further advocacy or use the one that you selected in the previous activity.

1. Write a letter to one of your state legislators (preferably the individual from your home district) about your selected issue.

2. Use the tips provided in this chapter.

3. Ask your instructor to read your letter and provide feedback.

4. Revise your letter and send it to your legislator.

5. Include a copy in the Resource Access and Management section of your portfolio.

Making an Advocacy Resource List

Create an advocacy resource list that includes the names, titles, and contact numbers of individuals within your community who can publicize and garner support for certain health issues.

Planning a Social Media Strategy for Advocacy

Use Appendix C, "Planning a Social Media Strategy for Advocacy," to develop a social media strategy that enhances an advocacy campaign related to a health issue and organization of your choice.

13

Resource Access
and Management

You have just been hired as a health education specialist for a local community health center. One of your first assigned tasks is to develop a digital health clearinghouse that will provide local, national, and international educational resources to the residents in the county on a variety of health issues. Your job description uses the phrase, "serve as a community health resource person," to describe the overarching nature of your work. So, as a health professional, what does that mean? Are you expected to have an answer for everything? Health is so dynamic and wide-ranging that it's impossible to know everything, and to *think* you know everything is precarious. Perhaps what is most important as a resource person is to identify what you don't know and what sources to access for help.

Chapter Objectives

1. Describe what it means to be a resource person in a health setting.
2. Explore online sources of health information.
3. Discuss the importance of recruiting and maintaining volunteers as resources within health organizations.
4. Evaluate the credibility and quality of health information.
5. Analyze parameters of effective consultative relationships.
6. Explain why networking is a necessary skill to develop and maintain consultative relationships.
7. Provide examples of government agencies that serve as health resources.
8. Contrast health care and insurance terms.
9. Locate online sources of information using the Internet, library databases, and online journals.

What Does It Mean to Be a Resource Person?

Regardless of the health setting (i.e., school, hospital, state agency, nonprofit, or corporate), one of your responsibilities as a community health professional will be to know (a) how to get information, (b) where to find available services, and (c) who will be able to help in a given situation. A good resource person doesn't have to know everything but, rather, knows where to find information and services. In this chapter we discuss several types of resources, including people, computer and digital technologies, and organizations.

People as Resources

People are the world's most valuable resources. The wisdom, knowledge, and skills that a diverse group of individuals can bring to a project are considerable. We encourage you to explore and leverage the wealth of available human resources.

Health and Allied Health Professionals

Reaching out to other health professionals who may have the information, skills, or insights you are looking for is a practical first step. Chances are, you are already working inter-professionally and know several colleagues who could assist you. Although competencies, standards, credentialing, and training differ among the myriad of health occupations, there is a common goal that unites all health professions, which is to improve health and quality of life.

You can learn more about the wide variety of health professions on the U.S. Bureau of Labor and Statistics (BLS) Occupational Outlook Handbook website at http://www.bls.gov/ooh/. Exploring the occupations and reading the descriptions of each health profession will give you a better idea of the range of human resources and potential allies who can help support your work.

While it can be argued that all health professionals serve as resource persons in some capacity, there are a growing number of job titles and positions that focus largely on one's ability to help individuals locate, understand, and coordinate health information and resources. FYI 13.1 provides a few examples of job titles used to describe careers that focus on serving as a resource person in health as found on popular job search websites or professional organization's social networks.

13.1   Sample Job Titles for Health Resource Specialists

• Health educator	• Medical social worker
• Patient navigator	• Public health information specialist
• Community health worker	• Health information manager
• Health coach	• Medical librarian
• Patient support specialist	• Health communications specialist

Serving as a Health Resource Person

According to the National Commission for Health Education Credentialing (NCHEC, 2015), one of the primary responsibilities of a health education specialist is to serve as a "resource person." So what exactly does that mean? Below are just a few of the competencies associated with acting in the role of a community health resource person as outlined by NCHEC:

- Obtain and disseminate health-related information
- Assess needs for health-related information
- Identify valid information resources
- Evaluate resource materials for accuracy, relevance, and timeliness
- Adapt information for consumers

- Train others to use health education/promotion skills
- Assess training needs of potential participants
- Develop a plan for conducting training
- Conduct formative and summative evaluations of training
- Provide advice and consultation on health education/promotion issues
- Apply ethical principles in consultative relationships

Two of the authors of this book were reminded of the value of health professionals as resources recently when we sought specific information on the dollar value of lives saved through early detection of breast cancer. We searched the online databases and the Internet but could not find the specific information we needed. We mentioned the problem to one of our students, a radiology technician. She had the information we needed within five minutes. What an incredible resource we had without realizing it!

Another example we offer relates to serving as a resource person for the process of grant writing. In developing a community grant-funded program to increase breast cancer screening and follow-up care for uninsured or low-income Hispanic/Latina and African American women in Denton County, Texas, it was necessary for the director to collaborate with staff from a nearby clinic and medical practice. They would serve as the health care providers and interpret the screening results for the women participating in the free and reduced-cost mammogram services. Otherwise, the funding source would not award the grant. Ethically, it would not be responsible for an organization to offer free or low-cost mammograms without having a physician or other medical specialist review the results with the client and refer her to the appropriate treatment if needed. One could also argue that providing screenings without access to treatment is also inhumane.

The health education specialist in this example contacted the director of a local nonprofit health clinic that was funded by multiple grants and provided a number of medical services to low-income and uninsured persons in the county. The clinic's existing funding did not provide for culturally relevant breast health education services that would encourage more women in the community, especially those from ethnic minority backgrounds, to participate in early detection. It seemed like both sides could benefit from a partnership.

Consequently, the collaboration between the health education specialist and the director of the clinic was advantageous for all involved: the clinic director could connect patients to breast health information and mammography services offered through the health education specialist's grant-funded program and the health education specialist could offer women without a primary care physician an opportunity to receive the results and any follow-up referrals through the clinic; and uninsured or low-income minority women in the community would have access to a more comprehensive breast health program and potentially life-saving service (i.e., screening, follow up, and treatment). To be effective in your role as a community health professional, you must be resourceful enough to not only access general health information, but also to recognize other health professionals who might serve as allies in locating specific information or coordinating services. The old saying is true: Together everyone achieves more (TEAM)!

Volunteers

Almost any health-related agency for which you will work will depend on volunteers. In 1998, Penner and Finkelstein wrote, "If the trend toward fewer government services for disadvantaged and ill individuals continues, the need for unpaid volunteers will increase" (p. 525). Although decades have passed, the statement is still relative and timely given the political efforts in the U.S. to end the Affordable Care Act and replace it with something that reduces funding for Medicaid.

Lack of money to purchase health care coupled with societal forces and sociodemographic factors limit the ability of many individuals and families to achieve and maintain adequate health status" (Beardain & Grantham, 1993, p. 2). Volunteers, including formally trained health professionals and non-degreed lay individuals, help increase the volume of health-related services provided by community programs (Penner & Finkelstein, 1998). Moreover, they may be the only hope for some agencies to make a difference in the health status of people in their community.

There are many reasons beyond financial savings to utilize volunteers. The more connected to a community people feel, the more likely they are to take responsibility for the community and engage themselves in its growth and overall health. Mobilizing community resources and expanding capacity through volunteers may also enhance an organization's general profile, which can attract more volunteers, participants, and funding.

As noted in *Successful Strategies for Recruiting, Training, and Utilizing Volunteers*, a manual compiled by the U.S. Department of Health and Human Services (2004), other potential benefits of using volunteers include the following:

- An increased ability to serve clients and respond to the needs of the community (e.g., increased services, expanded hours of operation, shorter wait times)
- Greater staff diversity (e.g., age, race, social background, income, education)
- Increased skill set (volunteers have a diverse array of talents)
- Expanded community support
- Networking that may lead to greater resources and cost savings for the organization

Sometimes the magnitude of dismal news in the media gives the impression that few people choose to be helpful and giving. However, volunteerism is alive and well in this country. According to a report from the Bureau of Labor Statistics (BLS, 2016), almost 63 million people volunteered for an organization between September 2014 and September 2015, with the adult volunteer rate holding steady at approximately 25%. This included a median of 52 hours of service by each volunteer annually during this period, with increasing hours spent by those 65 and older.

It is also important to note *who* volunteers. The demographic profile of volunteers indicates that more women than men volunteer, approximately 28% versus 22% (BLS, 2016). People with higher education also volunteer at a greater rate, reaching almost 39% for college graduates, compared to 27% for persons with some college or an associate's degree, and 16% for high school graduates. Among age groups, persons 35 to 54 were most likely to volunteer (less than 28%). Finally, married persons volunteered at a higher rate (29%) in 2015 than those who had never married (20%) or indicated "Other" status. (BLS, 2016). See FYI 13.2 for additional details.

13.2   Who Volunteers in America?

• About 63 million people in the U.S. volunteer annually (almost 20% the U.S. population).

• Volunteers donate an average of 52 hours of time a year.

• About 28% of women volunteer compared to 22% of men.

• People 35 to 54 years old are most likely to volunteer, while individuals ages 20 to 24 have the lowest volunteer rates.

• More married persons (29%) volunteer at a greater rate compared to those non-married (20%).

People with higher education also volunteer at a greater rate, reaching almost 39% for college graduates, compared to 27% for persons with some college or an associate's degree, and 16% for high school graduates

• Volunteers are most likely to work with religious groups, and with youth or community service organizations

• The most common volunteer activities performed are preparing food, teaching, coaching, and general labor.

Source: *Volunteering in the United States—2015*, Bureau of Labor Statistics, U.S. Department of Labor. Press Release: Thursday, February 25, 2016. USDL-16-0363.

To successfully recruit and retain volunteers, it is important to know *why* people volunteer. People volunteer for various reasons and are attracted to different kinds of organizations. Some of the reasons people give for choosing to volunteer include personal satisfaction, professional responsibility, perceived community need, desire to help others (Ward, 1998); commitment to service, business networking, career development (Ellis, 1993); recreation, a desire to make friends (Glascoff, Baker, & Glascoff, 1997); and recognition.

In addition, people are often attracted to specific organizations for volunteer opportunities. Religious organizations attract many volunteers (33%), followed by educational/youth services organizations (25%), and finally community or social service organizations (15%) (BLS, 2016).

Moreover, volunteers have broadly reported serving in distinct activities. Preparing and serving food was cited often: 11% of volunteers reported this as their main activity. Teaching, tutoring, and coaching were also popular at approximately 9%, as well as general labor. Participation rates in these activities reflected gender and educational differences. Volunteers with higher education worked more often as tutors or mentors, while persons with less education were more involved with food service or general labor. Male volunteers were most likely to engage in general labor (12%) or supervise sports teams (9%). Those who identified themselves as female were more likely to collect, prepare, distribute, or serve food (13%); tutor or teach (11%); or fund raise (10%) (BLS, 2016). This data is helpful to those developing plans for recruiting and retaining volunteers.

If, in the future, you need volunteers in your work, we encourage you to tailor recruitment and retention efforts for specific types of individuals. Creating an environment where volunteers can make a difference in health status requires more than just providing an opportunity to volunteer. A comprehensive understanding of why people volunteer, what barriers prevent them from volunteering, and what keeps them motivated to continue to volunteer may improve the volunteer experience and have a powerful impact on the effectiveness of volunteer services. Volunteers will also need training and development opportunities. We hope you will accept the challenge of maximizing your volunteer resources through a respectful understanding of them as individuals. Some helpful tips for recruiting and working with volunteers are listed in FYIs 13.3 and 13.4 (on the next page).

Consultants

Consultants, people you hire to assist with a specific project or program, can offer a combination of five abilities: expertise, perspective, authenticity, friendship, and accomplishment (Bellman, 1990). Let's discuss these abilities in a little more detail.

FYI

13.3   Strategies for Recruiting Volunteers

- Contact your local volunteer center.
- Use current volunteers—they are convincing salespeople because they are dedicated to your cause and believe in your organization.
- Use the mass media (e.g., television, radio, the Internet, newspapers, billboards), as well as neighborhood newspapers, newsletters, and organizational bulletins.
- Make announcements at services, educational sessions, meetings, and social gatherings of your congregation or organization.
- Post volunteer opportunities on appropriate websites.
- Make personal appearances at schools, senior centers, career fairs, and community events.
- Generate personal interest stories based on volunteer experiences.
- Staff booths and exhibits at special events.
- Use mass mailings or personalized, handwritten notes.
- Get referrals from staff, ministers, friends, and lay leaders.
- Register with volunteer referral organizations.
- Volunteer in other organizations' projects.
- Collaborate with schools that require community service hours for graduation.
- Ask people to volunteer; most people volunteer because they are asked.
- Create print materials such as flyers and brochures about your organization and include descriptions of the volunteer opportunities available.

Source: *Successful Strategies for Recruiting, Training, and Utilizing Volunteers: A Guide for Faith- and Community-Based Service Providers* [online manual], U.S. Department of Health and Human Services, 2004.

13.4   How to Write a Volunteer Position Statement

If your agency, company, or organization depends largely upon volunteers, you may be asked to recruit them. As part of this task, you may need to develop descriptions of the volunteer position. Some things to consider when developing a written description are outlined below:

1. **Position Title**

   A specific, descriptive title provides the volunteer with a sense of identity and ensures that salaried staff and other volunteers understand this particular role. Steer away from descriptions that have to do with the presence of lack of pay. For example, why call the receptionist a "volunteer" receptionist? You don't say "paid" receptionist for a staff member.

2. **Work Location**

   Where will the individual be working? Can the work be done at home or only on site, or at a particular site? Make sure that there is public transportation near your work site so you can recruit people who might not have their own transportation.

3. **Purpose of the Position**

   How will the volunteer's work affect the project's outcome, clients, or mission? It is important to identify the expected impact for both direct service and administrative assignments so that volunteers will understand how important their work is.

4. **Responsibilities and Duties**

   Specifically identify the volunteer position's responsibilities and duties. Define what is expected from the volunteer.

5. **Qualifications**

   It pays to be clear and concrete in listing qualifications for any volunteer position. Include education, personal characteristics, skills, abilities and/or experience required.

6. **Commitment Expected**

   What do you expect of the volunteer? Include length of service, hours per week, hours per day. Include any special requirements such as weekend work.

7. **Training**

   List what training the volunteer will receive. Include general training that all positions receive plus any position-specific training for this assignment.

8. **Other**

   Include the date the description was written or the date that it was updated. List the volunteer supervisor's name and his/her contact information. Include information about how to get more information and who to call if interested. You might want to include signature lines for the volunteer manager and the site supervisor if appropriate.

Source: *Successful Strategies for Recruiting, Training, and Utilizing Volunteers: A Guide for Faith- and Community-Based Service Providers* [online manual], U.S. Department of Health and Human Services, 2004.

EXPERTISE

This ability pertains to a special knowledge or skill. You might, for example, want to hire a consultant to help you evaluate a specific program. According to Bellman (1990, p. 129), you may want to use a consultant's expertise for one or more reasons:

1. You may not have the knowledge and skills yourself.
2. You may have the knowledge and skills but not the time.
3. You may not be in the right position to do the work.
4. You may not want to do the work yourself.

Be honest with consultants about why you are hiring them. If you happen to be serving as a consultant yourself, be sure to find out why you are being hired.

PERSPECTIVE

This ability involves seeing the world in a new way, or bringing a fresh perspective to a situation. Sometimes, an organization or program isn't running smoothly because an individual or individuals are not performing as they should. For example, your authors were helping public health personnel access information and found that they rarely used the Internet as a tool. We made the assumption that they lacked the skills to use the Internet. According to Bellman (1990, p. 131), however, the lack of performance isn't usually lack of skills, as normally perceived by supervisors, but instead faulty perceptions about the use of skills. For example, such people:

- see the situation in a way that precludes using the skills that would be appropriate to the situation.
- don't understand that the skills might be necessary.
- are scared to use the skills they have because of perceived consequences.
- don't want to use their skills because they think it would be inappropriate.
- don't know when to use their skills because no one has indicated that the skills are needed.
- suffer in some way when they use their skills.

In our case, the individuals with whom we were working mistakenly believed that they were not allowed to use the Internet. Whether your organization needs a new perspective or requires help in pinpointing a lack of training, a consultant can assist.

AUTHENTICITY

A consultant can help people in an agency recognize the true nature of the organization. The previous section talked about seeing the world in a new way, but authenticity is "seeing" reality. The consultant must be personally authentic (know and understand self) in order to add this dimension to the consulting process.

FRIENDSHIP

Bellman (1990) notes that characteristics we expect from our friends are the same characteristics we should expect in a consulting relationship:

- We want friends to be honest.
- We expect our friends to allow us to take responsible risks.

- We want to be able to talk about what is important to us with our friends and to be taken seriously.

- We want to accomplish things, reach goals shoulder to shoulder, and enjoy our accomplishments with our friends.

- We want be able to talk with friends about concerns, knowing that they will be supportive.

Although friendship might seem out of place in a business relationship, the elements of friendship we have listed are necessary to honest appraisal and true teamwork.

ACCOMPLISHMENT

The normal expectation from a consulting relationship is that results will be achieved. Obviously, results are the bottom line for hiring a consultant. We caution you, however, to be careful in the way you define *results*. Sometimes we have personal agendas for accomplishments that are not based in reality. For example, if you hire someone to help you evaluate a program, you cannot demand that the results show the program in a completely positive light. Accomplishment in this case is gaining information that will help you improve your program. You might also want to think in terms of small successes, much like advocacy work. Give yourself and your programs credit for the process of improvement, not just the final outcome.

The costs associated with hiring a consultant need to be considered. Yet, in cases where you are "stuck" due to overwork, lack of skills, or inability to gain perspective, the benefits of hiring a consultant may far outweigh the costs. A good consultant can save a program or project.

Currently, there is very little research published about the opportunities or trends in consulting within the field of community health. As the health care system continues to evolve, with increasing emphasis on prevention and on program accountability and sustainability, the opportunities for consulting should multiply.

Networking

Do you hear people talking about networking but still wonder what it involves? Networking is an important tool for serving as a community health resource person. Look at Figure 13.1 and you will see the potential connections generated through meeting and getting to know people. For example, if you meet and share information with person A, you have the potential of gaining resources from persons A, B, C, and E. Person A knows and talks with B, C, and E; and if you ask, he or she will most likely be willing to pass along your name, needs, or skills. Networking can take you even further because each individual knows other individuals. The key to networking is that you place yourself in situations where you can meet and talk with other professionals. You must be willing to discuss your needs as well as those skills you are willing to share with others. Professional conferences, workshops, and other professional development activities are good places to start networking.

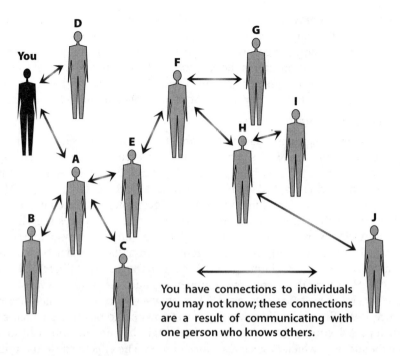

You have connections to individuals you may not know; these connections are a result of communicating with one person who knows others.

Figure 13.1　Networking.
Networking is a key factor when you are serving as a resource person and when you are seeking resources. Communicating with a couple of key individuals could be of great benefit to you and your agency.

Computers as Resources

Technology is a powerful tool for acquiring and sharing health information. Through the click of a button, people from any side of the world can now access health information 24 hours a day, 7 days a week on the Internet. Acting as a health-related resource person requires you to possess the computer skills necessary to not only search and find health information through the Internet, but to be able to determine its accuracy and credibility. Some commonly used terms and strategies for sharing and evaluating online health information are discussed next.

Search Tools

WEB BROWSER

A Web **browser** is software that helps you view the World Wide Web on your computer. Popular Web browsers include: Firefox (Mozilla); Internet Explorer (Microsoft); Chrome (Google), and Safari (Mac). Full-screen browsers display only text on the screen. The others show text and graphics and provide other services. As a World Wide Web (e.g., Internet) user, you travel from one **Uniform Resource Locator** (URL) to another using a browser. The URL is a Web address, and knowing this can connect you to health information instantly. Online resources that support community health abound. However, you need to make sure that the information you choose is indeed factual (see the discussion later in the chapter), and you can expect to get frustrated over the plethora of addresses, types of sites, and contradictory information. You probably have a favorite search tool; if not, try one of those mentioned in the following paragraphs.

SEARCH ENGINES

A **search engine** is a database created by software that searches the Web for titles and phrases. In other words, when you initiate a search using a search engine, you are not searching the Web itself but, rather, the search engine database. Without sophisticated search engines and without knowing a specific URL, it would be virtually impossible to locate anything on the Web. The numerous search engines all have similarities, but they differ in size and in the types of Web pages they list. Some of the most well-known search engines are Google (http://www.google.com) and Bing (http://www.bing.com). Google currently dominates all other search engines in the United States market, claiming 65.6% of the market share ("Share of Search Queries," 2018). However, there are other competitors such as Bing (www.bing.com), owned and operated by Microsoft, and Yahoo (www.yahoo.com), which has been around since 1994. Search engines that require site owners to pay to have their sites indexed, such as Ask.com, index fewer pages. Although they are all similar in ways, you must be the judge of which best serves your purpose. The effectiveness and utility of search engines depends largely upon the information you seek. FYI 13.5 provides a list of search engines that you may want to explore further.

A **meta-search engine** allows you to enter a query and search multiple search engines and their databases of Web pages simultaneously. Meta-search engines can speed up your ability to find credible, relevant information rather than sift through everything you might find from a search engine such as Google. Within a few seconds, you get results from all the search engines. Examples of meta-search engines include DeeperWeb (http://www.deeperweb.com), Dogpile (http://www.dogpile.com), Ehealthcarebot (www.ehealthcarebot.com) and PubMed (http://www.ncbi.nlm.nih.gov/pubmed). Some additional meta-search engines that are useful to health professionals are below in FYI 13.5.

DIRECTORIES

Although the terms *search engine* and *directory* are often used interchangeably, they are not the same thing. A **directory** is a database that usually organizes websites by topic and is managed by humans, unlike a search engine, which uses software (Kennedy, 1999). Websites are categorized by subject, date, and even format. Some well-known directories are YouTube (http://www.youtube.com), About.com (http://www.about.com), and LookSmart (http://www.looksmart.com). In early 2006, YouTube emerged as one of the ten most popular websites on the Internet (Burke, Snyder, & Rager, 2009). The world's largest online video directory, YouTube, gives individuals the ability to watch homemade and professionally produced video clips or upload their own video content to share on a wide range of topics. FYI 13.5 includes a listing of popular search engines and health directories. We encourage you to try them all and compare your results.

13.5 Popular Internet Search Engines and Health Directories	
Search Engines	**Health-Related Directories**
Google https://www.google.com/	Science Direct http://www.sciencedirect.com/
Bing https://www.bing.com/	Google Scholar http://scholar.google.com/
Yahoo https://www.yahoo.com/	Health6.com http://www.health6.com/
Dog Pile http://www.dogpile.com/	Healthfinder https://healthfinder.gov/
AOL Search http://www.aolsearch.com/	National Institutes of Health Library https://nihlibrary.nih.gov/
Hotbot http://www.hotbot.com/	Health.gov https://health.gov/
DeeperWeb http://www.deeperweb.com/	HealthData.gov http://www.healthdata.gov/
	CDC Wonder http://wonder.cdc.gov/
	Highlight Health http://www.highlighthealth.info/
	Medlineplus https://medlineplus.gov/
	Public Library of Science Medicine http://journals.plos.org/plosmedicine/
	Web MD http://www.webmd.com/
	Web of Science http://www.webofknowledge.com/

INTELLIGENT SOFTWARE AGENTS

An **intelligent software agent** (i.e., "agents" or "intelligent agents") is a software tool that you can download to your computer that will help you find information on the Internet in less time (Sullivan, 2005). These agents will automatically do certain jobs on the Internet according to what you ask them to do. For example, a search agent will send your search question to all of the best ranked search engines simultaneously and rank the results so you quickly find what you need. There are agents that speed up your computer downloads, ones that remove ads from your computer screen or block "pop up" advertising or "spyware." Search agents are commonly used to sort your e-mail or scan it for spam or junk mail. There are also **data mining agents** that will find trends and patterns in an abundance of information from many different sources. So, for example, if you were looking for particular news articles on a certain topic or for the most relative foundations that provide grants on a particular issue, a data mining agent could assist. It's also not hard to find examples specific to public health and health care. Take, for instance, the Agency for Healthcare Research and Quality (AHRQ). AHRQ is helping patients and their doctors find answers to health-related questions by pioneering innovative ways to gather and analyze multiple sources of health care data for evidence about what care works. According to a AHRQ brief, "This 'mining of health data' has already led to practice changes that, for example, have reduced repeat knee replacement surgery among seniors and enabled children with inflammatory bowel disease to play with their friends three times as many days each month" (AHRQ, 2015a, para. 1). Data mining can help individuals locate and sort information that improves health decision making, makes personalized health care possible, and improves efficiency which leads to cost savings.

LISTSERV

A **Listserv** is an e-mail discussion group or mailing list that is bound by a common interest. Although not as popular today as they once were, they still continue to be used because of their ease. Transcripts of a Listserv can be saved and the archives can be reviewed. An example of a Listserv relating to health is the **HEDIR** (Health Education Directory) that was developed and copyrighted by Dr. Mark J. Kittleson. In addition to sharing messages, a Listserv could be a portal for sharing health information and ideas with your peers. For example, are you interested in finding out how many health education specialists work in school settings versus corporations? Or, perhaps you'd like to discuss the current Master Certified Health Education Specialist (MCHES) requirements? The HEDIR Listserv could be a valuable medium for collecting this information in a short span of time, particularly if some of the intended audience is not using social media.

Online Communities of Practice (OCPs)

Online communities of practice provide a critical resource to health professionals who want and need recommendations, pointers, tips and tricks, best practices, or insights and innovations. Part of what makes a community practice effective is the aggregation of relevant and credible knowledge; that is, people and information related to a coherent set of topics which certain people will find interesting, useful, and potentially profitable. Online communities of practice are usually moderated and facilitated through technology and easy to access for those seeking to connect to others in their profession or interested in a particular issue. Some OCPs require memberships or subscriptions. For example, some professional organizations, such as the American Public Health Association (http://www.apha.org), offer a wide variety of OCPs to members on a variety of topics, from asthma to vision care.

Online Databases for Peer-Reviewed Literature

Don't forget about professional and peer-reviewed journals when you are seeking information. Sometimes the ease of gathering information electronically makes seeking and reading professional journals less attractive. However, as you will learn in a later section of this chapter, the information you collect should be verified through research. Because peer-reviewed journals are generally the means by which research is disseminated, it is vitally important that you stay abreast of what they report.

Locating professional articles has become as simple as searching the Web. Large databases that archive articles and abstracts exist for most professions. For example, Medline is a database compiled by the U.S. National Library of Medicine that archives articles and abstracts from approximately 5,630 medical journals. Other databases that health education specialists might find useful include CINAHL (the Cumulative Index to Nursing and Allied Health Literature), Psychlit (psychology-related journals), and ERIC (educational journals). Most databases for professional journals can be accessed via the Internet, but we suggest that you visit your university library and speak with a reference librarian to gain more information. Or, you may want to attend a library workshop on database searching or tour your library's Web pages to learn more about searching the databases available to you. There are more than you can imagine.

There are also growing numbers of online health-related professional journals; some of the most popular peer-reviewed periodicals relating to community health are:

- *Journal of Community Health*
- *American Journal of Health Education*
- *Journal of Family and Community Health*
- *American Journal of Public Health*
- *Health Promotion Practice*
- *Journal of School Health*
- *The International Electronic Journal of Health Education*
- *The Internet Journal of Allied Health Sciences and Practice*
- *Pedagogy of Health Promotion*
- *Journal of Community Health Nursing*

More than likely, you will have access to these journals through your university library. In fact, your library may actually have a directory of all electronic journals related to health as well as other subjects. As with hard-copy journals, electronic journals also require subscriptions, and there is a schedule for publication. Although you have the option of printing a hard copy of a journal article if necessary, you will not have to store or dispose of a pile of journals. This plays a small but important role in preserving the environment in which we live.

Web 2.0 and Web 3.0 Technology

The Internet has rapidly evolved over the two decades, making it easier for people to share information quickly and with tools that allow for more personalization. This evolution of user capabilities and creativity is often referred to as "**Web 2.0.**" The number 2 does not denote a "second version" of the Internet but rather a second generation of Internet tools and communities (O'Reilly, 2005) that make it easier to interact and create. Blogs, wikis, podcasts, and mobile apps, are just a few examples of Web 2.0 technology that can be sources of health information. The technology of today is now moving toward "**Web 3.0**," which provides capabilities for more tailored web searches and uses artificial intelligence agents (think Siri and Alexa) to get context from the user and provide an individual with the most useful information.

BLOGS

As defined by *Webster's New Millennium Dictionary of English* (2007), a **blog** is a frequently updated online diary or personal chronological log of thoughts published on a Web page. Blogs are typically published by individuals, and their style is personal and informal. Anybody with an Internet connection can publish his or her own blog. Blogging has evolved from its origins as a medium for the online publication of personal diaries to a respected vehicle for editorials on specific topics including social, economic, and political issues (Oomen-Early & Burke, 2007). The quality, content, and ambition of blogs varies greatly, and they may have anywhere from a handful to tens of thousands of daily readers (Lenhart & Fox, 2006). Some blogs are explicitly or implicitly fictional, though the standard genre expectation, particularly for health and education-based sites, is nonfiction. (Educause Learning Initiative, 2005; Lenhart & Fox, 2006).

In 2016, over 18 million people worldwide were publishing blogs on either blog websites or through their social media (Liubarets, 2016). Blogs have become a popular information channel for health consumers. In fact, according to a survey conducted by the American Press Institute in 2014, almost 47% percent of Americans access blogs as an information source along with other channels such as TV, radio, print newspapers and magazines, etc. (American Press Institute, 2014). You may even be hosting your own blog on a popular blog site such as Wordpress, Blogger, or LiveJournal. In addition to providing opportunities for personal expression, blogs are an effective strategy for delivering health information, connecting health professionals, raising social conscience, and advocating for the field and specific health issues (Oomen-Early & Burke, 2007).

WIKIS

The term *Wiki* is a Hawaiian term meaning "super fast" (Tonkin, 2006). A **Wiki** is a piece of server software that allows users to freely create and edit Web page content using any Web browser. According to the original creator, Ward Cunningham, "a Wiki is the simplest online database that could possibly work" (Tonkin, 2006, p. 43). Wikis support hyperlinks and have a simple text syntax for creating new pages and cross-links between internal pages that are user-friendly. A Wiki is unique compared to other collaborative communication mechanisms in that it allows all users to contribute and edit the content (Tonkin, 2006). Wikis can be used for such things as sharing helpful websites on specific topics (also called webliographies); comparing fieldwork notes; presenting and reviewing favorite articles, pictures, or papers within groups; collecting peer feedback; scheduling events or appointments; and a multitude of other tasks. Like many simple concepts, "open editing" has some profound and subtle effects on Wiki usage. "Allowing everyday users to create and edit any page in a Web site is exciting in that it encourages democratic use of the Web and promotes content composition by nontechnical users" (Herman, 2005, para. 2). The most widely used Wiki to date is **Wikipedia** (see FYI 13.6). One of the disadvantages of using Wikis to find or present health information is that you do not always know who is authoring or editing a Wiki; therefore, you cannot guarantee that the information you find is accurate or unbiased.

13.6   Wikipedia: The Online Encyclopedia

Wikipedia is an online encyclopedia that can be edited by anyone. It was based on Nupedia, an earlier prototype by Jimmy Wales. Larry Sanger built upon Wales' ideas and launched Wikipedia on January 15, 2001. The concept behind Wikipedia was to establish a free, "living" encyclopedia that could quickly build upon global knowledge and perspectives (Wikipedia: Size Comparisons, n.d., para. 2). Information is therefore accessible and "controlled" by anyone and everyone. Wikipedia includes over 5 million articles, with over 38 million pages, and it is published in 250 languages. The English Wikipedia gains a steady 1,700 articles a day, and the wikipedia.org domain name ranked as one of the busiest on the Internet (Wikipedia: Size Comparisons, n.d., para. 3).

Wikipedia continues to garner visibility by the press and has steadily gained some acceptance as a secondary source. In fact, in 2005, a British science journal, Nature, published results from a content analysis and argued that Wikipedia was as accurate on entries related to science as the Encyclopedia Britannica (Giles, 2005). However, even though credibility of Wikipedia is growing as its quality assurance and fact checking improves, people should still be cautious in using it as a sole source of information. The fact that it is an "open source" means that it is only as credible as the authors who contribute to it. In fact, some critics of Wikipedia have called it "garbage, an incoherent hodge-podge of dubious factoids that adds up to something far less than the sum of its parts" (Orlowski, 2005). In fact, co-founder Larry Sanger, who is no longer a part of Wikipedia, has openly urged former colleague Wales to seek more "established sources of expertise" (Orlowski, 2005, para. 2).

Wikipedia also acknowledges its need for improvement on its own website. "Many of the articles are of poor quality and some mainstream encyclopedia topics are not covered adequately. The average article length is only a little over half the size of that in Encyclopedia Britannica. When searching for health information, you might consider Wikipedia as a first stop or springboard to lead you to other sources or ideas on the topic. As with any source, it is always important to think critically about what is presented and be judicious in the application of this information based on its apparent credibility and accuracy.

Sources: "Internet Encyclopedias Go Head to Head: Jimmy Wales' Wikipedia Comes Close to Britannica in Terms of the Accuracy of Its Science Entries," by J. Giles, 2005, Nature 438(7070): 900–1; "Wikipedia Day: 15 Interesting Facts You Didn't Know about the Online Encyclopedia," (n.a.), 2006, International Business Times. Retrieved from http://www.ibtimes.co.uk/wikipedia-day-15-interesting-facts-you-didnt-know-about-online-encyclopedia-1538018; "Wikipedia Founder Admits to Serious Quality Problems," by A. Orlowski, 2005 [Newsbrief], The Register. Retrieved from http://www.theregister.co.uk/2005/10/18/wikipedia_quality_problem; "Wikipedia: Size Comparisons," (n.d.). Retrieved from http://en.wikipedia.org/wiki/Wikipedia:Size.comparisons.

PODCASTS

A **podcast** is an audio broadcast that has been converted to a file type called *MP3* or other audio file format for playback in a digital music player or computer. The "pod" in podcast was coined from iPod, the predominant portable, digital music player by Apple on which the podcasts can be downloaded and played. Podcasts are not just limited to MP3 players or iPods, however. You can listen to a podcast from your computer by accessing them through a website or a mobile app such as iTunes, iTunes U, the App Store (on Apple devices), Google Play, or open sources such as the Internet Archive (http://archive.org) or Ted Radio Hour on NPR (http://www.npr.org/programs/ted-radio-hour).

A podcast is distinguished from other digital media formats by its ability to be syndicated, subscribed to, and downloaded automatically when new content is added (PCMag.com, n.d.). Podcasting has become a popular medium for presenting information because of its immediacy, archiving capabilities, and ability to reach a global audience. For example, the National Institutes of Health (NIH) uses podcasting to disseminate health information. Individuals can subscribe to NIH Radio and receive free podcasts on a variety of health presentations by some of the nation's leaders in health. You can browse the NIH Radio archives and listen to a variety of podcasts by visiting https://www.nih.gov/allofus-research-program/podcasts or downloading their mobile app.

MOBILE APPLICATIONS

According to the World Health Organization (2011), the use of mobile and wireless technologies (mHealth) to support the achievement of health objectives has the potential to transform the face of health education and service delivery across the globe. A **mobile app** is a software application designed to run on mobile devices such as smartphones and tablet computers. You actually might be reading this text through some kind of mobile app. The use of mobile health-related apps is becoming increasingly popular.

The ability to download health and medical apps on mobile devices has made a wealth of mobile resources available to health professionals. Health promotion and medical apps for many purposes have been developed, including ones for weight loss, tracking physical activity, electronic prescribing, diagnosis and treatment, practice management, coding and billing, and health education. A broad choice of apps that assist with answering clinical practice and other questions at the point of care exist, such as: drug reference guides; medical calculators; clinical guidelines; and other decision support aids, textbooks, and literature search portals (Ventola, 2014). There are even mobile apps that simulate surgical procedures or that can conduct simple medical exams, such as blood pressure monitoring, hearing, or vision tests.

WEBINARS AND WEBCASTS

A **webinar** is a seminar broadcasted on the Internet that may be interactive. It can contain both audio and video elements. Webinars connect people synchronously and are superior to teleconferencing in that participants can be anywhere on the planet and participate in the presentation. Presenters have the ability to use presentation slide shows, videos, or links to places on the Internet while facilitating the webinar. GoToMeeting, Adobe Connect, Zoom, Google Hangouts, and Skype are just a few of the synchronous platforms that currently offer the ability to connect live with large or small groups. Webinars may be archived to be viewed later, at which time they may become webcasts. **Webcasts** differ from webinars in that data is transmitted one way and does not allow interaction between the presenter and the audience. Webinars and webcasts are powerful tools for health professionals because they can connect people from all points of the globe and serve a multitude of purposes, including training, simulations, focus groups, meetings, lectures, and press conferences.

Analyzing Computer Resources

Think about a time when you used information from the Internet for a paper or other class assignment. How did you know that the information you used was accurate, objective, and appropriate? Did the author or authors seem credible? Was the content thorough? The Internet provides massive amounts of information, but, unfortunately, some of the easiest Internet sources to access don't provide reliable, unbiased information. You may recall that the issue of "fake news" was of significant concern in the 2016 U.S. presidential election (and still is). Discerning fact from fiction and communicating credible information are critical skills that impact the health of individuals and populations locally and globally. There are actually five categories to consider when analyzing a source of information: accuracy, authority, objectivity, currency, and coverage. FYI 13.7 provides guidelines for analyzing your computer sources of information.

13.7   Five Criteria for Evaluating Web-Based Content

Evaluation of Web documents	How to interpret the basics
1. Accuracy • Who wrote the page and can you contact him or her? • What is the purpose of the document and why was it produced? • Is this person qualified to write this document? • Is the information reliable and error free?	• Make sure the author provides e-mail or a contact address/phone number. • Know the distinction between author and Webmaster.

2. Authority
 • Is there an author listed?
 • Who published the document and is this entity separate from the "Webmaster"?
 • Check the domain of the document. What institution publishes this document?
 • Is the author qualified? An expert?
 • Does the author list his or her qualifications?
	• If the page includes neither a signature nor indicates a sponsor, is there any other way to determine its origin?
	   + Look for a header or footer showing affiliation.
	   + Look at the URL: http://www.fbi.gov
	   + Look at the domain: .edu, .com, .ac.uk, .org, .net
	 • What credentials are listed for the authors?
	 • Where is the document published? Check URL domain.

3. Objectivity • What goals/objectives does this page meet? • How detailed is the information? • What opinions (if any) are expressed by the author? • Does the information show a minimum of bias? • Is the page designed to sway opinion? • Is there any advertising on the page?	• Determine if the page is a mask for advertising; if so, information might be biased. • View any Web page as you would an infomercial on television. Ask yourself why was this written and for whom?

(continued)

Evaluation of Web documents	How to interpret the basics
4. Currency • When was it produced? Is there a date listed? • When was it updated? • How up-to-date are the links (if any)? • Have some expired or moved?	• How many dead links are on the page? • Are the links current or updated regularly? • Is the information on the page outdated?
5. Coverage • What topics are covered? • What does this page offer that is not found elsewhere? • How in-depth is the material? • Are the links (if any) evaluated and do they complement the documents' theme? • Is it all images or a balance of text and images? • Is the information presented cited correctly?	• If the page requires special software to view the information, how much are you missing if you don't have the software? • Is it free or is there a fee to obtain the information? • Is there an option for text only, or frames, or a suggested browser for better viewing?

Putting It All Together

Accuracy—If a Web page lists the author and institution that published the page and provides a way of contacting him/her and . . .

Authority—If the page lists the author credentials and its domain is preferred (.edu, .gov, .org, or .net), and . . .

Objectivity—If the page provides accurate information with limited advertising and it is objective in presenting the information, and . . .

Currency—If the page is current and updated regularly (as stated on the page) and the links (if any) are also up-to-date, and . . .

Coverage—If you can view the information properly—not limited to fees, browser technology, or software requirement, then . . .

From "Evaluation Criteria," *The Good, The Bad & The Ugly: Or, Why It's a Good Idea to Evaluate Web Sources* [online presentation], by Susan E. Beck, 1997. Retrieved from http://lib.nmsu.edu/instruction/eval.html. Used with permission of the author.

ACCURACY

The term **accuracy** refers to the correctness of the information. We can all agree that you need to present the most accurate information possible. If you are a member of HEDIR (the Listserv mentioned earlier), you have read discussions about **urban myths**. These myths are anecdotes and supposed facts that are widely disseminated but have no accuracy. An example of such a myth is the claim that antiperspirants cause cancer. The assertion sounds somewhat plausible. You might read that an antiperspirant can block sweat glands and, further, that a blocked sweat gland might result in cellular changes that, in turn, could possibly result in cancer. Despite the apparent plausibility of the claim, however, current research does not document a relationship between antiperspirants and cancer.

Unfortunately, much online information is presented as fact, even though it has no empirical basis. Empirical research would involve an experimental study design. Recall from chapter 3 that an experimental design is a type of research study that uses at least two groups of subjects, one for the intervention and another for comparison. When you present information, be sure to identify the experimental studies that document what you are saying.

Sometimes research alone isn't enough to document the accuracy of information because of the presence of bias or flaws in some research designs. In cases like these, it may be wise to check the opinions of experts in the field to verify information you are presenting. To find expert opinion, check the databases for peer-reviewed journals; experts will have published articles on their area of concentration.

AUTHORITY

When evaluating online content, one must also question the authority who is sponsoring the information. For example, is the website produced by a pharmaceutical company? A physician? A governmental organization like the Centers for Disease Control? An angry blogger? Would your reaction to the information be different if you knew the document was written from the perspective of one of these? Knowing who is generating the information will allow you to put what you are reading into proper context and consider the bias or objectivity in delivery of the content. When examining the authority of a Web page or website, consider such things as its domain (e.g., .org, .edu, or .com); the credentials of the author(s); headers or footers that provide information about the sponsoring agency; and where the document or website is published (i.e., China, U.S., the UK, etc.).

OBJECTIVITY

The **objectivity** of information can be determined by assessing its source. If the source presents two or more different perspectives accompanied by citations, it may be more appropriate than sources offering just one perspective. You can be more confident that the information is not based on one biased viewpoint. But look for evidence of bias if the source is a for-profit organization or is funded by an organization that wishes to propound a specific viewpoint.

CURRENCY

Currency of information is also important. You usually need the most timely information or enough background material for a historical perspective. Determine your specific needs, but make a deliberate decision about the time issue rather than accept information no matter when it was written.

COVERAGE

The **coverage** of information has to do with its depth. For example, the statement "Smoking causes health problems" has meaning by itself. It can be backed by research that is current and independent. It is not likely to be misconstrued even if it stands alone. Some statements need to be supported by additional information that is also accurate and appropriate in order to have meaning. For example, the statement "Herbal preparations can enhance health" does not stand alone. Many herbal preparations haven't even been studied. If you are discussing herbs, you will want to give supporting evidence. Frequently, it's difficult to determine the extent of coverage of a topic from a Web page. The page may or may not include links to other Web pages or print references that might provide the full picture of the issue. Sometimes Web information is "just for fun," a hoax, someone's personal expression that may be of interest to no one, or even outright silliness. It is up to you to make certain that the information is adequate either by itself or in combination with additional information.

EVALUATING PODCASTS, BLOGS, AND MOBILE APPS

As you know, websites are not the only sources of health information. As mentioned earlier, podcasts, blogs, and mobile apps can be helpful in disseminating health content. According to the American Heart Association (AHA), a number of clinical and quasi-experimental studies have reported that mobile apps can improve health outcomes and effectively enhance health education, simulations, screening, and monitoring (AHA, 2015). Apply the same standards mentioned in FYI 13.7 in reviewing the content contained in these sources and consider questions outlined in FYI 13.8–13.10 as well.

13.8   Questions to Ask When Evaluating Blogs

- Does the title of the blog provide information about its content?
- Is the purpose of the blog stated on the blog page?
- Is there a link to lead you to further information about the blog creator?
- Can you determine the credentials of the creator from the blog content?
- If you conduct a search on the creator's name in a search engine or in Google Groups, can you find out what provides the creator with the authority to write about the blog topic?
- Can you tell from the comments on the blog that others treat the creator as an expert in the topic that the blog covers?
- Do many other blogs link to this one? (Conduct a URL search in a blog search engine like Google BlogSearch or Technorati.)
- When looking at the blogger's posts, can you recognize any bias?
- Is the content found in the blog written in a readable manner, with correct grammar/spelling?
- Does the content in the blog contradict information found in another source?
- Is the information on the blog updated on a regular basis?

From "Critical Evaluation of a Blog," *Kathy Schrock's Guide for Educators* [online manual], by K. Schrock, 2006. Retrieved from http://discoveryschool.com/schrockguide/. Used with permission.

13.9 Questions to Ask When Evaluating Podcasts

- Did the podcast include content that appeared accurate? Timely? Appropriate?
- Were the technical qualities (audio, slides, etc.) acceptable in the production?
- Was a written transcript of the podcast available?
- Was the podcast linked from a site that included subject tags?
- Who was the sponsor of the podcast? Did it appear to be credible?
- Was the podcast linked from a site that included links to other resources?
- Did the podcast adhere to the copyright guidelines in its use of music, pictures, etc.?
- Was the length of the podcast appropriate for its content? (20 min. or less)
- Was the podcast part of a regularly scheduled series?
- Did the presenter in the podcast keep you interested?
- What were the presenter's credentials?
- Did the presenter seem biased?
- Did the podcast flow smoothly (introduction, content, summary)?
- Was it obvious how to add the podcast feed to your aggregator? (RSS)
- If the item was an enhanced podcast, did the use of slides enhance the content?
- If the item was an enhanced podcast, was it available in various file formats to allow viewing on various hardware devices?

From "What Makes a Good Podcast?" *Kathy Schrock's Guide for Educators* [online manual], by K. Schrock, 2006. Retrieved from http://discoveryschool.com/schrockguide/. Used with permission.

13.10 Criteria for Evaluating a Mobile App

Content quality

1	Does it make the function that you expected?	1 2 3 4 5
2	Can you do the same without the application?	1 2 3 4 5
3	Does the application receive updates regularly?	1 2 3 4 5
4	Do you think the data are reliable?	1 2 3 4 5
5	Can you identify with this application health problems?	1 2 3 4 5
6	Do you have possibility to send information about your status to your doctor?	1 2 3 4 5
7	Do you have better quality of life by using this application?	1 2 3 4 5

Security

10	Do you think that this application has appropriate security methods to protect data that are introduced?	1 2 3 4 5
11	Do you think that the data obtained with this application are sufficiently protected?	1 2 3 4 5

(continued)

Ease of use

12   Do you find what you need?   1 2 3 4 5

13   Do you think that the traditional method used so far is more difficult   1 2 3 4 5
     or does not exist?

14   Is this application useful for monitoring the disease?   1 2 3 4 5

Availability

15   Do you have the guarantee of access to the application and its data at   1 2 3 4 5
     any time?

Performance

16   Do you think you might have a more optimized performance?   1 2 3 4 5

17   Do you find some kind of error or problem while using the application?   1 2 3 4 5

Appearance

18   Do you find adequate the appearance of this application?   1 2 3 4 5

19   Would you change or add something from this application?   1 2 3 4 5

Learning

20   Do you think that the time for learning the use of the application   1 2 3 4 5
     is appropriate?

Precision

21   Do you think the calculations done by this application are correct?   1 2 3 4 5

From "Development and Evaluation of Tools for Measuring the Quality of Experience (QoE) in mHealth Applications," by B. Martínez-Pérez, I. de la Torre-Díez, S. Candelas-Plasencia, and M. López-Coronado, 2013, *Journal of Medical Systems, 37*(5): 9976. Doi. 10.1007/s10916-013-9976. Copyright © 2013, Springer Science Business Media, New York. Used with permission.

≡ Organizations as Resources

We introduced the importance of health organizations in chapter 2. These organizations can have a powerful impact on the health of a community. It will be important to familiarize yourself with the organizations in your community and network with the professionals staffing them.

Voluntary Health Organizations

Voluntary health organizations are powerful allies for community health professionals and help to build healthier communities. Brief descriptions of a few of the many voluntary health organizations follow.

- *The American Cancer Society.* This organization is dedicated to helping people who face cancer through research, patient services, early detection, treatment, and education. The national office is located in Washington, DC, but the organization has state and local affiliates.

- *The American Heart Association.* The mission of this organization is to help people build healthier lives, free of heart disease and stroke, through health education and advocacy. It is divided physically into the National Center (located in Dallas, Texas) and nine affiliate offices that cover the United States and Puerto Rico.

- *The American Lung Association.* Fighting lung disease for more than 90 years, the American Lung Association is a leader in tobacco education and regulation. It has a strong focus on the prevention of lung diseases like asthma, tuberculosis, pneumonia, and emphysema.

- *March of Dimes.* Four major problems threaten the health of America's babies: birth defects, infant mortality, low birth weight, and lack of prenatal care. The March of Dimes has adopted goals to bring us closer to the day when all babies will be born healthy. The goals include a commitment to "reduce birth defects by 10%, reduce infant mortality to 7 per 1,000 live births, reduce low birth weight to no more than 5% of all live births, and increase the number of women who get prenatal care in the first trimester of their pregnancy to 90%" (March of Dimes, 1999, p. 1).

- *Muscular Dystrophy Association.* This voluntary health agency is working to defeat 40 neuromuscular diseases through worldwide research, comprehensive services, and public health education.

- *National Kidney Foundation.* The National Kidney Foundation seeks to prevent kidney and urinary tract diseases. It also seeks to improve the health and well-being of individuals and families affected by these diseases and increase the availability of all organs for transplantation.

- *Cystic Fibrosis Foundation.* The mission of the Cystic Fibrosis Foundation is ongoing improvements in the quality of life for individuals with this disease.

- *American Red Cross.* This organization has multiple functions and services. The primary mission, however, is to help prevent, prepare for, and cope with emergencies. Approximately 30 million people are assisted each year.

- *The National Academies of Practice.* This organization is dedicated to quality health care for all. The members, nominated by individuals in their respective fields, have spent a significant portion of their careers in direct health care delivery to consumers. The NAP serves as an interdisciplinary policy forum, addressing public policy, education, research, and inquiry.

Government Agencies

We discussed the National Institutes of Health (NIH) and the Centers for Disease Control and Prevention (CDC) in chapter 2. These two agencies have a powerful influence on the health of the nation. You will find more detailed information about each in the paragraphs that follow. Keep in mind, however, that even government agencies that don't seem to be directly health-related can have an impact on health.

NATIONAL INSTITUTES OF HEALTH

The NIH mission is "to uncover new knowledge that will lead to better health for everyone" (NIH, 1999, p. 1). The NIH, housed in Bethesda, Maryland, has over 20 institutes (or more by the time you read this text) and six centers. It is one of the eight agencies of the Public Health Service, which is part of the Department of Health and Human Services. The institutes work toward their mission by conducting research in their own laboratories; supporting research at universities, medical centers, and other institutions; and assisting in the training of research investigators.

According to the NIH website (2018),

> the NIH invests nearly $37.3 billion annually in medical research. More than 80% of this funding is awarded through almost 50,000 competitive grants to more than 300,000 researchers at more than 2,500 universities, medical schools, and other research institutions in every state and around the world. (para. 1)

NIH funding has supported research in the following accomplishments:

- **An expanded map of the human brain.** A high-resolution map of the human brain provides new insights and tools for understanding the roles of specialized brain regions in health and disease.

- **How breast cancers resist chemotherapy.** Researchers discovered an unexpected way that breast cancers cells with mutant BRCA1 or BRCA2 genes become resistant to treatment—a crucial step toward improving therapies.

- **Stem cells grown on scaffold mimic hip joint cartilage.** In work that could lead to new approaches to treat joint surfaces damaged by osteoarthritis or injury, stem cells were grown on a 3-D scaffold to mimic a hip joint surface.

- **Molecule may impact Gaucher, Parkinson's disease.** Scientists identified a molecule that restores the activity of a Gaucher disease-related enzyme and decreases the buildup of a protein that's a hallmark of Parkinson's disease.

- **Structure of rhinovirus C revealed.** Researchers determined the structure of a rhinovirus C, a virus linked to severe asthma attacks, colds, and other respiratory infections. The finding may aid in the development of antiviral therapies and vaccines.

- **Approach targets autoimmunity.** Researchers developed a strategy to treat a rare autoimmune disease called *pemphigus vulgaris*, and demonstrated its potential in a mouse model.

- **Omega-3s linked with lower risk of fatal heart attacks.** Researchers found that blood with higher levels of seafood- and plant-based omega-3 fatty acids were associated with a lower risk of dying from heart attacks.

- **Biomarker signatures of prostate cancer.** Biomarkers in urine suggest a noninvasive approach to diagnosing prostate cancer and assessing tumor progression.

- **How the spleen keeps blood healthy.** Researchers used computer modeling to show how the spleen maintains the quality of red blood cells in the bloodstream.

CENTERS FOR DISEASE CONTROL AND PREVENTION

As you may recall from chapter 2, the CDC's mission is to "promote health and quality of life by preventing and controlling disease, injury, and disability" (CDC, 2008a, para. 1). Its main office is in Atlanta, Georgia. The CDC seeks to accomplish its mission by working with partners throughout the nation and the world to:

- monitor health
- detect and investigate health problems
- conduct research to enhance prevention
- develop and advocate sound public health policies

- implement prevention strategies
- promote healthy behaviors
- foster safe and healthful environments
- provide leadership and training

Organizations That Impact Health Care Delivery

Most of us are aware of the typical organizations that deliver health care: hospitals with emergency rooms, community outreach clinics or health centers, and doctors' offices. Much education is provided by these organizations. Unfortunately, health information is not always presented appropriately or in a culturally sensitive manner. Moreover, the timing of information presentation is not always beneficial to the patient. For example, providing education during a crisis in the emergency room is not generally effective. Nevertheless, these organizations can be valuable health information resources.

Even schools can serve as health-related resources. Public Law 94-142 requires that all children in the United States be provided free and appropriate public education. Because some children need health care in order for education to be meaningful, schools have implemented many health services. Among them are physical therapy, occupational therapy, counseling, speech therapy, and nursing services (Rodman et al., 1999).

Health Care and the Role of Insurance

In becoming an effective community resource person, it is important to have a basic understanding of the health care environment in the United States. However, we offer the caveat that health care policy can change with each government administration, so it's important to stay "tuned into" what's happening politically. While the information below is helpful to your foundational and historical understanding of health policy in the U.S., we recognize that this information may change; additionally, this is a brief overview and more information on each topic is available online. Therefore, be sure to refer to the http://www.healthcare.gov site for the most current information.

To fully comprehend how a health system operates, one must first understand how it's paid for and by whom. In the United States, both the government and insurance companies play important roles in determining appropriate care for individuals as well as payments to health care providers.

The 2010 Affordable Care Act (ACA), formally known as the Patient Protection and Affordable Care Act (and popularly known as Obamacare), was one of the most landmark health care reforms to date. Stated goals of the ACA are to make health care more affordable, accessible, and of a higher quality for families, seniors, businesses, and taxpayers alike. This includes previously uninsured Americans, and also those with insurance that didn't provide adequate coverage. For the health care industry itself, the traditional fee-for-service payment model is evolving toward value-based care and quality goals characteristic of managed care programs. Key features and benefits of the ACA include:

- Preventive care
- Rx discounts for seniors
- Support for pre-existing conditions
- Small business tax credits
- Expanded benefits for women
- Expanded coverage for young adult
- Consumer protections

Under the original ACA, individuals were required to enroll in a health care program or face a tax penalty. Options for individuals to meet the requirement included: enrolling in a government health program such as Medicare or Medicaid, or acquiring private health insurance offered by an employer or in the marketplace.

One of the anchoring concepts to ACA is that when more people are paying into the system, overall health costs are reduced, making premiums lower for people over time and health care more assessable to all. This was approaching a **single-payer health system** where the state, financed by taxes, covers basic health care costs for all residents regardless of income, occupation, or health status. In 2017, under executive order of President Donald Trump, the ACA's non-enrollment tax penalty ended.

The federal **Medicare** program offers health plans and services to people 65 or older, and people under 65 with certain disabilities. Medicare offers different types of coverage:

- **Part A Hospital Insurance**. Most people don't pay a premium for Part A. Part A covers inpatient care in hospitals, including critical access hospitals, and skilled nursing. It also helps cover hospice care and some home health care.

- **Part B Medical Insurance**. Most people pay a monthly premium for Part B. It covers doctors' services and outpatient care, and some services that Part A doesn't cover, such as some of the services of physical and occupational therapists.

- **Prescription Drug Coverage**. Most people will pay a monthly premium for this coverage. Everyone with Medicare can get this coverage that may help lower prescription drug costs.

For further information, refer to the government's website at https://www.medicare.gov/.

Medicaid is a program created by the federal government and administered by state to provide payment for medical services to low-income earning individuals. For example, in California this program is called *Medi-Cal*. People qualify for Medicaid by meeting federal income and asset standards and by fitting into a specified eligibility; additional rules vary by state. Medicaid information is available at local county social services, welfare, or human services office. For further information, refer to the governments website at https://www.medicaid.gov/.

People eligible for both Medicare and Medicaid (dual eligibility), can have both. Medicaid generally provides inpatient and outpatient health care coverage, including prescription drugs, diagnostic and preventive care, and eyeglasses. The amount of coverage, however, varies from state to state. In some states, Medicaid charges consumers small amounts for certain services.

Individuals with children who earn too much to qualify for Medicaid may be eligible for the federal **Children's Health Insurance Program**, or CHIP. Requirements for this program also vary by state. To learn more about the program and check on current legislative outcomes, visit https://www.medicaid.gov/chip/chip-program-information.html.

Common plan features of **private health** insurance,[1] include the following:

- Exclusive Provider Organization (EPO): A plan where services are covered only if you use doctors, specialists, or hospitals in the plan's network (except in an emergency).

- Preferred Provider Organization (PPO): A type of health plan where you pay less if you use providers in the plan's network. You can use doctors, hospitals, and providers outside of the network without a referral for an additional cost.

- Point of Service (POS): A type of plan where you pay less if you use doctors, hospitals, and other health care providers that belong to the plan's network. POS plans require you to get a referral from your primary care doctor in order to see a specialist.

- Health Maintenance Organization (HMO): A type of plan that usually limits coverage to care from doctors who work for or contract with the HMO, except in an emergency. HMOs often provide integrated care and focus on prevention and wellness.

Volunteers and Health Care Privacy

Volunteers who come into contact with individuals' health information should also be aware of privacy issues. Privacy issues affect patients and their medical information, as well as health care providers and insurance companies. Federal laws collectively known as HIPAA[2] identify many patient rights, and create a legal framework for health care organizations.

Though HIPAA rules are complex, volunteers should know that any health care organization, such as a hospital, clinic, small doctor's office, or insurance company, is included under the HIPAA umbrella and should be following these rules. Volunteers should follow these rules too, and may ask the health care organization for information or directions regarding patient privacy or HIPAA. In fact, many health care organizations will have a formal HIPAA Awareness Training program that applies to volunteers. In short, the health care organization will lead compliance in this area, and volunteers should follow.

For patients, HIPAA specifies certain rights, such as the right for a patient to have a copy of his or her medical record in certain circumstances. Again, the health care organization where a patient receives treatment has knowledge of these patient rights, and should be able to provide information to the patient, or to any volunteers in their employment. One key element in HIPPA is the Privacy Notice[3] document, which most all health care providers make available either on their website or posted in their office. This explains many patient rights. The health care provider can answer further questions.

---

[1] "Private" health insurance plans are offered by private companies such as United Health, Aetna, or Humana, but also include nonprofits such as Blue Cross Blue Shield.

[2] Officially, the Healthcare Insurance Portability and Accountability Act

[3] Officially known as the Notice of Privacy Practices

13.11   Common Health Care Terms

Term	Definition
Exclusive Provider Organization (EPO)	A plan where services are covered only when people use doctors, specialists, or hospitals in the plan's network (except in an emergency).
Preferred Provider Organization (PPO)	A type of health plan where people pay less when they use providers in the plan's network. Doctors, hospitals, and providers outside of the network may be used for an additional cost.
Point of Service (POS)	A type of plan where fees are less when using providers that belong to the plan's network. POS plans require individuals to get a referral from their primary care doctor in order to see a specialist.
Health Maintenance Organization (HMO)	A type of plan that usually limits coverage to care from doctors who work for or contract with the HMO, except in an emergency. HMOs often provide integrated care and focus on prevention and wellness.
Case managers	Insurance company employees who manage treatment for an individual receiving health care.
Copayment fees	Predetermined fee for which the insured is responsible.
Deductibles	Predetermined amount of money that the insured will pay before insurance coverage begins.
Fee for service	Payment after the delivery of health care services.
Managed care	An organized plan for supervising the delivery of health care services. Under the Affordable Care Act, these plans are developed by the government and insurance companies working together.
Preventive medicine	Health care services provided before health problems occur.
Private Insurance	Private insurance plans are offered by private companies such as United Health, Aetna, or Humana, but also include not-for-profits such as Blue Cross Blue Shield. (but does not include government plans such as Medicare or Medicaid).
Provider	A health care professional such as a doctor (and their office), nurse, hospital or lab.
Primary care physician	A doctor who authorizes specialty health care.
Single Payer Healthcare System	The state, financed by taxes, covers basic health care costs for all residents regardless of income, occupation, or health status.
Utilization review	Review and management of treatment, normally conducted by an insurance company under ACA guidelines.

In general, it is important to remember that any person's medical information is subject to very specific rules and regulations. (Note that medical information can exist on paper or in electronic form, such as on a computer, or can even be verbal.) Volunteers should always regard medical information with respect and professionalism, and seek out guidance from any organization they serve. Further details are available at http://www.hhs.gov/hipaa/.

≡ In Conclusion

Although you do not need to know everything and everyone related to health, you do need to be able to access and use health resources. Begin by understanding your most valuable resource: people. Other health care professionals can offer knowledge and skills that you alone cannot hope to attain in one lifetime. They may serve as volunteers or form a vital resource network for you. Devoting time and attention to your relationships with other health professionals is a wise career investment.

In addition to people, technology is a vital resource. In today's world, technology enables people to find information quicker than ever before. Your ability to locate and present information depends on your mastery of current computer technology and your efforts to keep up-to-date with innovations.

Finally, organizational resources are abundant, whether they are voluntary health organizations, health care facilities, or government agencies. Your understanding of their missions and roles will guide your search for information and enable you to use it effectively. So, how do you manage all of this information? A resource inventory is a tool that can help community health professionals manage and locate resources expeditiously. Appendix D provides a template for you to use. Serving as a resource person is a key responsibility for those working within a community setting. People need to have accurate, credible information as well as know how to apply this information and where to go for additional help or services. Navigating people toward essential information, community agencies, organizations, or health services is key to building healthier, empowered communities.

REVIEW QUESTIONS

1. Identify three health professionals working in community health and describe how each might serve as a resource for a health education specialist.

2. List three to four reasons people might volunteer. What can you do to help maintain volunteers?

3. Reflect on consulting within the field of health and list three things one might consider before beginning consulting work.

5. Define networking and discuss its importance.

6. Compare strengths and limitations of at least three different sources of health information.

7. Evaluate the quality and credibility of a blog, podcast, and mobile app using criteria included in this chapter.

8. List resources you can use to find further information about the Affordable Care Act and changes in health care policy and delivery.

FOR YOUR APPLICATION

Locating Health Information on a Select Topic

Select a health-related topic and search the Internet using two sources described in this chapter to collect information about it. Write several paragraphs in summary of what you found, comparing findings from the two sources. Explain any differences you found and whether you found one source was easier to use than the other.

Recruiting and Keeping Volunteers

Imagine that you work for a voluntary health association. Select a specific agency and create a hypothetical activity in which that agency might be involved. Develop a list of methods you will use to recruit volunteers for the activity you have chosen. Make a second list of methods you will use to keep those volunteers.

Evaluating Electronic Information

Choose a health topic to explore. Locate an online article, blog, wiki, archived or live webcast, podcast, or mobile app related to this health issue. Using the criteria included in this chapter, evaluate the reliability, credibility, and overall effectiveness of the health material presented.

Subscribing to a Health Listserv or Health Blog

Learn more about health-related Listservs and blogs in your field such as the HEDIR (www.hedir.org), The HEDIR Blog (http://hedir.hpcareernetwork.com/), or HPCareer.Net. If the membership is free (like it is for the HEDIR), consider joining it for at least a week. Keep track of the kinds of discussion and information sent through this Listserv or posted on the blog. What is the quality of the discussion? Overall, do you think this is an effective way to share health information?

Creating a Resource File or Resource Web Page

Imagine that you are a college campus health education specialist or a clinical health education specialist in a hospital setting. Using Appendix D, create an electronic resource list of health materials and resources that could be used for planning and implementing campus-based or hospital health education events and/or workshops on various topics. Or, approach this as a group activity and work with your peers to compile information about a select health issue in a wiki or on a Web page you design. Share a link to the wiki or Web page with your peers or on professional social media channels to contribute to your field.

14

Trends in the Global Community

As you sit down to enjoy your favorite Thai cuisine at a local restaurant, a scrolling head-line on the television screen within your view captures your attention: "Soaring cost of rice from drought leads to social unrest and violence internationally." As you dive into your meal, you ponder how such a common staple, like the one on the plate in front of you, could be causing such mayhem worldwide. The television images of chaos, violence, and starvation in places like the Sudan and Yemen jump out at you and generate even more questions: What social, political, and ecological factors influenced these situations? What impact does climate change and food security have on communities and countries around the globe? How does it affect you personally?

Chapter Objectives

1. Define the terms *globalization, quality of life, human development index, sustainable environment,* and *global capacity.*

2. Analyze trends and projections relating to globalization, world demographics, dis-ease, and health.

3. Explain how technology may serve as both a barrier and as an asset to building healthier global communities.

4. Describe predicted changes in health care systems and their potential influence on community health.

5. Examine predicted job-market growth patterns as they relate to community health and the health workforce world-wide.

6. Explain the importance of promoting community empowerment at the local and global levels.

7. Describe strategies for career development and lifelong learning that will increase one's ability to work successfully in the field of community health.

≡ Global Health and Quality of Life

In a world full of uncertainties, these things are inevitable: death, taxes, and *change.* The world is evolving at an accelerating, dizzying pace. Globalization has become a buzzword for the 21st century to describe this change process. The World Health Organi-zation defines **globalization** as "a comprehensive worldwide process involving the inter-nationalization of communication, trade, and economic organization. It involves parallel rapid social, economic, and political change" (WHO, 2004, p. 5). Ongoing changes in these socio-ecological factors (refer to chapter 1, Figure 1.8) can put the health of a com-munity in a state of constant flux. Though globalization benefits many parts of the world, it can exacerbate disparities and significantly impact health and quality of life for poor and marginalized populations in developed and undeveloped economic regions.

Isn't that how we began this textbook—with a discussion about the meaning of health and quality of life? Now we have come full circle. Yet we dare not simply repeat what we said at the beginning of the textbook. There is so much more that you need to know as a health professional and citizen of the world to be equipped for the global changes ahead. The pace of change in the world and within health professions compels us to describe in this final chapter some future trends, global change, and recommendations for professional development. We begin this venture with brief comments about these topics within the context of a global future.

Global Health Concepts

Type in the words *global health* into any Internet search engine, and an avalanche of links to websites with information will appear. The plethora of choices will be overwhelming, particularly if you are trying to focus on only a few key concepts. Finding a simple, concise definition that encompasses the broad spectrum that global health represents is also a challenge. Instead, we offer five characteristics of global health based on a variety of sources (Global Health Council, n.d.; Skolnik, 2008) and our own experiences. Each characteristic, in isolation, is an insufficient description of all that comprises global health. Collectively, however, these descriptive statements begin to paint the broader picture.

- *Global health is* a process through which public health and community health promotion principles are applied across national boundaries.
- *Global health is* a goal that stretches beyond the mere absence of disease and embraces the concepts of total wellness and quality of life for all.
- *Global health is* a worldview in which individual members are seen as interdependent for survival and well-being.
- *Global health is* a partnership in which "countries work together not only to understand critical health issues but also to solve them" (Skolnik, 2008, p. 7).
- *Global health is* the common ground where individuals and nations can meet from across a complex array of boundaries (geographic, political, ideological, etc.) to share a common goal.

≡ Quality of Life and Human Development on a Global Scale

Public health scholars Larry Green and Marshall Kreuter (2005) describe **quality of life** as "the perception of individuals or groups that their needs are being satisfied and that they are not being denied opportunities to pursue happiness and fulfillment" (p. 34). A measure that relates to quality of life is the **Human Development Index [HDI]**. HDI is a composite statistic of life expectancy, education, and income first introduced by the United Nations in the first *Human Development Report* in 1990 (UNDP, 2010). HDI can be viewed as an index of "potential" human development and quality of life which could be achieved if there were no inequality. Quality of life and HDI comparisons on a global scale reveal that people living today are healthier, wealthier and better educated than before; however, there are still enormous inequalities related to daily needs and human development opportunities. Surprisingly, income is not necessarily a deciding factor. A rigorous review of trends from 1970 to 2010 by the United Nations (UN) showed that "there is no significant correlation between national economic performance and achievement in the HDI areas of health and education" (UNDP, 2010, p. E-1-1).

The United Nations Development Programme's (UNDP, 2013) *Human Development Report* also revealed that there is much that countries can do to improve peoples' quality of life, even in adverse conditions. Data showed that developing countries Oman, China, Nepal, Algeria, and Morocco made the "Top Movers" list in terms of investing in health and public education, which improved their HDI the greatest over the last forty years. The UNDP states, "The rise of the South is unprecedented in its speed and scale. Never in history have the living conditions and prospects of so many people changed so dramatically and fast" (UNDP, 2013, p. E-1-1).

On a global scale, over the last 40 years, HDI has largely improved. Life expectancy at birth climbed from 59 years in 1970 to 71 in 2017, school enrolment rose from just 55% of all primary and secondary school-age children to 70%, and per capita GDP doubled to more than US$10,000 (UN, 2017). The world is witnessing a global "rebalancing." The UNDP describes it this way:

> The rise of the South and developing countries in the 21st Century is much like what took place in the early part of the 20th Century with Europe and North American as a result of the Industrial Revolution and two World Wars. Now another "tectonic shift" has put developing countries on an upward curve. (UNDP, 2013, p. E-1-2)

The UNDP predicts that the "Rise of the South" should continue and even accelerate as the 21st century progresses. Tables 14.1 and 14.2 (on pp. 354–355) list the countries with the highest and lowest HDI rankings in 2015.

However, despite these huge gains, and the increase of a "middle class" worldwide, there are still enormous inequities related to satisfied needs and denied opportunities. As the UNDP reports, many countries from sub-Saharan Africa and the former Soviet Union lag behind due to the impact of AIDS, conflict, economic upheaval, and other factors. Life expectancy actually declined over the past 40 years in three countries of the former Soviet Union (Belarus, Ukraine and the Russian Federation) and six in sub Saharan Africa (the Democratic Republic of the Congo, Lesotho, South Africa, Swaziland, Zambia, and Zimbabwe) (UNDP, 2013). Contributing factors and potential solutions for these inequities in quality of life can be viewed within the context of the trends we describe in the following sections.

≡ Trends in the Global Community

As we mentioned earlier, our world is evolving at lightning speed. The populations, languages, cultures, economies, technologies, and diseases of the 19th and 20th centuries are markedly different than those in the 21st. This continual metamorphosis will have a profound impact on the quality of life and prosperity of people in every corner of the world. Established in 1948, the World Health Organization has expanded its focus over the last six decades to include improving overall well-being rather than just survivorship. In fact, it reports that due to socioeconomic development, increased

Table 14.1 Twenty Countries with Very High Human Development 2015

HDI rank	Human Development Index (HDI) Value 2015	Life expectancy at birth (years) 2015	Expected years of schooling (years) 2015[a]	Mean years of schooling (years) 2015[a]	Gross national income (GNI) per capita (2011 PPP $) 2015	GNI per capita rank minus HDI rank 2015	HDI rank 2014
VERY HIGH HUMAN DEVELOPMENT							
1 Norway	0.949	81.7	17.7	12.7	67,614	5	1
2 Australia	0.939	82.5	20.4[b]	13.2	42,822	19	3
3 Switzerland	0.939	83.1	16.0	13.4	56,364	7	2
4 Germany	0.926	81.1	17.1	13.2[c]	45,000	13	4
5 Denmark	0.925	80.4	19.2[b]	12.7	44,519	13	6
5 Singapore	0.925	83.2	15.4[d]	11.6	78,162[e]	-3	4
7 Netherlands	0.924	81.7	18.1[b]	11.9	46,326	8	6
8 Ireland	0.923	81.1	18.6[b]	12.3	43,798	11	8
9 Iceland	0.921	82.7	19.0[b]	12.2[c]	37,065	20	9
10 Canada	0.920	82.2	16.3	13.1[f]	42,582	12	9
11 United States	0.920	79.2	16.5	13.2	53,245	1	11
12 Hong Kong, China (SAR)	0.917	84.2	15.7	11.6	54,265	-2	12
13 New Zealand	0.915	82.0	19.2[b]	12.5	32,870	20	13
14 Sweden	0.913	82.3	16.1	12.3	46,251	2	15
15 Liechtenstein	0.912	80.2[g]	14.6	12.4[h]	75,065[e,i]	-11	14
16 United Kingdom	0.909	80.8	16.3	13.3	37,931	10	16
17 Japan	0.903	83.7	15.3	12.5[c]	37,268	10	17
18 Korea (Republic of)	0.901	82.1	16.6	12.2	34,541	12	18
19 Israel	0.899	82.6	16.0	12.8	31,215	16	19
20 Luxembourg	0.898	81.9	13.9	12.0	62,471	-12	20

[a]Data refer to 2015 or the most recent year available; [b]In calculating the HDI value, expected years of schooling is capped at 18 years; [c]Updated by HDRO using Barro and Lee (2016) estimates; [d]Based on data from the national statistical office; [e]In calculating the HDI value, GNI per capita is capped at $75,000; [f]Based on Barro and Lee (2016); [g]Value from UNDESA (2011); [h]Calculated as the average of mean years of schooling for Austria and Switzerland; [i]Estimated using the purchasing power parity (PPP) rate and projected growth rate of Switzerland.

Adapted from "Human Development Report 2016 'Human Development for Everyone.'" Human Development Report Office, United Nations Development Programme. Retrieved from hdr.undp.org.

Table 14.2   Countries with the Lowest Human Development Index 2015

HDI rank	Human Development Index (HDI) Value 2015	Life expectancy at birth (years) 2015	Expected years of schooling (years) 2015a	Mean years of schooling (years) 2015a	Gross national income (GNI) per capita (2011 PPP $) 2015	GNI per capita rank minus HDI rank 2015	HDI rank 2014
LOW HUMAN DEVELOPMENT							
148 Swaziland	0.541	48.9	11.4	6.8n	7,522	−33	149
149 Syrian Arab Republic	0.536	69.7	9.0	5.1s	2,441t	13	145
150 Angola	0.533	52.7	11.4	5.0q	6,291	−27	150
151 Tanzania (United Republic of)	0.531	65.5	8.9	5.8	2,467	10	152
152 Nigeria	0.527	53.1	10.0	6.0q	5,443	−23	151
153 Cameroon	0.518	56.0	10.4	6.1c	2,894	2	154
154 Papua New Guinea	0.516	62.8	9.9k	4.3f	2,712	4	153
154 Zimbabwe	0.516	59.2	10.3	7.7	1,588	20	158
156 Solomon Islands	0.515	68.1	9.6m	5.3d	1,561	19	155
157 Mauritania	0.513	63.2	8.5	4.3f	3,527	−12	155
158 Madagascar	0.512	65.5	10.3	6.1n	1,320	25	157
159 Rwanda	0.498	64.7	10.8	3.8	1,617	14	162
160 Comoros	0.497	63.6	11.1	4.8q	1,335	22	160
160 Lesotho	0.497	50.1	10.7	6.1f	3,319	−12	161
162 Senegal	0.494	66.9	9.5	2.8m	2,250	3	163
163 Haiti	0.493	63.1	9.1k	5.2c	1,657	9	164
163 Uganda	0.493	59.2	10.0	5.7m	1,670	8	165
165 Sudan	0.490	63.7	7.2	3.5	3,846	−22	165
166 Togo	0.487	60.2	12.0	4.7q	1,262	18	167
167 Benin	0.485	59.8	10.7	3.5c	1,979	1	168
168 Yemen	0.482	64.1	9.0	3.0c	2,300	−4	159
169 Afghanistan	0.479	60.7	10.1	3.6f	1,871	1	169
170 Malawi	0.476	63.9	10.8	4.4f	1,073	16	170
171 Côte d'Ivoire	0.474	51.9	8.9	5.0f	3,163	−20	172

172 Djibouti	0.473	62.3	6.3	4.1[k]	3,216	-22	171
173 Gambia	0.452	60.5	8.9	3.3[f]	1,541	3	173
174 Ethiopia	0.448	64.6	8.4	2.6[q]	1,523	5	174
175 Mali	0.442	58.5	8.4	2.3	2,218	-9	175
176 Congo (Democratic Republic of the)	0.435	59.1	9.8	6.1	680	15	178
177 Liberia	0.427	61.2	9.9	4.4[f]	683	13	177
178 Guinea-Bissau	0.424	55.5	9.2[m]	2.9[k]	1,369	3	179
179 Eritrea	0.420	64.2	5.0	3.9[k]	1,490	1	181
179 Sierra Leone	0.420	51.3	9.5	3.3[f]	1,529	-1	176
181 Mozambique	0.418	55.5	9.1	3.5[q]	1,098	4	182
181 South Sudan	0.418	56.1	4.9	4.8[n]	1,882	-12	179
183 Guinea	0.414	59.2	8.8	2.6[q]	1,058	4	182
184 Burundi	0.404	57.1	10.6	3.0[c]	691	5	184
185 Burkina Faso	0.402	59.0	7.7	1.4[q]	1,537	-8	185

[a] Data refer to 2015 or the most recent year available; [b] In calculating the HDI value, expected years of schooling is capped at 18 years; [c] Updated by HDRO using Barro and Lee (2016) estimates; [d] Based on data from the national statistical office; [e] In calculating the HDI value, GNI per capita is capped at $75,000; [f] Based on Barro and Lee (2016); [g] Value from UNDESA (2011); [h] Calculated as the average of mean years of schooling for Austria and Switzerland; [i] Estimated using the purchasing power parity (PPP) rate and projected growth rate of Switzerland; [j] Estimated using the PPP rate and projected growth rate of Austria and Switzerland; [k] Based on cross-country regression; [l] HDRO estimate based on data from World Bank (2016a) and United Nations Statistics Division (2016a); [m] Updated by HDRO based on data from UNESCO Institute for Statistics (2016); [n] Based on data from United Nations Children's Fund (UNICEF) Multiple Indicator Cluster Surveys for 2006–2015; [o] Updated by HDRO based on data from ICF Macro Demographic and Health Surveys for 2006–2015; [p] Based on a cross-country regression and the projected growth rate from UNECLAC (2016); [q] Based on data from ICF Macro Demographic and Health Surveys for 2006–2015; [r] Value from WHO (2016); [s] Updated by HDRO based on Syrian Centre for Policy Research (2016); [t] Based on projected growth rates from UNESCWA (2016) and World Bank (2016a).

Adapted from "Human Development Report 2016 'Human Development for Everyone.'" Human Development Report Office, United Nations Development Programme. Retrieved from hdr.undp.org.

investment in education and health, and technological advances, the world as a whole is moving toward a healthier, longer life span (WHO, 2013). As you look forward and plan for the future, consider the emerging trends that will shape our global community as well as your role as a health professional. We offer them as issues to consider as you prepare to engage in promoting health within communities, locally, and globally.

Trend #1: World Population Continues to Grow

Though it might be hard to believe, the rapid growth of the world population is a fairly recent phenomenon. Population growth in the earliest centuries was relatively slow, and the number of people in the world did not significantly expand over periods of time. For those inhabitants of early civilization, life was harsh. Living conditions were poor and death rates were high. War, famine, disease, poverty, illiteracy, and lack of technological innovation kept the population in check. Because both fertility and mortality were high, the world census changed very little in the years leading up to 1800. It is estimated that two thousand years ago, the world's population was 300 million (about as large as the population of the United States today!); ten centuries later, it may have increased only by 10 million. It rose to about 500 million by 1500, and by 1800 the population had climbed to almost 1 billion.

With the advances brought on by the Enlightenment and the Industrial Revolution, the world's population nearly doubled between 1800 and 1900. Still, that gain is modest compared to the unprecedented population boom that occurred in the 20th century. With the introduction of scientific and technological innovations such as vaccines and medications, public health and epidemiological strides to control disease, better access to food and water, and the rise of modern industry and communications, world population nearly quadrupled! Over the course of 100 years, the world's population grew from 1.65 billion in 1900 to 6.11 billion in 2000, an increase of 4.46 billion (UN, 2009). Even more wondrous is the fact that well over half of this growth (80%) took place in the second half of the century, and from 2005 to 2017, the world population grew by another billion (UN, 2017).

According to the *World Population Prospects Key Findings Report* by the United Nations (2017), the population of the world is projected to continue to increase, but at a slower pace. By 2050, world population is expected to reach 9.8 billion and by 2100 it is projected to climb to over 11 billion (see Figure 14.1). The numbers of men and women are roughly equal, with the male population being slightly larger than the female population (see Figure 14.2). In 2017, there were 102 men for every 100 women.

The current population of the most developed regions is expected to remain relatively constant, from its present 1.23 billion to 1.27 billion by 2050. However, the UN (2017) reports that the 49 **least developed countries (LDCs)** as a whole still have the *fastest growing populations in the world*, at 2.3% per year. Although this rate of increase is expected to slow significantly over the next decades, the population of the LDCs is projected to double by mid-century, from 898 million in 2013 to 1.8 billion in 2050, and further increasing to 2.9 billion in 2100 (p. 4). Half of all population growth is concentrated in a small number of countries. From 2013 to 2100, many African countries as well as India and the U.S. will account for over half of the world's population increase (see Table 14.3 on p. 358). How will this growing census impact world

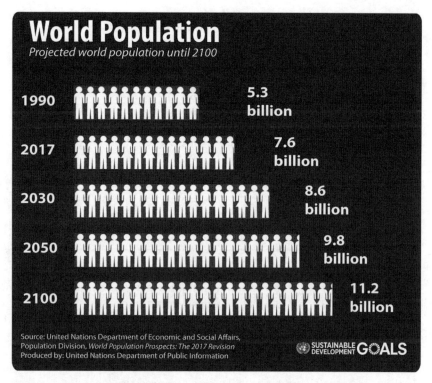

Figure 14.1   World Population Estimates and Projections: 1990–2100

From *World Population: Projected World Population until 2010*, by United Nations, Department of Public Information, copyright © 2017 United Nations. Reprinted with the permission of the United Nations.

**Figure 14.2
Distribution of the
World's Population by
Age, Sex 2017**

From *World Population Prospects: The 2017 Revision*, by United Nations, Department of Economics and Social Affairs, Population Division, copyright © 2017 United Nations. Reprinted with the permission of the United Nations.

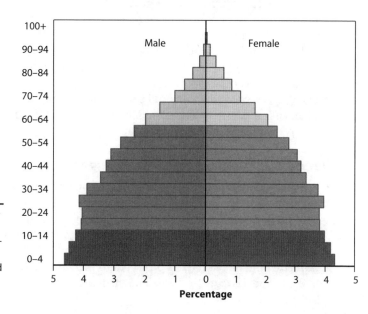

Table 14.3   The Ten Most Populous Countries by 2100

	Country	2100 Population (in billions and millions)
1	India	1,659,785,948
2	China	1,004,391,965
3	Nigeria	752,247,359
4	USA	450,384,823
5	Congo	388,732,857
6	Pakistan	364,282,652
7	Indonesia	313,648,122
8	Tanzania	299,132,889
9	Ethiopia	242,644,125
10	Niger	209,334,454

Source: *World Population Prospects: The 2017 Revision, Key Findings and Advance Tables,* United Nations Department of Economic and Social Affairs/Population Division, 2017, New York: Author.

resources, economies, and overall health? This is a hot topic of debate among world leaders, economists, sociologists, health scientists, and researchers across the world.

Related to the issue of increasing population is the world's rapid urbanization (UN, 2017). About 45% of the world's population lived in urban areas in 1995. By 2025, that proportion is expected to increase to over 60%. People are flocking to cities all over the world to be closer to jobs and other resources. As more children are born in those areas, city boundaries will expand by necessity.

This growth rate gives rise to growing concerns about our ability to maintain a sustainable environment for all those people. In a **sustainable environment**, such factors as housing, education, health and nutrition, and the use of natural resources keep adequate pace with population growth and distribution patterns (WHO, 2006a). In other words, a sustainable environment is one in which the people who live in it have access to what they need to live.

The downside of rapid urban growth is crowding and stress. Those who can afford to move out of crowded inner-city areas and into more attractive suburbs leave behind those who face poverty and marginalization. The result is often inadequate housing, poor waste disposal and sanitation systems, and stress-induced violence and accidents. It is possible that, as the urbanization phenomenon grows, so will the number of people living in this poverty gap.

Trend #2: People Are Living Longer

The average human life span is continuing to increase worldwide (Figure 14.3). This is true for both men and women. Life expectancy for men is expected to increase from 65.4 to 73.3 by 2050, and for women, it will increase from 69.8 to 77.9 (UN, 2017).

The **median age**, or the age that divides the population in two halves of equal size, is an indicator of population aging. At the world level, the United Nations (2017) reports that the median age is projected to increase from 29 to 36 years between 2017 and 2050, and 41 years by 2100. The median age is higher in countries or regions that

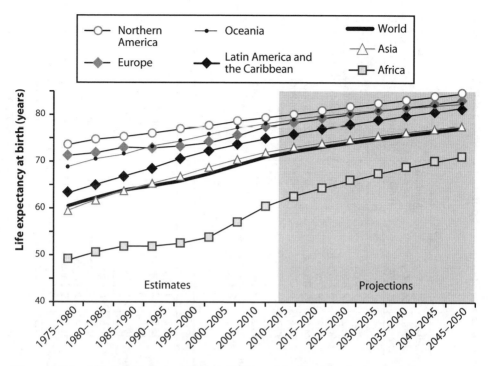

Figure 14.3   Life Expectancy at Birth (in Years) by Region: Estimates 1975–2015 and Projections 2015–2050

From *World Population Prospects: The 2017 Revision,* by United Nations, Department of Economic and Social Affairs, Population Division, copyright © 2017 United Nations. Reprinted with the permission of the United Nations.

have been experiencing low fertility for a long time. Europe today has the oldest population, with a median age of 41 years in 2017, which is expected to reach 46 years in 2050 and then 47 years in 2100. Within countries with the oldest populations, this will increase to 55.8

In 2017, members of the United Nations reported that the average life expectancy globally was 70.1 years, with wide differences across regional groups: 59.1 years in countries with low HDI, and 80.1 years in very high HDI. Differences across countries are even wider, with a low of 48.1 years in Sierra Leone and a high of 83.6 years in Japan. In sub-Saharan Africa, life expectancy stagnated at 49.5 years between 1990 and 2000, a result of the HIV and AIDS pandemic. Between 2000 and 2012, however, it increased 5.5 years (UN, 2017). According to the United Nations (2017), North America currently has a life expectancy of 79 years and this will increase to 84 by 2050.

Population aging will occur for both industrialized as well as developing countries (Table 14.4). Slow population growth brought about by reductions in fertility leads to population aging; that is, "it produces populations where the proportion of older persons increases while that of younger persons decreases" (WHO, 2013, p. xvii) In the more developed regions, 23% of the population is already aged 60 years or over and that proportion is projected to reach 32% in 2050 and 34% in 2100 (UNPF, 2017). In

Table 14.4 Ten Countries or Areas with the Oldest and Ten Countries with the Youngest Populations, 1950, 1980, 2015, 2030, and 2050

	1950		1980		2015		2030		2050
Country or area	Median age (years)	Country or area	Median age (years)	Country or area	Median age (years)	Country or area	Median age (years)	Country or area	Median age (years)
A. Oldest populations									
1. Channel Islands	35.7	1. Germany	36.4	1. Japan	46.5	1. Japan	51.5	1. Other non-specified areas	56.2
2. Austria	35.7	2. Sweden	36.2	2. Germany	46.2	2. Italy	50.8	2. Republic of Korea	53.9
3. Belgium	35.5	3. Austria	35.0	3. Martinique	46.1	3. Portugal	50.2	3. Japan	53.3
4. Germany	35.3	4. Luxembourg	35.0	4. Italy	45.9	4. Spain	50.1	4. Bosnia and Herzegovina	53.2
5. Luxembourg	35.0	5. Latvia	35.0	5. Portugal	44.0	5. Greece	48.9	5 Singapore	53.0
6. United Kingdom	34.9	6. Channel Islands	34.9	6. Greece	43.6	6. China, Hong Kong, SAR	48.6	6. China, Hong Kong, SAR	52.7
7. France	34.7	7. Switzerland	34.6	7. Bulgaria	43.5	7. Germany	48.6	7. Portugal	52.5
8. Sweden	34.2	8. Hungary	34.4	8. Austria	4.32	8. Other non-specified areas	48.1	8. Greece	52.3
9. Switzerland	33.2	9. United Kingdom	34.4	9. China, Hong Kong, SAR	43.2	9. Slovenia	48.1	9. Cuba	51.9
10. Norway	32.6	10. Denmark	34.3	10. Spain	43.2	10. Republic of Korea	47.5	10. Poland	51.8
WORLD	23.5	WORLD	22.5	WORLD	29.6	WORLD	33.1	WORLD	36.1
B. Youngest populations									
1. Niger	15.2	1. Kenya	15.0	1. Niger	14.8	1. Niger	15.2	1. Niger	17.8
2. St. Vincent and the Grenadines	15.4	2. State of Palestine	15.1	2. Uganda	15.9	2. Somalia	17.7	2. Somalia	20.8
3. Tonga	15.5	3. Yemen	15.3	3. Chad	16.0	3. Angola	17.7	3. Angola	21.0
4. Grenada	16.3	4. Mayotte	15.4	4. Angola	16.1	4. Chad	17.9	4. Zambia	21.4
5. Paraguay	16.5	5. Jordan	15.5	5. Mali	16.2	5. Mali	17.9	5. Mali	21.4
6. Djibouti	16.5	6. Zimbabwe	15.5	6. Somalia	16.5	6. Uganda	18.1	6. Chad	21.7
7. Samoa	16.6	7. Swaziland	15.6	7. Gambia	16.8	7. Gambia	18.3	7. Burundi	21.8
8. Fiji	16.6	8. Syrian Arab Republic	15.6	8. Zambia	16.9	8. Burundi	18.5	8. Uganda	21.9
9. Vanuatu	16.8	9. Zambia	15.9	9. Dem. Republic of the Congo	16.9	9. Zambia	18.5	9. Gambia	22.1
10. United Republic of Tanzania	16.9	10. Rwanda	16.0	10. Burkina Faso	17.0	10. Dem. Republic of the Congo	18.6	10. United Republic of Tanzania	22.2
WORLD	23.5	WORLD	22.5	WORLD	29.6	WORLD	33.1	WORLD	36.1

Note: Only countries or areas with 90,000 persons or more in 2015 are considered. From *World Population Prospects: The 2015 Revision*, by United Nations, Department of Economic and Social Affairs, Population Division, copyright © 2017 United Nations. Reprinted with the permission of the United Nations.

developed countries as a whole, the number of older persons (over 15 years old) has already surpassed the number of children (persons under age 15 years old), and by 2050 the number of older persons in developed countries will be *nearly twice* the number of children.

Population aging is less advanced in developing countries. Nevertheless in developing countries as a whole, 9% of the population today is aged 60 years or over, but that proportion *will more than double* by 2050, reaching 19% that year, and triple by 2100, reaching 27% (UN, 2015). Figure 14.4 depicts the world population by age groups between 1950 and 2050 and the upswing in the percentage of people ages 60 and older. Note how the number of persons over age 60 will actually exceed more than those from any other age group.

According the UN (2017), the number of persons aged 60 years or over is expected to more than triple between 2013 and 2100, increasing from 841 million in 2013 to 2 billion in 2050 and close to 3 billion in 2100. Now, for the first time in human history, older persons will outnumber the population of children ages 0 to 14. In 2017 nearly 1 in 4 people (23.5%) in the world were over the age of 60 (UN, 2017). Table 14.5 depicts trends for the countries with the most percentage of people living over 60.

As more people live longer, the primary challenge will be to help individuals develop and sustain their well-being into old age as well as address the shortage of caregivers and health care professionals trained to help manage a graying society. The

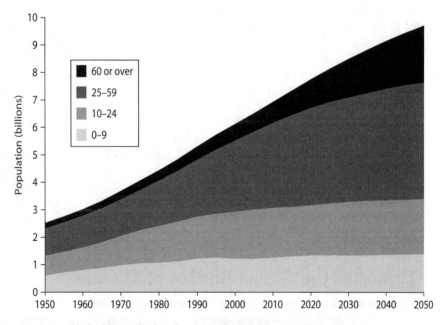

Figure 14.4   Global Population by Broad Age Group, 1950–2050

From *World Population Prospects: The 2015 Revision, Key Findings and Advance Tables,* by United Nations, Department of Economic and Social Affairs, Population Division, copyright © 2017 United Nations. Reprinted with the permission of the United Nations.

Table 14.5   Countries with the Most People Aged 60 Years and Older, 2000, 2015, and 2030*

Rank	2000 Country or area	Percentage aged 60 years or over	2015 Country or area	Percentage aged 60 years or over	2030 Country or area	Percentage aged 60 years or over
1	Italy	24.1	Japan	33.1	Martinique	38.5
2	Japan	23.3	Italy	28.6	Japan	37.3
3	Germany	23.1	Germany	27.6	Italy	36.6
4	Greece	22.8	Finland	27.2	Germany	36.1
5	Sweden	22.2	Portugal	27.1	Portugal	34.7
6	Bulgaria	22.2	Greece	27.0	China, Hong Kong SAR	33.6
7	Belgium	22.0	Bulgaria	26.9	Spain	33.5
8	Croatia	21.8	Martinique	26.2	Greece	33.2
9	Portugal	21.7	Croatia	25.9	Slovenia	32.7
10	Spain	21.4	Latvia	25.7	Austria	32.4

*Of 201 countries or areas with at least 90,000 inhabitants in 2015.

From *World Population Prospects: The 2015 Revision*, by United Nations, Department of Economic and Social Affairs, Population Division, copyright © 2017 United Nations. Reprinted with the permission of the United Nations.

focus will continue to rest on healthy lifestyle behaviors such as physical activity, diet, and abstinence from tobacco, but expanding needs will center on efforts to help the elderly remain active in their communities, live independently, maintain and develop new social contacts, and engage in intergenerational activities (UN, 2017).

This aging of our global society will undoubtedly have an impact on not only the health care system, but other facets of society. For example, with more people living longer, active lives, the age of retirement will continue to increase, businesses and entertainment will continue to tailor services and advertising to this growing segment of the population, and our entire notion of "growing old" will evolve. Perhaps 60 will be the new 50 by 2025? With declining birth rates in many industrialized countries, will we have enough trained individuals to care for the elderly in these regions? How will models of caregiving evolve to accommodate for increases in this segment of the population as well as shortages in health care and social services? These questions must be answered within the next 10 to 15 years, and it will take a "village" of practitioners, scholars, and community members working together to find effective solutions.

≡ Trends in the Global Burden of Disease

As the world population grows and life expectancy increases, we will continue to battle diseases both infectious and chronic. Global surveillance, modern medicine, and health education and prevention will play important roles in battling and preventing worldwide epidemics and pandemics.

Trend #3: Infectious Diseases Are Making a Comeback

In this era of globalization, medicine, and technology, it might seem paradoxical to think that many of the infectious diseases that plagued populations in centuries past are now resurging—and with a vengeance. According to the *Global Report for Infectious Disease and Poverty* by the World Health Organization, each year infectious diseases kill almost 9 million people, many of them children under five, and they also cause enormous burdens through life-long disability. As described in chapter 3, an **infectious disease** is a communicable disease, including parasitic and zoonotic diseases, and some forms of respiratory infections and diarrheal disease (WHO, 2012a). A communicable disease spreads from individual to individual or from insects, animals, or other carriers to humans. Infectious diseases are sometimes called **tropical diseases** because they are endemic and epidemic infections that cause disease and disability for people living or visiting warmer climates of the world (WHO, 2008a). However, it is important to note that tropical diseases are not necessarily *caused* by climate or geography. They are actually due in part to poor and disenfranchised people having limited or no access to a public health infrastructure (WHO, 2013).

While epidemiologists, medical scientists, health organizations, and governments have made great strides in controlling some of history's most pestilent infectious diseases in developed countries—such as guinea worm, leprosy, onchocerciasis ("river blindness"), lymphatic filariasis, Chagas disease, and rabies—these diseases still plague some of the world's poorest and the most marginalized populations. These diseases, which are less common in industrialized parts of the world, are deemed **Neglected Tropical Diseases** (NTDs) by the World Health Organization because they have faded from focus in terms of research and support. NTDs affect more than 1 billion people worldwide, primarily poor populations living in tropical and subtropical climates. They are frequently clustered together geographically and individuals are often afflicted with more than one parasite or infection. More than 70% of countries and territories that report the presence of NTDs are low-income or lower middle-income economies (WHO, 2012a). Even though an estimated 1 in 7 people globally are affected by NTDs, less than 1% of all drugs registered between 1975 and 2007 were for these tropical diseases (WHO, 2013). For some of these NTDs, the cost of treatment is mere pennies. However, for other NTDs such as Chagas disease, Buruli ulcer, or human African trypanosomiasis, cost effective tools do not exist and they are more challenging to contain (WHO, 2012a). For those who reside in more isolated areas, an NTD may prove fatal before it can be diagnosed because the currently available diagnostic tools require skilled health workers and hospital care.

There is reason to be optimistic, however. Many neglected tropical diseases can be prevented, eliminated, or even eradicated with improved access to existing safe and cost-effective tools. Control relies on simple interventions that can be carried out by non-specialists—for example, schoolteachers, village leaders, and local volunteers—in community-based preventive action. NTDs are now on the global health agenda as the WHO and other health organizations realize that the programs to combat such treatable diseases must be expanded and made accessible to the poor.

Likewise, attention must also be given to acute infectious diseases, diseases which spread from one individual to another. Examples of infectious diseases include malaria, cholera, tuberculosis, HIV, Ebola, SARS (Severe Acute Respiratory Syndrome), avian flu, meningitis, hepatitis, and dengue fever and they pose great health, economic, and security threats to modern society. According to the WHO (2013), most deaths by infectious diseases, almost 90%, are caused by only a handful of diseases. The diseases are: pneumonia, tuberculosis, diarrheal diseases, malaria, measles, and HIV/AIDS. Figure 14.5 below provides a snapshot of the burden of disease by disease and injury.

HIV/AIDS remains a global killer; in fact, it is one of the leading causes of death inclusive of both infectious and chronic diseases, especially among poor countries. According to the WHO (2018), in 2016 there was an estimated 36.7 million people worldwide living with HIV. This represents an increase in those living with HIV from previous years. However, this increase is due to increased longevity for individuals who have the virus, *not new infections*. In fact, new HIV infections declined by 33% between 2001 and 2017 globally (UNDP, 2016). If access to antiretroviral therapy in low- and middle-income countries improves (an estimated 17 million people in such countries have received treatment over the last decade, with 2 million receiving treatment in 2016), it is expected that the population living with HIV will continue to grow as fewer people die from AIDS-related causes since access to retroviral medications has improved (see Figure 14.6).

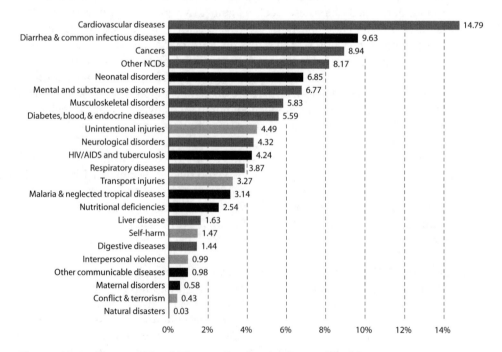

Figure 14.5   Share of Total Disease Burden by Cause, World, 2016

Disease burden by cause as a share of total disease burden. Disease burden is measured in DALYs (Disability-Adjusted Life Year). DALYs are used to measure total burden of disease—both from life lost and years lived with a disability. One DALY equals one lost year of healthy life.

Adapted from *Burden of Disease*, by Max Roser and Hannah Ritchie, 2018a, published online at OurWorldInData.org. Retrieved from https://ourworldindata.org/burden-of-disease

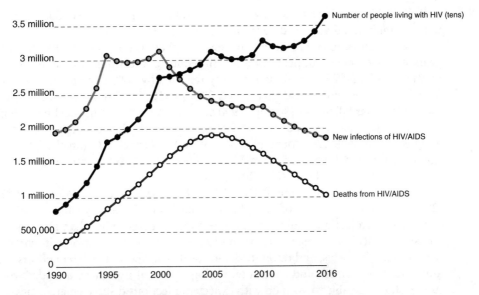

Figure 14.6   Prevalence of HIV: New Cases and Deaths, World

Total number of deaths from HIV/AIDS (not including deaths from tuberculosis), new cases of HIV infection per year, and total number of people living with HIV. The total number of people living with HIV is measured in tens (i.e. equal to 36 million in 2016).

Adapted from *HIV / AIDS*, by Max Roser and Hannah Ritchie, 2018b, published online at OurWorldInData.org. Retrieved from https://ourworldindata.org/hiv-aids

The continent hit hardest by the ravages of HIV/AIDS is Africa, which accounts for 69% of cases globally. In Southern Africa, the region with the highest prevalence of the disease, life expectancy has fallen from 62 years in 1990 through 1995 to 52 years in 2005 through 2010, and is only recently beginning to increase. Unfortunately, the WHO (2013) reports that "life expectancy in the region is not expected to recover to the level where it was in the early 1990s until the year 2030" (p. xx).

It is essential that sustained global efforts continue to help those populations and regions out of reach to antiviral treatments gain access to them. Reduced costs will not resolve the problem entirely; culture, religion, gender, education, and politics also play significant roles in access to treatment.

Other infectious nemeses such as malaria, cholera, and tuberculosis were once under control in industrialized countries during the early part of the 20th century, but they re-emerged in the latter part of the 20th century as the world population became increasingly mobile, transcontinental travel became commonplace, and new strains of diseases emerged as a result of antibiotic resistance. These infectious diseases are still causing significant damage in the 21st century despite having made great strides in vaccine development and immunization programs. However, a number of bacteria strains have become resistant to medicines, and new and reemerging microbes are still a problem. For example, tuberculosis (TB), a disease that had largely been contained by the earlier half of the 20th century, has reemerged with more aggressive strains

(WHO, 2013). TB is second only to HIV/AIDS as a global infectious killer; more than 1.4 million individuals died from it in 2013 (WHO, 2013).

Despite some re-emergent threats, however, there is good news: Over the last few years we have made significant progress in reducing infectious disease. For example, between 2000 and 2010, malaria mortality rates fell by 26% around the world. In the WHO African Region, the decrease was 33% (WHO, 2012a). Also, mortality due to tuberculosis has fallen by 41% since 1990 and continues to steadily decline with global efforts. Ending the TB epidemic by 2030 is among the health targets of the newly adopted Sustainable Development Goals. WHO has set a 2035 target of 95% reduction in deaths and a 90% decline in TB incidence—similar to current levels in low TB incidence countries today (WHO, 2013).

Another report from the WHO, *Global Report for Infectious Disease and Poverty* (2012a), shows projections of mortality and burden of disease by cause from 2004 to 2050. These projections indicated that infectious diseases, other than HIV and tuberculosis, will decline at faster rates than diseases that are more chronic in nature (i.e., heart disease, diabetes, and respiratory illnesses). They point to current efforts such as antibiotic development and control technologies that, if rigorously attended to in the future, should be able to keep up with expected infectious disease emergencies.

Furthermore, the WHO's initiatives, such as Roll Back Malaria, STOP TB, antimicrobial resistance monitoring, partnerships with global NGOs, epidemic and pandemic alert response systems, and modifications of protocols in world travel, trade, land use, and ecology around the world have helped to prevent and reduce the spread of disease. These successes represent a tremendous reduction in human suffering and are a clear success of the former **Millennial Development Goals (MDG)** (which are now the **Sustainable Development Goals**) and efforts related to them. However, we cannot become complacent.

Worldwide recession over the past several years has decreased funding of these efforts and threatens to slow progress. There is still much work to be done. Our global society must continue efforts such as: helping all regions gain access to clean drinking water, improving infrastructure for energy and sanitation in less developed countries, creating and improving regional and international networks and partnerships, developing and improving disease monitoring systems, and strengthening on-the-ground programs and services in order to further reduce the burden of infectious disease.

Trend #4: Chronic Diseases Are Leading Killers across the Globe

As mentioned earlier, it is good news that life expectancy across the globe is increasing and many are enjoying socioeconomic improvements (UN, 2012a). However, the bad news is that as people live longer and adopt unhealthy lifestyle habits (such as smoking, sedentary living, and high-fat diets), a global epidemic of chronic diseases such as heart disease, cancer, diabetes, obesity, and depression is unfolding (UN, 2012a). The UN (2012a) reports that each year, non-communicable diseases (NCDs) cause more than 36 million deaths worldwide, representing around 63% of all mortality. Four categories of NCDs are responsible for more than 80% of NCD deaths globally: cardiovascular diseases, cancers, diabetes, and chronic respiratory diseases. Exposures to risk factors that accumulate over the life course, such as tobacco use, unhealthy diets, physical inactivity, and harmful use of alcohol, increase the risk of morbidity and mortality due to NCDs. The World Health Organization (2013) estimates that over 20 million deaths could be prevented each year by reducing the level of exposure to these modifiable risk factors.

Chronic diseases are now among the leading causes of death for people in high-, middle-, and low-income countries (see Figure 14.7). In low-income countries less than a quarter of all people reach the age of 70, and more than a third of all deaths are among children under 14 (WHO, 2013). Although cardiovascular diseases are among the leading causes of death in these countries, the combined toll of infectious diseases (especially HIV/AIDS, lung infections, tuberculosis, diarrheal diseases, and malaria) claims more lives. In middle-income countries, nearly half of all people live to age 70 and chronic diseases are the major killers. In high-income countries, more than two thirds of all people live beyond age 70 and predominantly die of chronic diseases (WHO, 2013). We have at our disposal the knowledge to combat the lifestyle choices that contribute to chronic disease. The exciting news is that you, as a future community health professional, are part of the solution!

Rank 2012	Rank 2000	Cause of death	Deaths per 100,000 population
1	1	Ischaemic heart disease	104.0
2	2	Stroke	94.3
3	4	Chronic obstructive pulmonary disease	43.9
4	3	Lower respiratory infections	43.1
5	9	Trachea, bronchus, lung cancers	22.6
6	6	HIV/AIDS	21.7
7	5	Diarrhoeal diseases	21.2
8	10	Diabetes mellitus	21.2
9	12	Road injury	17.7
10	16	Hypertensive heart disease	16.1
11	8	Preterm birth complications	16.0
12	13	Cirrhosis of the liver	14.4
13	7	Tuberculosis	13.2
14	17	Kidney diseases	12.2
15	14	Self-harm	11.4
16	11	Birth asphyxia and birth trauma	10.5
17		Liver cancer	10.5
18	18	Stomach cancer	10.4
19		Colon and rectum cancers	10.2
20		Alzheimer's disease and other dementias	9.9

Noncommunicable diseases
Infectious and parasitic diseases
Injuries

2012

2000

Figure 14.7   Top 20 Leading Causes of Death Worldwide, 2000–12

From *Top 20 Leading Causes of Death Worldwide, 2000–12*, Oxford Analytica Daily Brief, 2016. Retrieved from https://dailybrief.oxan.com/Analysis/GI214168/Top-20-leading-causes-of-death-worldwide-2000-12. Data from World Health Organization.

≡ Trends in Global Capacity

Have you ever heard the phrase, "health is wealth"? It's not just catchy—it's true. A country's economic prosperity, stability, or decline has a momentous impact on the health of its citizens. Simply put, the health status of each country's citizens will impact their ability to add to their country's **gross national product (GNP)**, or the sum of all goods and services a country produces for a given year. Health is a resource that enables more individuals to work, generating productivity and economic activity. In turn, the wealth generated helps stabilize a country economically and politically and improves the standard of living or quality of life for those living there. As countries in the 21st century harness new technologies, expand their sources of industry and revenue, maximize their natural resources, educate and train those in the labor force, and respond to demands from the global economy, they will strengthen their ability to establish and uphold a stable or expanding economic environment, which is also known as **global capacity**. Conversely, those countries which lack natural resources, industry, education, political stability, internal peace, and a strong labor force will be vulnerable to widespread poverty, disease, and violence.

Trend #5: Educating Women and Girls Raises a Country's GDP and Health Status

Education is the key to increasing a country's global capacity, and the education of women, especially, improves more than just literacy rates—it saves millions of lives. Educated women tend to use health services more and often make better choices on hygiene, nutrition, and parenting. As female education rates rise, fertility, population growth, and infant and child mortality fall, and family health improves (UN, 2011). There is significant evidence to support this. For example, American researchers at the University of Washington analyzed 915 censuses and surveys from 175 countries tracking education, economic growth, HIV infection rates, and child deaths from 1970 to 2009. Results showed that for every extra year of education a woman achieved, the death rate for children under five dropped by almost 10 percent! The researchers estimated that 4.2 million fewer children died in 2009 than in 1970 because women of child-bearing age in developing countries were more educated. The world has begun to take notice. Global Campaigns, such as the United Nation's Before 10 Campaign, the UN Campaign for Women, the Malala Fund, and GirlRising.org are just a few of the many efforts globally to increase gender equality and education. In fact, in 2017, the UN's *Population Prospectus* focused solely on the importance of supporting girls at age 10. The report emphasized the importance of the new SDGs and was the first time in history that a UN agenda explicitly committed countries to leaving no one behind as they seek to develop.

Why age 10? According to the United Nations Population Fund's (2017) *State of the World Population* report:

> At 10, a girl arrives at a vulnerable point in her life. She must negotiate a tricky transition to adulthood, with its rapid changes in body and brain, and dramatic shifts in family and social expectations. Although risks abound for both girls and boys, gender discrimination makes these worse for girls in almost every way. Public

policies often focus on young children or older adolescents, failing to adequately manage the potential risks 10-year-old girls might face. (para. 5)

More than 35 million of today's 10-year-old girls live in countries with high levels of gender inequality, measured by a Gender Inequality Index.

> Relative to their brothers, these girls are less likely to stay in school, more likely to be engaged in child labor, more likely to be married before they turn 18, more likely to experience intimate partner violence, more likely to suffer from complications related to pregnancy and childbearing, and less likely to have a substantive say in household decisions, including about their schooling or health care. If her rights are not well protected, through appropriate laws, services and investments, the chance to bloom in adolescence and become a fully fledged adult forever slips away. The implications for these patters can also extend to families, communities and countries. (UNFPA, 2017, para. 7)

Addressing gender equity and factors that impact girls' access to education also has an impact on maternal health. Maternal mortality represents the largest health inequity in the world, and it relates to both Goals 1 & 3 of the UN's **Sustainable Development Goals** (Figure 14.1).

Even in this Millennial society, maternal mortality is still a pressing issue. Every year, more than half a million women die during pregnancy and childbirth, largely from problems that can be prevented. And for every woman who dies, 20 other women suffer injuries and disabilities that can last a lifetime and rob them of energy and productivity (UNFPA, 2013b).

Early pregnancy takes a toll on a girl's health, education, and rights. As reported in the *State of World Population 2013* produced by the United Nations Population Fund (UNFPA), out of the 7.3 million births globally, 2 million are to girls who are 14 or younger. Many of these young women will suffer serious long-term health and social consequences from pregnancy (UNFPA, 2013b). Too often, society blames only the young woman for getting pregnant. However, as the executive director of the United Nations Population Fund explains,

> The reality is that adolescent pregnancy is most often not the result of a deliberate choice, but rather the absence of choices, and of circumstances beyond a girl's control. It is a consequence of little or no access to school, employment, quality information and health care. (UNFPA, 2013a, par. 5)

To tackle maternal mortality and adolescent pregnancy, the UN urges countries to adopt a holistic approach which does not dwell on changing girls' behavior, but seeks to change attitudes in society so girls are encouraged to stay in school, child marriage is banned, girls have access to sexual and reproductive health including contraception, and young mothers have better support systems.

Educating women is also a smart economic decision that benefits everyone. The success of achieving the Millennial Development Goal of reducing the number of individuals who live on less than $1.90 (MDG #1) (mentioned in Trend #7 below) was met *ahead of time* because of the efforts made by large developing countries, such as China and Brazil, investing more in education, especially among young women (UNFPA, 2017). Achieving equity in education results in more equity in the workforce and a stronger, more productive economy. It also reduces a country's financial costs associated with illness, early child and maternal mortality, and early pregnancy.

Educating girls and women improves lives for everyone. The Ghanaian scholar, Dr. James Emmanuel Kwegyir-Aggrey, once wrote, "If you educate a man you educate an individual, but if you educate a **woman** you educate a nation." In addition to improving the status of women worldwide, it elevates everyone's quality of life and human capacity. Children of educated mothers, especially daughters, are more likely to be enrolled in school and to attain higher levels of education. Educated women are also more politically active and better informed about their legal rights and how to exercise them. The education of women improves health, results in greater likelihood for peace, reduces poverty, and strengthens economies. According to the United Nations Development Programme (2013), "Educating women through adulthood is the closest thing to a 'silver bullet' formula for accelerating human development" (p. E-1-3).

Trend #6: Mobile Health Technology Is Reducing Poverty and Disease

It seems almost absurd to think that individuals in low-income or developing countries who often have little or no access to running water, much less a computer or any other technology, could be "lifted from poverty" by something as ubiquitous as a cell phone. However, there are a growing number of economists who maintain that cell phones and other communication technology can restructure developing countries. The possibilities afforded by a proliferation of cell phones are potentially revolutionary. In just the last 10 years, diffusion of cell phone use in developing countries has increased tremendously. According to the International Telecommunication Union (ITU, 2011), in 2011 there were over 5 billion wireless subscribers; over 70% of them reside in low- and middle-income countries. Conversely, less than 30% of populations in developing nations had access to Internet technology, but that number is expected to rise over the next decade (WHO, 2011). Even the smallest improvements in communication and efficiency in developing countries could raise their GDP significantly and reshape the global economy in ways that we are just beginning to understand.

The ideal case study of this antipoverty innovation comes from Bangladesh, once the poorest country in the world. In 1990 the Grameen Bank, an unconventional enterprise that makes **microloans** to the poor, provided a loan to Grameen Telecommunications, a nonprofit organization that provides low-cost phone services in rural areas. Using the borrowed money, village entrepreneurs purchased mobile phones which they then used to sell phone services to other villagers. This led to a rise of mobile phone entrepreneurs, of which 95% were female. Villagers reaped the benefit of instant communication, and village entrepreneurs earned a steady income. Even the poorest of the poor could use the phones to communicate with family, sell their goods to others who lived out of the area, find employment elsewhere, check prices in other markets before selling their goods, and have more options during emergency situations (Corbett, 2008). This mobile phone enterprise created a domino effect, spurring other economic activities, moving people above the poverty line, and replacing feelings of fatalism with hope. Most importantly, this case study has shown that even individuals living in the most abject poverty have proven themselves to be more technologically savvy and more enterprising than people would have believed.

The use of mobile technology is impacting more than just economies, it is also reshaping global health and health care. As mentioned in chapters 11 and 13, **mobile health** (mHealth) is "the medical and public health practice supported by mobile devices, such as mobile phones, patient monitoring devices, personal digital assistants (PDAs), and other wireless devices" (World Health Organization, 2011, p. 15). It is a new frontier which has altered the way in which health information is delivered and to whom, how health data is retrieved and stored, and ways in which people communicate.

Examples of mHealth span continents and health issues. For example, EpiSurveyor is a free, mobile software program that has been used in developing countries by community health workers to collect public health data using their cell phones. Another example is SexInfo, a sexual health text message service developed by the Internet Sexuality Information Services (ISIS) in partnership with the San Francisco Department of Public Health to reduce rising rates of gonorrhea among African American youth. mHealth is expanding our reach as a global society; in fact, commercial wireless signals cover over 85% of the world's population, extending far beyond the reach of the electrical grid (WHO, 2011). Governments are expressing interest in mHealth as a complementary strategy for strengthening health systems and achieving the Sustainable Development Goals in low- and middle-income countries.

Mobile technology is now and will continue to be the future of health. Undoubtedly, it will evolve from primarily tracking or gaming devices to more sophisticated health tools, such as patient home-monitoring devices to help reduce hospital re-admittance or as mobile screening tools that can transform your phone into an ultrasound scanner.

As health professionals, we can harness technology to our advantage to improve not only individual and community health, but also our discipline and professional competencies. Keeping up with this technology is a constant challenge, of course. In fact, by the time you read this statement, there will have likely been thousands of health apps launched since the inception of this paragraph. Perhaps you've already created one?

Trend #7: Depleting Natural Resources Require "Green Solutions"

One could argue that finding alternatives and solutions to protecting the earth's resources is the most pressing challenge of the new millennium. In the opening of Thomas Friedman's op-ed, "The Earth Is Full" (one of the most shared pieces on *The New York Times* website), he writes:

> You really do have to wonder whether a few years from now we'll look back at the first decade of the 21st century—when food prices spiked, energy prices soared, world population surged, tornados plowed through cities, floods and droughts set records, populations were displaced and governments were threatened by the confluence of it all—and ask ourselves: "What were we thinking? How did we not panic when the evidence was so obvious that we'd crossed some growth/climate/natural resource/population redlines all at once?" (2011, par 1)

The link between the environment and human health has been established for centuries. Why is it, as Friedman writes, are we, as a global society, not reacting as quickly to the warning sirens? There are a myriad of factors, such as politics, economics, education, urbanization, war, apathy, uncertainty, and cynicism, that slow our global response to addressing environmental threats. However, to Paul Gilding, former executive director of Greenpeace, Australian environmentalist, and author, there is just one reason: denial. Gilding notes, "When you are surrounded by something so big that requires you to change everything about the way you think and see the world, then denial is the natural response" (Romm, 2011, par. 3).

The phrase "Going Green"—using the earth's resources wisely and trying to improve the overall health of the planet—used to represent a preferred way of living, but now it represents a required change for human survival. The World Health Organization, American Public Health Association, Environmental Protection Agency, and a number of other health and environmentally focused organizations maintain that a new approach to urbanization offers us the opportunity to develop healthy cities by pooling our concentrated resources to create positive environments. WHO refers to it as the **preferred future** and describes it as follows:

> We create an environment in which everyone's health is promoted and protected—whether this is in schools, workplaces, or the home. An environment in which the air is clear, the water safe, and where health, transport, and waste management services are well managed and effective. An environment in which everyone enjoys access to social amenities such as safe play areas for children. An environment in which the different "players"—civilians young and old, industries and companies, municipal authorities, nongovernmental organizations, and public utilities—work together to optimize use of the resources, skills, and capacities that are often abundant in urban areas. In short, a healthy city that meets needs for work, learning, rest, and play. (WHO, 1999)

Former U.S. vice president Al Gore, a 2007 Nobel Peace Prize winner for his environmental advocacy, awakened the political and social consciousness of America to the impending energy and climate crisis. In a 2008 speech at a national convention, Gore warned that the United Sates and the rest of the world were "facing unprecedented problems, including growing demand for electricity, dangerous changes in the climate driven largely by emissions of carbon dioxide, and political instability in regions that produce much of the world's oil" (Broder, 2008, para. 5). "The survival of the United States of America as we know it is at risk," he warned, and "the future of human civilization is at stake" (Broder, 2008, para. 5).

Years after Gore's speech, we have seen even more in the headlines and published scientific journals about the human imprint on Earth. As a global society, we are overdue to take action to reverse this trend. As the world population grows and urbanization spreads, the earth's natural resources, habitats, and climates will be increasingly imperiled unless we can learn to balance our need to industrialize and modernize with the future sustainability of the earth. In fact, the issue of water (or lack thereof) was the focus of the 137th 2009 Annual Conference of the American Public Health Association whose theme was "Water and Public Health: the 21st Century Challenge." Managing water, in addition to other natural resources, has become an important part of many national agendas, and is a vital part of achieving Sustainable Development Goals (UN, 2016).

Have we reached a point in history where our urbanization and global population has reached maximum capacity? According to Friedman, and many others, "the earth is full." But this is not science fiction, nor should it come as a surprise. According to Gilding:

> If you cut down more trees than you grow, you run out of trees. If you put additional nitrogen into a water system, you change the type and quantity of life that water can support. If you thicken the Earth's CO^2 blanket, the Earth gets warmer. If you do all these and many more things at once, you change the way the whole system of Planet Earth behaves, with social, economic, and life support impacts. This is not speculation; this is high school science. (Romm, 2011, par. 3).

This vision of a healthy community requires more than just a village to actualize. It requires a forward-thinking, global citizenry working together. This vision may seem idyllic, but many scientists, environmentalists, activists, educators, and concerned citizens say it *is* achievable. Even small changes now will result in big environmental and global health gains for years to come. Those individuals working on the front lines (or trenches) of community health play a key role in helping others to understand the complete picture and how those socio-ecological factors impact everyone. But we must act quickly. As Gilding (2011) warns, "The longer we wait, the bigger the response required" (para. 4).

Trend #8: Abject Poverty Has Declined, but Poverty and Hunger Still Persist

When it comes to the issue of poverty, there is good news and bad. Let's start with the good news: According to the World Bank (2018), there are less people living today on $1.90 a day than there were a decade ago. In fact, since 1990, more than 1 billion people no longer live in extreme poverty. In 2015, there were 702 million people, or 9.6% of the global population, living in extreme poverty in comparison to 1.75 billion in 1990 (World Bank, 2018). Furthermore, the former Millennial Development Goal #1 to reduce extreme poverty rates by half was met five years *ahead* of the 2015 deadline. Despite these remarkable gains, the number of people living in extreme poverty may not be falling fast enough to reach the new MDG target of ending extreme poverty by 2030. Most of those living in poverty and hunger are women and children (World Bank, 2015). After a prolonged decline, world hunger appears to be on the rise again due to political conflicts, climate change, and economic recessions (Food and Agriculture Organizations of the United Nations [FAOUN], 2017). According to the World Bank (2015), one in eight people on the planet are going hungry. The estimated number of undernourished people increased to 815 million in 2016, up from 777 million in 2015 (FAOUN, 2017).

Food insecurity, starvation, and abject poverty impact all of us as a global society. Poverty and hunger are like weapons of mass destruction, unjustly claiming billions of lives each year and destroying human potential and peace.

As explained by the World Bank (2014):

> Children who are malnourished when they reach their second birthday could suffer permanent physical and cognitive damage, thereby affecting their future health, welfare, and economic well-being. For developing countries, the impact on their ability to raise a productive workforce can last for generations, while in the shorter term rising food prices can exacerbate inequality and lead to conflict and political instability. (para. 1)

Hunger and poverty malign one's opportunity for education, and increase political unrest, violence, terrorism, and gender inequalities. It is within our grasp to eradicate hunger and poverty within the next decade. According to the World Bank (2014), we can do this by:

- investing in agriculture
- creating jobs
- expanding social safety nets
- expanding nutrition programs that target children under two years of age
- universalizing education
- promoting gender equality
- protecting vulnerable countries during crises

If there is any war worth fighting, and one in which we had the best odds of winning and saving lives in the process, it is the war on poverty. Reducing poverty has been a slow and steady process, with reductions within some groups and parts of the world, and increases in others. For example, in the United States, since 1970, there has been steady progress in reducing poverty, especially among persons over 65, largely due to Social Security. However, between the years 2007 and 2011, those numbers increased due to economic recession. According to a U.S. Census Bureau report by Semega, Fontenot, and Kollar (2017), progress has been minimal among all other age groups, almost stagnant. These numbers might look a little different if you use a different measure of poverty, or include health care benefits, but not by much. However, the numbers begin to look more optimistic when you view this issue globally, especially in developing countries. Extreme poverty has decreased and is projected by the World Bank to continue to shrink if countries continue to invest in people's education, health, and social safety nets (World Bank, 2015). Jim Young Kim, World Bank group president, speaking at an annual meeting in 2013, said:

> This is the best story in the world today—these projections show us that we are the first generation in human history that can end extreme poverty. This new forecast of poverty falling into the single digits should give us new momentum and help us focus even more clearly on the most effective strategies to end extreme poverty. It will be extraordinarily hard, especially in a period of slower global growth, volatile financial markets, conflicts, high youth unemployment, and the growing impact of climate change. But it remains within our grasp, as long as our high aspirations are matched by country-led plans that help the still millions of people living in extreme poverty. (World Bank, 2015, para. 5)

Trends in the Global Health System

The World Health Organization (2008c) defines a health system as "all the organizations, institutions, resources, and people whose primary purpose is to improve health" (para. 1). Two trends in the global health system that might impact your future as a health professional are the global health worker shortage and the increasing emphasis on global health promotion.

Trend #9: The Health Worker Shortage Is Increasing

According to a WHO (2013) report entitled, *A Universal Truth: No Health Without a Workforce*, the world needs to train more health professionals—and fast. In this report, the WHO warns that the world will be short 12.9 million health care workers by 2035; in 2013, that figure stood at 7.2 million. "If the shortage of healthcare workers, is not addressed now, it will have serious implications for the health of billions of people across all regions of the world" (WHO, 2013, para. 1). A more recent report by Darzi and Evans (2016) shows that the situation is worsening. The authors cite the WHO in reporting that the shortage is actually higher than predicted in 2013, increasing to 18 million shortfall by 2030.

While shortages exist across all continents, Asia and Africa are currently experiencing the greatest shortage of health care workers. Sub-Saharan Africa is a region where the shortage is most acute: "In the 47 countries of sub-Saharan Africa, just 168 medical schools exist. Of those countries, 11 have no medical schools, and 24 countries have only one medical school" (WHO, 2013, para. 7). This shortage is driven by a number of factors, according to the WHO report including:

- Populations are living longer in high-income countries, which are struggling with increasing rates of heart disease, diabetes, and other chronic conditions.

- In addition, millions of health care workers are reaching retirement age and replacement is a challenge.

- Many health workers (such as nurses) are leaving their profession due to burn-out, stress, and/or job dissatisfaction.

- Advanced practitioners, midwives, nurses and other health professionals (such as health educators) are insufficiently used in many settings.

- Availability and accessibility of health workers continue to vary widely within countries because of regional conditions which make it difficult to attract and retain workers. For example, there are far more health professionals working in urban vs. rural areas.

- There is a pressing need to revisit educational requirements and increase the volume of academic programs to sustain ageing and increasing populations;

- Health worker turnover must be addressed in order to improve motivation and retention of trained health professionals.

- Performance assessment and quality of care must be priorities

- The capacity to predict human resources for health needs is lacking in many countries including those considered modernized. (2013, p. 4)

The workforce shortage and migration trends are also true within the United States, where dwindling numbers of primary care providers in medicine and dentistry cannot meet the demands of a growing and aging population (Darzi & Evans, 2016). In addition, the implementation of the Affordable Care Act in the U.S. and a focus on improving primary care means more health care workers are needed to support the demand since the population's access to health care has improved. In addition, an increased focus on prevention will expand opportunities for a number of health professions including health educators. According to the U.S. Bureau of Labor and Statistics, the demand for trained health educators will increase by nearly 19% over the next decade (BLS, 2014).

In addition, a public health workforce crisis is also looming (ASPH, 2008; Perlino, 2006). According to a 2008 report from the Association of Schools of Public Health (ASPH), this workforce has decreased by over 50,000 employees since 1980, is expected to dwindle an additional 23% by 2012, and will not be able to meet the expected demand for an additional 250,000 workers by 2020.

Consequences of these worker shortages are already beginning to reverberate in the U.S. and around the world (ASPH, 2008; Darzi & Evans, 2016). Addressing this global crisis will require not only national policy changes but international cooperation and will also underscore the need for more intra-professional collaboration (as we discussed in chapter 1). Improving individual and population health necessitates health professionals working together at all levels of care. We encourage you to think of the global health challenge as an opportunity for you to use your training in community health to make a significant impact.

The key to becoming part of the global health solution is to think beyond what can be seen at the moment. BigPictureSmallWorld, Inc. (www.BigPictureSmallWorld.com) creates Web movies for the United Nations Environmental Programme and other organizations that inspire and challenge the world to think creatively. In a quote from the Web movie, *America America*, Medard Gabel (2006) reminds us that:

> What you do matters.
> Every person is a suggestion of what they should be.
> Every country is the seed of what it could be.
> We walk as prophesies of the next age. (frames 12–13)

Trend #10: Global Health Promotion Is the New Horizon

As mentioned in chapter 1 and throughout this text, health and well-being are heavily influenced by social, economic, political, and ecological factors outside of the individual as well as the health care system. These forces largely shape the circumstances in which people grow, live, work, and age as well as the systems put in place to deal with health needs ultimately leading to inequities in health between and within countries. Consequently, the attainment of health for all depends on a comprehensive, holistic, and culturally relative approach which goes beyond traditional medical care, and involves communities, health providers, and other stakeholders. This holistic approach captures the essence of **global health promotion**: "a process that can empower individuals and communities to take actions that will improve their well-being, foster leadership for public health, promote inter-sectoral action to build healthy public policies and create sustainable health systems in the global society" (Kumar & Preetha, 2012, para. 3).

You may recall from earlier chapters that *Healthy People 2020* are a set of goals and objectives for the U.S. that guide health promotion and strategies to improve quality of life for individuals across all stages of life (U.S. Department of Health and Human Services, 2010). At the global level are the former United Nation's **Millennium Development ment Goals (MDGs)**, which are now the **Sustainable Development Goals (SDGs)**. In 2000, at the beginning of the new millennium, global leaders signed the **United Nations Millennium Declaration**, a commitment "to combat poverty, hunger, disease, illiteracy, environmental degradation, and discrimination against women" (WHO, 2008b, para. 1). These leaders developed the (then) eight Millennium Development Goals (MDGs) with a target year of 2015 to achieve goals addressing issues such as: hunger and extreme poverty, universal primary education, gender quality and empowerment, reducing child mortality, and improving maternal health. You can read more about the former MDGs on the UN website at http://www.un.org.

So what happened in 2015? Were all of the MDGs achieved? Unfortunately they were not. Yet over the last two decades, there has been remarkable progress in achieving of some of them. As mentioned earlier in this chapter, extreme poverty and hunger were reduced significantly. The number of children attending primary school increased, the mortality rate for children under the age of five (globally) dropped in most countries, and women and girls are major drivers of development. However, we are still behind in many ways. As explained by the United Nations General Assembly,

> Progress has been insufficient and highly uneven. Rural areas and marginalized groups continue to lag behind on virtually all goals and targets. Countries in or emerging from conflict, disaster or instability face significant challenges. In addition, the economic and financial crisis in recent years has complicated efforts, including by putting pressure on official development assistance. (2013, p. 5)

MDGs have evolved into the SDGs. *Transforming Our World: The 2030 Agenda for Sustainable Development* outlines the SDGs, which are a set of 17 "Global Goals," and includes 169 targets created to support goal success. The 17 goals are illustrated in Figure 14.8.

Figure 14.8   Sustainable Development Goals (SDGs)

Reprinted from World Health Organization. Retrieved from http://www.who.int/mediacentre/events/meetings/2015/sdgs-icons-950.jpg?ua=1

The SDGs were developed by representatives from 70 countries working in open discussion groups (Lee, et al., 2016). In addition, the UN conducted a series of "global conversations" (UN, 2015). These included 11 thematic and 83 national consultations, and door-to-door surveys. The UN also launched an online *My World* survey asking people to prioritize the areas they'd like to see addressed in the goals. The results of the consultations were fed into the working group's discussions and reflected in the SDGs. Which of these SDGs do you feel most impact your own health and well-being?

It would be too simplistic for us to imply that everything we have covered in this textbook will work in all global health situations. In fact, whether you apply this textbook content in a country that differs from your own or in your local community, adaptation to population interests, needs, cultures, and unique situations is always warranted. Nevertheless, leaders of the International Union for Health Promotion and Education (IUHPE, 2007) have pointed out that the general principles and framework of health education and health promotion are embedded in the former MDGs and current SDGs. Health promotion is already a recognized professional paradigm in many countries of the world. The IUHPE recommends that future workers in the global health arena possess tools for "developing the knowledge and skills for advocacy and mediation with politicians and the private sector, assessing the impact of policies on health and its determinants, accessing and using available information and evidence, and evaluating interventions" (2007, p. 5) in global health settings.

Looking ahead, beyond the SDGs and targets, the UN's vision must lean on global collaboration with sustainable development at the center:

> The articulation of a post-2015 development agenda provides an opportunity to place sustainable development where it should be: at the core of humankind's pursuit of shared progress. With a new sustainable development agenda, the world can make many historic achievements: eradicating extreme poverty by 2030, protecting the environment and promoting social inclusion and economic opportunities for all. Ultimately, the aspiration of the development agenda beyond 2015 is to create a just and prosperous world where all people realize their rights and live with dignity and hope. (UN General Assembly, 2013, p. 12)

To this end we offer some advice in FYI 14.1 that may seem contradictory at a glance but really isn't. The first paired set of recommendations in that FYI, "Think globally. Act locally," can truly be accomplished simultaneously if you master the art of addressing local communities within the context of global perspectives. Furthermore, FYI 14.2 lists important health organizations and resources that will be valuable guides as you seek to learn more and expand your view of the global landscape.

14.1   Insights and Approaches for Future Success

These insights and approaches are not as contradictory as they may seem at first glance.

Think globally	Act locally
Remain current	Know your history
Know a lot	Assume you don't know much
Be patient	Be assertive
Be flexible	Be consistent
Use creativity	Honor tradition
Be a team player	Be a leader
Work hard	Have fun

FYI

14.2   Global Health Organizations and Resources

Centers for Disease Control and Prevention (CDC) Coordinating Office for Global Health	www.cdc.gov/cogh
The Clinton Global Initiative	www.clintonglobalinitiative.org
Department of Commerce—U.S. Census Bureau	www.census.gov
Food and Drug Administration (FDA) Office of International Programs	www.fda.gov/oia/homepage.htm
Bill and Melinda Gates Foundation	www.gatesfoundation.org
The Global Fund to Fight AIDS, Tuberculosis, and Malaria	www.theglobalfund.org
Global Health Council	www.globalhealth.org
Global Health Education Consortium	www.globalhealthedu.org
Global Partnerships	www.globalpartnerships.org
One Campaign	www.one.org
Pan-American Health Organization (PAHO)	www.paho.org
Partners in Health (PIH)	www.pih.org
UNICEF	www.unicef.org
United Nations	www.un.org
U.S. Agency for International Development (USAID)	www.usaid.gov
U.S. State Department	www.state.gov
World Health Organization	www.who.org

≡ In Conclusion

As discussed in this chapter and throughout this text, we live in a rapidly evolving society in which change is the only true constant. Staying abreast of global trends and needed information and skills will require an ongoing commitment on your part, particularly after you graduate. Some health professionals who are working in the field find it difficult to carve out of their busy schedules the time needed for professional development. In light of the rapid pace at which our profession and the world are changing, we urge you to view continual renewal as a necessity rather than a luxury. To be adequately equipped for success in the field of community health, we encourage you to:

- Reach beyond the confines of course expectations and grade incentives, and view learning as the lifeline to your professional future.

- Adopt and implement a plan for professional development beyond graduation.

- Develop a deep-rooted understanding of community health within the context of global social structures and quality of life.

- Pay close attention to predicted trends, and embrace new ideas and technologies as they develop.

- Assume that there is always more to learn, and take the frequent initiative to do so. Establish a regular period (at least one day a month) in which you read professional literature and visit reliable Internet sources.

- Broaden your community perspective; visit and revisit community organizations and information sources, attend community events, remain actively involved in the community, and listen to its members.

- Be patient when working toward community goals since wide-sweeping change, especially at the policy level, can take time. When necessary, initiate small tasks with reachable objectives at the beginning of each community effort.

- Be willing to try something new if you think it will appeal to targeted members of a community, but be sure to always consider and respect the culture and unique characteristics of your community.

- Remember that it really does "take a village." Community health is about working together and empowering people to help themselves. It is not a didactic process where professionals, who claim to know what is best, reign over those who are most in need. Everyone plays an important role in improving quality of life on a global scale. We challenge you to adopt this mind-set, and as you work with others toward this common goal, lead in the spirit of unity:

> **Tao of Leadership**
>
> Go to the people
> Live with them
> Love them
> Learn from them
> Start with what they have
> Build on what they know.

But of the best leaders
When their task is accomplished
Their work is done
The people will all remark
We have done it ourselves.

—Lao Tzu, from *The Tao of Leadership* (ancient Chinese text)

REVIEW QUESTIONS

1. Analyze the concept of quality of life from a global perspective.

2. Discuss the health needs that may arise in the future as a result of what is happening in the world and in U.S. communities today.

3. Describe predicted changes in world demographics, health care systems, and their potential influence on community health education and promotion.

4. Explain how chronic diseases have overtaken infectious diseases as the world's leading killers.

5. Discuss why many infectious diseases, such as TB, are making a comeback.

6. Explain the role technology plays in improving individual and global health.

7. Recount three to four factors which have led to an increasing shortage of health care professionals worldwide.

8. Justify how the Sustainable Development Goals play an important role in global health promotion.

9. Provide suggestions for lifelong learning and career development in community health.

FOR YOUR APPLICATION

Addressing Quality-of-Life Issues

Interview three people whose age, culture, and lifestyle differ from one another. Ask each to describe his or her personal definition of quality of life and the specific health issues that affect it. Use the results to:

- compare responses across interviews and identify similarities and differences,

- identify at least two professional disciplines outside of your own that could help enhance the quality of life of your interviewees, and

- brainstorm efforts that could involve representatives of these disciplines in a collaborative effort.

Global Impact of Disease

Research a chronic or infectious disease that is a major concern for the 21st century. Explain the historical trend of the disease globally as well as the projected impact of the disease in geographic, economic, social, and political terms. Highlight the role community health professionals can play in reducing the impact of the disease worldwide.

Global Health Promotion

Identify a global health organization, campaign, non-profit, and/or NGO that is working to improve an area of health related to the Sustainable Development Goals. Describe the organization's mission, its goals and objectives, and activities that it has implemented to achieve its goals. What are the organization's achievements to date, and what can other organizations learn from it? How is this organization contributing to global health promotion?

Polishing Your Portfolio

Review the narrative of your philosophy of health (chapter 1, "For Your Application"). Critique it in light of what you have learned from this textbook, particularly from this chapter, about quality of life for our *global* community and future trends. Revise the narrative to more accurately reflect your current perspectives about health, health education, and your role as a future health educator. Ask two health professionals who are working in your targeted employment area to review your entire portfolio (see Appendix B) and suggest format and content changes. Continue to add portfolio content as you progress through your degree program. Don't wait until graduation to seek out profession-related work and volunteer experiences. Carve time from your busy schedule to prepare yourself for the job market of the future.

Appendix A

Community Assessment Project Guide

 ## Part 1

1. **Describe the makeup and history of the community to provide a context within which to collect data on community members' current concerns as well as collective capacity** (Community Description)

   a. Comment on the type of information that best describes the community (e.g., demographic, historical, political, civic participation, key leaders, past concerns, geographic, assets).

   b. Describe the sources of information used (e.g., public record, local people, Internet, map, phone book, library, newspaper).

   c. Include pictures of the community to provide evidence of both resources and barriers to quality of life.

2. **Seek out community "gatekeepers" for perceptions on community health issues.**

   a. Identify at least two community gatekeepers (respected individuals, with or without positions of authority, who have some influence on the community).

   b. Interview the gatekeepers.

   c. Describe who you listened to and why.

   d. Describe how you arranged to listen to community leaders and members.

   e. Describe the methods (e.g., listening sessions, public forums, interviews, concerns surveys, focus groups) you used to listen to the community.

   f. Address whether the problems identified by the gatekeepers match epidemiological data and research information relating to the community.

   g. Describe the issues of concern to people in the community (i.e., do they care about safety, education, housing, access to health care, etc.).

   h. Discuss how important these issues are to the community.

   i. Discuss how satisfied community members are with past and current efforts to address the issues.

   j. List priority concerns based on issues of high importance and low satisfaction.

≡ Part II

3. **Describe the health problem identified and the methods (e.g., public forums, listening sessions, focus groups, interviews, surveys, observation) used to collect descriptive information from the community.**

   a. Describe the community-level indicators—the incidence (new cases) or prevalence (existing cases) of disease, and the social indicators related to the disease (i.e., rate of poverty in the community, unemployment, etc.).

   b. Report how frequently the problem (or related behavior) occurs (i.e., current statistics).

   c. Describe how many people are affected by the problem and the severity of its effects.

   d. Conduct a PRECEDE analysis of the identified health issue (predisposing, enabling, and reinforcing factors).

   e. Explain how feasible it is to address the issue.

   f. Discuss the possible impact and/or consequences of solving it.

   g. Indicate the intended populations and subgroups identified by stakeholders as particularly likely to benefit from the effort.

   h. Identify the method used to collect data from the identified target group.

   i. Describe any existing health assessment surveys available to use in data collection with the target group.

   j. Select the instrument (i.e., survey) used to collect the information.

   k. Describe the instrument in detail (authors, purpose, how it was developed). Include entire survey in an appendix.

   l. Explain how you selected the intended group or groups to take the survey.

   m. Describe your procedures (e.g., surveys, interviews) to gather information.

   n. If using a focus group or community forum in lieu of or in addition to a survey, list the question you used as well as the characteristics of the group you're interviewing (i.e., role in community, age, ethnicity, occupation, etc.).

≡ Part III

4. **Compile and describe the evidence suggesting that identified issues should be a priority.**

   a. Analyze data collected.

   b. Explain methods used to analyze data.

   c. Present findings (use descriptive statistics, charts, and graphs).

   d. Describe the barriers and existing community resources for addressing the identified issue(s) and achieving the goal (e.g., denial, discounting the problem). Describe how they can be minimized (e.g., reframing the issue).

5. **Provide suggestions for health education program developers.**

   a. Address how health education can address the predisposing, enabling, and reinforcing factors related to the health issue.

   b. Recommend a health education theory that can be used as a foundation for program planners.

   c. Indicate what resources and assets are available and where.

   d. Identify the community leaders. Describe the individuals and organizations with influence in the community who might support (or oppose) efforts to address this issue.

   e. Describe the community projects currently in progress. Identify strengths and weaknesses of these sources and propose how these efforts might be supported with future health education efforts based on this community health assessment.

Table A.1   Components to Include in a Formal Community Needs Assessment Report

Title Page	Title of your assessment project, name of author/s, and date.
Executive Summary or Abstract	A brief (250 words or less) summary of the purpose of the assessment, methods used, and findings.
Table of Contents	List all of the paper content sections with appropriate first page number.
Introduction and Community Description	Overview of the community (history, demographics, geographic boundaries, etc.). Provide facts collected through secondary data.
Data-Collection Methods	Discuss the data collection strategy/ies used along with the step-by-step protocol.
Data Analysis	Explain how the data collected was analyzed.
Findings	Illustrate and discuss results from the data analyses. Include graphs and charts to display your findings.
Community Assets	Identify community assets that would be helpful in program development, coordination, implementation, evaluation, and maintenance.
Implications for Health Education and Program Development	Discuss the implications of what you found, explain emergent health priorities, segment health needs by group, provide suggestions for health education and health interventions, and suggest guiding theoretical frameworks.
Conclusion	Provide a few summary statements and offer some of the limitations of the needs assessment. Explain how the results of the study will help plan or assist programs within the community.
References	Be sure to list all references in a format such as APA and provide parenthetical reference citations throughout.
Appendixes	You may want to include copies of the surveys or questions you used for data collection, articles or handouts relating to the community, and any miscellaneous documents you feel enrich the community assessment.

Appendix B

Community Health Professional E-Portfolio Guide

Content Area/Competency	Artifacts
Assessing Community Needs and Assets	• Community needs assessment report • Community description • PRECEDE analysis • Community health survey/s • Community asset inventories • Focus group questions and summaries • Community gatekeeper interviews (written transcripts and summaries or audio/video) • Photovoice application • Videos • Web pages (linked on E-portfolio)
Communicating Health Information	• Press Release • Brochure • Social marketing campaign (plan) • Blog/newspaper/journal article • Literature reviews • Website or Web page (linked on E-portfolio) • Podcast • Wiki/s (linked on E-portfolio) • Video or public service announcement • Event flyers and handouts • Posters • Social media • Examples of media evaluations and peer critiques • Materials created for those with lower literacy • Training manuals

Planning for Evidence-Based Programs	• Formal program plan; written critiques of program plans • Examples of health education strategies • Application of a planning model • Written mission statement, goals, and objectives • Evaluation plan • Research grant proposals • Related presentations and handouts
Implementing and Coordinating Community Health Programs	• Evidence of public presentations or teaching (text, photos, audio, video, Web page) • Lesson/presentation plans; presentation critiques • Case studies • Evidence and photos of volunteer experience or service learning • Related presentations and handout • Supervisor, instructor, or preceptor critiques • Thank-you letters or certificates of appreciation
Resource Access and Management	• Community resource directory • Asset map/inventories • Webliography and/or wikis • Spotlights on professional organizations and agencies • Case studies • Related presentations and handouts
Evaluation and Research	• Formal program evaluation report • Examples of program evaluation strategies and objectives • Literature reviews • Research proposals/reports • Published research articles/abstracts • Market research • Evaluation surveys/instrumentation • Presentation of data (graphs, charts, tables) • Peer and self-critiques • Self-constructed exams or rubrics • Photos • Pod or vodcast
Health Advocacy	• Letters to the editor, Congress, or community leaders • Op-ed pieces • Media advocacy plan • Local media contact directory • Public service announcement • Pod or vodcast • Blog/s • Examples of community forums attended or facilitated • Digital Stories

Resources for creating E-portfolios

McKenzie, J., Cleary, M. J., McKenzie, B., & Stephen, C. S. (2002). E-portfolios: Their creation and use by pre-service health educators. *International Electronic Journal of Health Education*, 4: 79–83.

http://www.eduscapes.com

http://www.electronicportfolios.org

Appendix C

Planning a Social Media Strategy for Advocacy

Use this worksheet to help you strategize about your audience, and the potential social media tools and channels you may want to use for your campaign or communication activity.

1. Target Audience

   Describe the person(s) you want to reach with your communication; be as specific as possible. More than one audience may be listed. Include a primary and secondary (influencers) audience if appropriate. (Examples: Mothers of children younger than two years old living in Atlanta, Pediatricians practicing in Nevada.)

   I.

   II.

   III.

2. Determine Your Objective

   What do you want to achieve in terms of advocacy through your social media outreach and communication? This could include something you want your target audience to do as a direct result of experiencing the communication. Objectives may include (but are not limited to) the following:

   a) Provide information to raise awareness
      • Highlight a campaign
      • Encourage a health behavior
      • Reinforce health messages
      • Encourage interaction
      • Obtain feedback/exchange ideas
      • Collaborate with partners
      (Example: Increase awareness of immunization campaign.)

   I.

   II.

   III.

b) Restate your objectives in SMART terms:

<u>Specific</u>—State in concrete, detailed and well-defined terms—What exactly are we going to do for whom?

<u>Measurable</u>—Should be quantifiable and the source of measurement has been identified.

<u>Attainable/Achievable</u>—Can the objective be achieved in the proposed time frame with the resources available?

<u>Relevant/Realistic</u>—Is the objective directly related to the overarching communication goal from your communication plan?

<u>Time-bound</u>—Have deadlines been set?

(Example: By December 2012 [time-bound], there will be a 5% increase [measurable] in recognition of the immunization campaign name [specific], as measured through surveying, by moms of children under two in the Metro Atlanta area [specific].)

   I.

  II.

 III.

Additional information on writing SMART objectives can be found at http://www.cdc.gov/healthyyouth/evaluation/pdf/brief3b.pdf and http://www.cdc.gov/dhdsp/programs/nhdsp_program/evaluation_guides/ smart_object ives.htm

3. Define Audience Communication Needs

People access information in various ways, at different times of the day, and for different reasons. If possible, define your audience needs by using market research or and other data. You can use the following resources:

- Pew Internet and American Life Project: http://www.pewinternet.org/
- Tools of Change Planning Guide: http://www.toolsofchange.com/en/planning-guide/ (This is a non-CDC site. This link does not imply endorsement.)

Describe your audiences and their health information needs.

   I.

  II.

 III.

4. Goal Integration

a) Describe how your social media objectives support your organization's mission and/or overall communications plan.

   I.

  II.

 III.

b) How does it support other online or offline components—what events (either national/state/local) present communication opportunities?

I.

II.

III.

5. Message Development

Develop the key messages based on the target audience and objectives identified. (Example: For moms of young children to encourage late season flu vaccination, "It's not too late to vaccinate.")

I.

II.

III.

6. Resources and Capacity

Determine who in your organization will be responsible for implementation, and determine the number of hours they can allocate for content creation and maintenance.

I.

II.

III.

7. Identify Social Media Tools

Determine what tools will effectively reach your target audience. Match the needs of the target audience with the tools that best support your objectives and resources. (Example: Because Facebook has a large population of young women who have children, is free, and requires minimal technical expertise, it may be a good tool for a mom-centered program while only requiring a small amount of funding for social media activities.)

I.

II.

III.

8. Define Activities

Based on all of the elements above, list the specific activities you will undertake to reach your communication goals and objectives. (Example: Develop and promote Facebook fan page for diabetes education program.)

I.

II.

III.

9. Identify Your Key Partners and Their Roles and Responsibilities

I.

II.

III.

10. Define Success for Evaluation
    What are your measures of success? Your measures of success may be different depending on your goals and objectives.

    I.

    II.

    III.

11. Evaluate
    Create an evaluation plan; see the Social Media Evaluation Plan for more information.

Excerpted from *The Health Communicator's Social Media Toolkit: Social Media Communications Strategy Worksheet*, Centers for Disease Control and Prevention, 2011, July. Retrieved from http://www.cdc.gov/socialmedia/tools/guidelines/socialmediatoolkit.html?

Appendix D

Creating a Resource Inventory for Community Health

No matter what setting you work in as a health professional (i.e., clinical, school, community, corporate, nonprofit) it is likely you will need to collect resources to help you develop effective health education programs. Use this worksheet as a guide to help you compile these resources.

Topic Area: _____   Date: _____

List helpful websites on your topic. (Remember to consider the accuracy, authority, currency, objectivity, and coverage of each website.)

List phone numbers for clearinghouses or "help" or "information" lines relating to the topic.

Identify community agencies or nonprofit organizations that may have information on the topic. (Provide name, address, phone number, and e-mail.)

List individuals who may serve as guest speakers on this topic. (Be sure you can justify their authority on this topic.)

Locate and list professional journal articles, reports, or books. (Include complete reference information, including the database you used.)

Search for podcasts or blogs that might provide helpful information. List these below. (Remember to apply the same evaluation criteria as other Web-based resources.)

References

Abramson, H. J. (1980). Religion. In S. Thernstrom (Ed.), *Harvard encyclopedia of American ethnic groups*. Cambridge, MA: Harvard University Press.

Agency for Healthcare Research and Quality. (2014a, March). *Community connections: linking primary care patients to local resources for better management of obesity*. Retrieved from http://www.ahrq.gov/professionals/prevention-chronic-care/improve/community/obesity-toolkit/obtoolkit3.html

Agency for Healthcare Research and Quality. (2014b, June). *Guide to clinical preventive services, 2014: Recommendations of the U.S. Preventive Services Task Force*. Retrieved from http://www.ahrq.gov/professionals/clinicians-providers/guidelines-recommendations/guide/index.html

Agency for Healthcare Research and Quality. (2015a, August). *AHRQ issue brief: Harnessing the power of data: How AHRQ is catalyzing transformation in health care*. Retrieved from https://www.ahrq.gov/sites/default/files/publications/files/databrief.pdf

Agency for Healthcare Research and Quality. (2015b, June). *Clinical-community linkages*. Retrieved from http://www.ahrq.gov/professionals/prevention-chronic-care/improve/community/index.html

Airhihenbuwa, C. O. (1990). A conceptual model for cultural appropriate health education programs in developing countries. *International Quarterly of Community Health Education, 11,* 53–62.

Ajzen, I. (1991). The theory of planned behavior. *Organizational Behavior and Human Decision Processes, 50,* 179–211.

Ajzen, I., & Fishbein, M. (1977). Attitude-behavior relations: A theoretical analysis and review of empirical research. *Psychological Bulletin, 84,* 888–918.

All As One. (2006, November 16). *Children of Sierra Leone still paying the price of "blood" diamonds.* [Press Release]. Retrieved from https://www.allasone.org/blogs/news

Almeida, J., Johnson, R., Corliss, H. Molnar. B., & Azrael, D. (2009). Emotional distress among LGBT youth: The influence of perceived discrimination based on sexual orientation. *Journal of Youth and Adolescents, 38*(7):1001–1014.

Alward, R. R., & Camunas, C. (1991). *The nurse's guide to marketing.* Boston: Delmar.

Amer, M., & Hovey, J. (2012). Anxiety and depression in a post-September 11 sample of Arabs in the USA. *Social Psychiatry & Psychiatric Epidemiology, 47*(3), 409–418.

American Academy of Pediatrics. (2003). Prevention of pediatric overweight and obesity. *Pediatrics, 112*(2), 424–430.

American Arab Institute. (2015). *Demographics.* Retrieved from http://www.aaiusa.org/demographics

American Cancer Society. (2015). *Cancer facts and figures 2015.* Retrieved from https://www.cancer.org/content/dam/cancer-org/research/cancer-facts-and-statistics/annual-cancer-facts-and-figures/2015/cancer-facts-and-figures-2015.pdf

American College Health Association. (2016). *Healthy Campus 2020.* Retrieved from http://www.acha.org/healthycampus/

American Heart Association News. (2015, August 13). *Mobile technology may help people improve health behaviors.* Retrieved at http://news.heart.org/mobile-technology-may-help-people-improve-health-behaviors/

American Medical Association. (2014, June 8). *AMA announces partnership with YMCA of the Greater Twin Cities, Minnesota physicians to prevent type 2 diabetes.* Retrieved from http://www.ama-assn.org/ama/pub/news/news/2014/2014-06-08-ama-partnership-ymca-type-2-diabetes.page

American Public Health Association. (n.d.). *APHA media advocacy manual.* Washington, DC.

American Press Institute. (2014, March 17). *How Americans get their news.* Retrieved from https://www.americanpressinstitute.org/publications/reports/survey-research/how-americans-get-news/

American Speech-Language-Hearing Association. (1999). *Language skill disorders.* Retrieved from http://www.healthtouch.com/levl/leaflets/aslha058.htm.

Anderson, J. A., & Adams, M. N. (1992). Acknowledging the learning styles of diverse student populations: Implications for instructional design. In L. L. B. Border & N. Van Note Chism (Eds.), *Teaching for diversity* (pp. 19–33). San Francisco: Jossey-Bass.

Anderson, M., & Jiang, J. (2018). Teens, social media, and technology 2018. *Pew Research Center: Internet and Technology.* Retrieved from http://www.pewinternet.org/2018/05/31/teens-social-media-technology-2018/

Anderson, L. W., & Krathwohl, D. R. (Eds.). (2001). *A taxonomy for learning, teaching and assessing: A revision of Bloom's taxonomy of educational objectives: Complete edition.* New York: Longman.

American Public Health Association. (2005). *APHA legislative advocacy handbook: A guide for effective public health advocacy.* Washington, DC: Author.

Association of Schools of Public Health. (2008, February). *Confronting the public health workforce crisis: ASPH statement on the public health workforce.* Washington, DC: Author. Retrieved from https://www.ncbi.nlm.nih.gov/pubmed/19006982

Association of Schools and Programs of Public Health. (2017a). *Discover: What is public health?* Retrieved from http://www.aspph.org/discover/

Association of Schools and Programs of Public Health. (2017b). *Framing the future.* Retrieved from http://www.aspph.org/educate/framing-the-future/

Association of Schools and Programs of Public Health. (2017c). *Study: Behavioral and social sciences.* Retrieved from http://www.aspph.org/study/social-behavioral-science/

Association of State and Territorial Health Officials. (2014). *ASTHO profile of state public health, volume three.* Retrieved from http://www.astho.org/Profile/Volume-Three/

Association for Supervision and Curriculum Development. (2017). *Whole school, whole community, whole child.* Retrieved from http://www.ascd.org/programs/learning-and-health/wscc-model.aspx

Baker, T. A., & Wang, C. C. (2006). Photovoice: Use of a participatory action research method to explore chronic pain experience in older adults. *Qualitative Health Research, 16*(10), 1405–1413.

Baker, J. (2017, April). Author Jean Kilbourne addresses sexualization of women in advertising. *The Michigan Daily.* Retrieved from http://www.jeankilbourne.com/jbp/pdfs/Michigan-Daily.pdf

Bandura, A. (1977). *Social learning theory.* Englewood Cliffs, NJ: Prentice-Hall.

Bauer, R. A. (1967). *Social indicators.* Cambridge, Massachusetts: M.I.T. Press.

Bean, J. C. (1996). *Engaging ideas: The professor's guide to integrating writing, critical thinking, and active learning in the classroom.* San Francisco: Jossey-Bass.

Beardain, R. P., & Grantham, J. B. (1993). The use of volunteerism in indigent health care. *Journal of Health and Social Policy, 5*(1), 1–7.

Bellman, G. M. (1990). *The consultant's calling: Bringing who you are to what you do.* San Francisco: Jossey-Bass.

Bernhardt, J. (2006, July). *Health marketing musings.* Retrieved from http://www.cdc.gov/print.do?url=http://www.cdc.gov/healthmarketing/blog_071306.htm#

Black, M. C., Basile, K. C., Breiding, M. J., Smith, S. G., Walters, M. L., Merrick, M. T., Chen, J., & Stevens, M. R. (2011). *The national intimate partner and sexual violence survey (NISVS): 2010 summary report.* Atlanta, GA: National Center for Injury Prevention and Control, Centers for Disease Control and Prevention.

Bloom, B. S., Englehart, M., Furst, E., Hill, W., & Krathwohl, D. R. (1956). *Taxonomy of educational objectives: The classification of educational goals. Handbook 1: Cognitive domain.* New York: Longmans.

Bornstein, D. (1996). *The blind men and the elephant: A Hindu fable by John Godfrey Saxe.* Retrieved from http://www.milk.com/random-humor/elephant_fable.html

Breckon, D. J. (1997). *Managing health promotion programs: Leadership skills for the 21st century.* Gaithersburg, MD: Aspen.

Bridges, D. R., Davidson, R. A., Soule Odegard, P., Maki, I. V., & Tomkowiak, J. (2011). Interprofessional collaboration: Three best practice models of interprofessional education. *Medical Education Online, 16,* 6035.

Brislin, R. W. (1986). The wording and translation of research instruments. In W. J. Lonner & J. W. Berry (Eds.), *Field methods in cross-cultural research* (pp. 137–164). Beverly Hills, CA: Sage.

Broder, J. M. (2008, July 18). Gore urges change to dodge an energy crisis. *The New York Times.* Retrieved from http://www.nytimes.com/2008/07/18/washington/18gore.html?_r=1&oref=slogin

Brooks, M. (2013, November 12). Report Warns of Worsening Global Healthcare Worker Shortage. *Medscape.* Retrieved from http://www.medscape.com/viewarticle/814221

Bryman, A. (1996). Leadership in organizations. In S. R. Clegg, C. Hardy, & W. R. Nord (Eds.), *Handbook of organizational studies* (pp. 276–292). Newbury Park, CA: Sage.

Bureau of Labor Statistics. (2014). Health educators and community health worker. In *Occupational outlook handbook.* Retrieved from http://www.bls.gov/ooh/community-and-social-service/health-educators.htm

Bureau of Labor Statistics. (2016). *Volunteering in the United States, 2015* [Press Release]. Retrieved from https://www.bls.gov/news.release/volun.nr0.htm

Bureau of Labor Statistics. (2018, April 13). Health educators and community health workers. In *Occupational outlook handbook.* Retrieved from https://www.bls.gov/ooh/community-and-social-service/health-educators.htm

Burke, S., Snyder, S., & Rager, R. (2009). An assessment of faculty usage of YouTube as a resource. *The Internet Journal of Allied Health Sciences and Practices, 7*(1). Retrieved from http://www.ijahsp.nova.edu/articles/Vol7Num1/burke.htm

Burman, R., & Evans, A. J. (2008). Target zero: A culture of safety. *Defense Aviation Safety Centre Journal, 2008,* 22–27. Retrieved from http://www.mod.uk/NR/rdonlyres/849892B2-D6D2-4DFD-B5BD-9A4F288A9B18/0/DASCJournal2008.pdf

Carnevale, A. P., Gainer, L. L., & Meltzer, A. S. (1990). *Workplace basics.* San Francisco: Jossey-Bass.

Carrington, P. J., Scott, J., & Wasserman, S. (2005). *Models and methods in social network analysis.* Cambridge, MA: Cambridge University Press.

CDCynergy. (n.d.). *Social marketing.* Retrieved from http://www.cdc.gov/dhdsp/CDCynergy_training/Content/activeinformation/example-social.htm

Centers for Disease Control and Prevention. (2006). *Bridging CDC to Congress and Washington-based partners.* Retrieved from http://www.cdc.gov/washington/

Centers for Disease Control and Prevention. (2007a, March). *CDC achieving greater health impact: Goals for the 21st century.* Washington, DC: Government Printing Office.

Centers for Disease Control and Prevention. (2007b). *Deaths, percent of total deaths, and death rates for the 15 leading causes of death: United States and each state, 1999–2004.* Retrieved from http://www.cdc.gov/nchs/data/dvs/LCWK92004.pdf

Centers for Disease Control and Prevention. (2008a). *About us.* Retrieved from http://www.cdc.gov/about

Centers for Disease Control and Prevention. (2008b). *Behavioral risk factor surveillance system.* Retrieved from http://www.cdc.gov/brfss/about.htm

Centers for Disease Control and Prevention. (2008c). *National health care surveys.* Retrieved from http://www.cdc.gov/nchs/nhcs.htm

Centers for Disease Control and Prevention. (2008d). *National notifiable diseases surveillance system.* Retrieved from http://www.cdc.gov/ncphi/disss/nndss/nndsshis.htm

Center for Disease Control and Prevention. (2011). *The health communicator's social media toolkit.* Retrieved from http://www.cdc.gov/socialmedia/tools/guidelines/socialmediatoolkit.html

Centers for Disease Control and Prevention. (2012). *Shawn's tip.* Retrieved from http://www.cdc.gov/tobacco/campaign/tips/resources/ads/tips-ad-shawn-full-v1a.pdf

Centers for Disease Control and Prevention. (2013a). *Bill's story.* Retrieved from http://www.cdc.gov/tobacco/campaign/tips/stories/bill.html

Centers for Disease Control and Prevention. (2013b, February 14). *Social capital.* Retrieved from http://www.cdc.gov/healthyplaces/healthtopics/social.htm

Centers for Disease Control and Prevention. (2014a, January 23). *About healthy places.* Retrieved from http://www.cdc.gov/healthyplaces/about.htm

Centers for Disease Control and Prevention. (2014b). *CDC social media tools, guidelines, and best practices.* Retrieved from https://www.cdc.gov/socialmedia/tools/guidelines/index.html

Centers for Disease and Control Prevention. (2014c). *Ebola (ebola virus disease).* Retrieved from https://www.cdc.gov/vhf/ebola/index.html

Centers for Disease Control and Prevention. (2014d, March 21). *Social determinants of health.* Retrieved from http://www.cdc.gov/nchhstp/socialdeterminants/definitions.html

Centers for Disease Control and Prevention. (2014e, May 29). *The public health system and the 10 essential public health services.* Retrieved from http://www.cdc.gov/nphpsp/essentialservices.html

Centers for Disease Control and Prevention. (2015a, August 18). *College health and safety.* Retrieved from http://www.cdc.gov/family/college/

Centers for Disease Control and Prevention. (2015b). Develop SMART objectives. *Communities of Practice Resource Kit.* Retrieved from http://www.cdc.gov/phcommunities/resourcekit/evaluate/smart_objectives.html

Centers for Disease Control and Prevention. (2015c, August 26). *Healthy schools: Whole school, whole community, whole child.* Retrieved from http://www.cdc.gov/healthyyouth/cshp/case.htm

Centers for Disease Control and Prevention. (2016a, January 7). *About NCCDPHP: Community health.* Retrieved from http://www.cdc.gov/nccdphp/dch/about/index.htm

Centers for Disease Control and Prevention. (2016b, June 13). *NCCDPHP: Community health.* Retrieved from http://www.cdc.gov/NCCDPHP/dch/index.htm

Centers for Disease Control and Prevention. (2016c, June 15). *Emerging infectious diseases.* Retrieved from http://www.cdc.gov/eid

Centers for Disease Control and Prevention. (2016d, May 31). *Health-related quality of life.* Retrieved from http://www.cdc.gov/hrqol/concept.htm

Centers for Disease and Control Prevention. (2016e). *HIV/AIDS. Basic statistics.* Retrieved from https://www.cdc.gov/hiv/basics/statistics.html

Centers for Disease Control and Prevention. (2016f, March 7). *Six tips for college health and safety.* Retrieved from http://www.cdc.gov/Features/CollegeHealth/index.html

Centers for Disease Control and Prevention. (2016g, October 21). *The community guide.* Retrieved from http://www.thecommunityguide.org/index.html

Centers for Disease Control and Prevention. (2017a, May 2). *10 Leading causes of death and injury: 2015.* Retrieved from https://www.cdc.gov/injury/wisqars/LeadingCauses.html

Centers for Disease Control and Prevention. (2017b, February 13). *About the CDC workplace health program.* Retrieved from http://www.cdc.gov/workplacehealthpromotion/about/index.html

Center for Disease Control and Prevention. (2017c, May 8). *Behavioral risk factor surveillance system.* Retrieved from http://www.cdc.gov/brfss/index.html

Centers for Disease Control and Prevention. (2017d). *Fast stats.* Retrieved from https://www.cdc.gov/nchs/fastats/heart-disease.htm

Centers for Disease Control and Prevention. (2017e, June 20). *Global health.* Retrieved from http://www.cdc.gov/globalhealth/index.html

Centers for Disease Control and Prevention. (2017f, July 10). *Mission, role, and pledge.* Retrieved from https://www.cdc.gov/about/organization/mission.htm

Centers for Disease Control and Prevention. (2018a). *About Zika.* Retrieved from https://www.cdc.gov/zika/about/index.html

Centers for Disease Control and Prevention. (2018b). *Diabetes report card 2017.* Atlanta, GA: Centers for Disease Control and Prevention, U.S. Department of Health and Human Services. Retrieved from https://www.cdc.gov/diabetes/pdfs/library/diabetesreportcard2017-508.pdf

Center for Health Care Strategies, Inc. (2013). *Fact sheet #1: What is health literacy.* Retrieved from https://www.chcs.org/media/CHCS_Health_Literacy_Fact_Sheets_2013_1.pdf

Chaskin, R. J., Brown, P., Venkatesh, S., & Vidal, A. (2001). *Community capacity and capacity building.* Hawthorne, NY: Aldine.

Child Trends Data Bank. (2016). *Teen births: Indicators of child and youth well-being.* Retrieved from https://www.childtrends.org/indicators/teen-births/

Clark, M. L., & Utz, S. W. (2014). Social determinants of type 2 diabetes and health in the United States. *World Journal of Diabetes, 5*(3): 296–304.

Clay, R. A. (2011, September). Muslims in America, post 9/11. *Monitor on Psychology, 42*(8): 72. Retrieved from http://www.apa.org/monitor/2011/09/muslims.aspx

Colby, S. L., & Ortman, J. M. (2015, March). Projections of the size and composition of the U.S. population: 2014 to 2060. *U.S. Census Bureau Report,* P25–1143., Retrieved from https://www.census.gov/content/dam/Census/library/publications/2015/demo/p25-1143.pdf

Connecticut Association of Non-Profits Advocacy. (2003). *Advocacy and lobbying toolkit.* Retrieved from http://www.ctnonprofits.org/Pages/NonProfitResources/Advocacy_Lobbying_Toolkit_WordVersions.asp

Corbett, S. (2008, April). Can the cell phone help end global poverty? *The New York Times.* Retrieved from http://www.nytimes.com/2004/04/13/magazine/13anthropology-html

Council on Education for Public Health. (2011). *Accreditation criteria: Public health programs.* Silver Spring, MD: Author.

Council on Education for Public Health. (2016a). *Accreditation criteria and procedures.* Retrieved from http://ceph.org/criteria-procedures/

Council on Education for Public Health. (2016b). *Search for a degree program.* Retrieved from https://ceph.org/accredited/search/

Cunningham, J., Salomone, J., & Wielgus, N. (2015). Project management leadership style: A team member perspective. *International Journal of Global Business. 8*(2), 27–54. Retrieved from http://web.b.ebscohost.com/ehost/detail/detail?vid=0&sid=91f29cdc-4792-4f6b-a6af-0829de46d43f%40sessionmgr120&bdata=JnNpdGU9ZWhvc3QtbGl2ZQ%3d%3d#AN=109299605&db=bsh

Cushner, K. (1994). Preparing teachers for an intercultural context. In R. W. Brislin & T. Yoshida (Eds.), *Improving intercultural interactions: Modules for cross-cultural training programs* (pp. 109–128). Thousand Oaks, CA: Sage.

D'Amour, D., & Oandasan, I. (2005). Interprofessionality as the field of interprofessional practice and interprofessional education: An emerging concept. *Journal of Interprofessional Care, Supplement 1*, 8–20.

Darzi, A., & Evans, T. (2016). The global shortage of health workers—an opportunity to transform care. *The Lancet, 388*(10060), 2576–2577.

Dearing, J. (2015). Social marketing and the diffusion of innovations. In D. W. Stewart (Ed.), *Handbook of persuasion and social marketing* (pp. 35–65). Santa Barbara, CA: Praeger. Retrieved from https://www.researchgate.net/publication/266613618_Social_Marketing_and_the_Diffusion_of_Innovations

DeConinck, J. B. (2013). The effects of leader–member exchange and organizational identification on performance and turnover among salespeople. *Journal of Personal Selling & Sales Management, 31*(1), 24–31. Retrieved from https://doi.org/10.2753/PSS0885-3134310102

Deloitte Center for Health Solutions. (2012). *mHealth in an mWorld: How mobile technology is transforming health care.* Retrieved from http://www.deloitte.com/view/en_US/us/Industries/life-sciences/2545b66b8dc4b310VgnVCM2000003356f70aRCRD.htm

DeSilver, D. (2017, May 15). U.S. trails most developed countries in voter turnout. Fact Tank: News in the Numbers. *Fact tank: News in the numbers.* Retrieved from http://www.pewresearch.org/fact-tank/2017/05/15/u-s-voter-turnout-trails-most-developed-countries/

Di Lima, N., & Schust, C. (1997). *Community health education and promotion: A guide to program design and evaluation.* Gaithersburg, MD: Aspen.

Doll, R. C. (1992). *Curriculum improvement: Decision making and process* (8th ed.). Boston: Allyn & Bacon.

Doyle, E. I. (2008). Toward a culturally competent health education work force. In M. A. Perez & R. Luquis (Eds.), *Cultural competence in health education and health promotion* (pp. 163–181). San Francisco: Jossey-Bass.

Doyle, E. I., Caro, C. M., Lysoby, L., Auld, M. E., Smith, B. J., & Muenzen, P. M. (2012). The National Health Educator Job Analysis 2010: Process and outcomes. *Journal of Health Education and Behavior, 39*(6), 69–708.

D'Souza, G., Kreimer, A. R., Viscidi, R., Pawlita, M., Fakhry, C., Koch, W. M., Westra, W. H., & Gillison, M. L. (2007). Case-control study of human papillomavirus and oropharyngeal cancer. *New England Journal of Medicine, 356*(19), 1944–1956. Retrieved from http://www.content.nejm.org/cgi/content/full/356/19/1944

Dunbar, E. (2006). Race, gender, and sexual orientation in hate crime victimization: Identity politics or identity risk? *Violence and Victims, 21*, 323–337.

Eck, D. I. (2001). *A new religious America: How a "Christian country" has become the world's most religiously diverse nation.* San Francisco: Harper.

Educational Testing Service. (2008). *Adult literacy.* Retrieved from http://www.ets.org/portal/site/ets/menuitem.d4640d54cfbd7becda20bc47c3921509/?vgnextoid=66f87862687da010VgnVCM10000022f95190RCRD

Educause Learning Initiative. (2005). *7 things you should know about blogs.* Retrieved from http://www.educause.edu/ir/library/pdf/ELI7006.pdf

Edutopia. (2016, July). *Multiple intelligences: What does the research say?* Retrieved from https://www.edutopia.org/multiple-intelligences-research

Elliott, J., Seals, B., & Jacobson, M. (2007). Use of the precaution adoption process model to examine predictors of osteoprotective behavior in epilepsy. *Seizure, 16*(5), 424–437.

Ellis, S. J. (1993). Volunteerism as an enhancement to career development. *Journal of Employment Counseling, 30*(3), 127–132.

Evans, C., & Cools, E. (2011). Applying Styles Research to Educational Practice. *Learning and Individual Difference, 21*(3), 249–254.

Fazal, F. (2017, June 13). *Somali health workers strive to educate during measles outbreak.* Retrieved from http://www.kaaltv.com/article/stories/S4511751.shtml?cat=10728

Federal Interagency Forum on Child and Family Statistics. (2015). *America's children: key national indicators of well-being, 2015.* Washington, DC: U.S. Government Printing Office. Retrieved from http://www.childstats.gov/pdf/ac2015/ac_15.pdf

Fielding, J. E., & Teutsch, S. M. (2009). Integrating clinical care and community health: Delivering health. *Journal of American Medical Association, 302*(3), 317–319.

Food and Agriculture Organizations of the United Nations. (2017). *The state of food security and nutrition in the world 2017. Building resilience for peace and food security.* Retrieved from http://www.fao.org/3/a-i7695e.pdf

Force Health Protection and Readiness. (2008). *The millennium cohort study offers the first comprehensive review of career-span military health.* Retrieved from http://www.deploymentlink.osd.mil/new.jsp?newsID=35

Fowler, F. J. (2002). *Survey research methods* (3rd ed.). Thousand Oaks, CA: Sage.

Free Press Release Center. (n.d.). *Sample Press Release.* Retrieved from http://www.free-press-release-center.info/sample-press-release.html

Friedman, T. (2001, June 8). The Earth is full. *The New York Times.* Retrieved from http://www.nytimes.com/2011/06/08/opinion/08friedman.html?_r=0

Friedson, E. (1988). *Profession of medicine: A study of the sociology of applied knowledge* (2nd ed.). Chicago: The University of Chicago Press.

Friis, R. H., & Sellers, T. A. (1999). *Epidemiology for public health practice* (2nd ed.). Gaithersburg, MD: Aspen.

Frohmann, L. (2005). The framing safety project: Photographs and narratives by battered women. *Violence Against Women, 11*(11), 1396–1419.

Gabel, M. (2006). *America America* [video]. *Big picture, small world.* Retrieved from http://www.bigpicturesmallworld.com/movies/america/america.html

Galer-Unti, R. A., Tappe, M. K., & Lachenmayr, S. (2004). Advocacy 101: Getting started in health education advocacy. *Health promotion practice, 5*(3), 280–288.

Gallup. (2016). *Islamophobia: Understanding anti-Muslim sentiment in the west.* Retrieved from http://news.gallup.com/poll/157082/islamophobia-understanding-anti-muslim-sentiment-west.aspx

Gardy, J. L., Johnston, J. C., Sui, S. J. H., Cook, V. J., Shah, L., Brodkin, E. . . . Tang, P. (2011). Whole-genome sequencing and social-network analysis of a tuberculosis outbreak. *New England Journal of Medicine, 1*(364), 730–739. DOI: 10.1056/NEJMoa1003176

Gardner, H. (1993). *Multiple intelligences: The theory in practice.* New York: Basic Books.

Gardner, H. (2003). *Multiple intelligences after twenty years.* Retrieved from http://www.pzweb.harvard.edu/PIs/HG_MI_after_20_years.pdf

Garrard, J. (1999). *Health sciences literature review made easy: The matrix method.* Gaithersburg, MD: Aspen.

Garson, D. G. (2006). *Public information technology and E-governance: Managing the virtual State.* Burlington, MA: Jones and Bartlett Learning.

Gilmore, G. D., & Campbell, M. D. (2005). *Needs and capacity assessment strategies for health education and health promotion* (3rd ed.). Boston: Jones & Bartlett.

Gilmore, G. D. (2012). *Needs and capacity assessment strategies for health education and health promotion* (4th ed.). Burlington, MA: Jones & Bartlett.

Ginsberg, Margery B., & Vlodkowski, R. J. (2009). *Diversity and motivation: culturally responsive teaching in college* (2nd ed.). Oxford: John Wiley.

Glanz, K., Rimer, B. K., & Viswanath, K. (Eds.). (2008). *Health behavior and health education: Theory, research, and practice* (4th ed.). San Francisco: Jossey-Bass.

Glanz, K., Rimer, B. K., & Viswanath, K. (Eds.). (2015). *Health behavior and health education: Theory, research, and practice* (5th ed.). San Francisco: Jossey-Bass.

Glascoff, M. A., Baker, J. B., & Glascoff, D. W. (1997). Successfully promoting volunteerism by offering extrinsic rewards in a personal health course: A pilot study. *Journal of School Health Education, 28*(4), 219–223.

Global Health Council. (n.d.). *Why does global health matter?* Retrieved from http://www.globalhealth.org/images/pdf/gh_message_box.pdf

Global Workforce Alliance & the World Health Organization. (2013). *A universal truth: No health without a workforce.* Retrieved from http://www.who.int/workforcealliance/knowledge/resources/hrhreport2013/en/

Godwin, M., Ruhland, L., Casson, I., MacDonald, S., Delva, D., Birthwhistle, R., . . . Seguin, R. (2003). Pragmatic controlled clinical trials in primary care: The struggle between external and internal validity. *BMC Medical Research Methodology, 3*(28). Retrieved from www.biomedicalcentral.com11471–12288/3/28

Gold, R. S., & Miner, K. R. (2002, January). Report of the 2000 joint committee on health education and promotion terminology. *Journal of School Health, 72*(1), 3–7.

Goodman, R. M., Speers, M. A., McLeroy, K. R., Fawcett, S., Kegler, M., Parker, E., . . . Wallerstein, N. (1998). Identifying and defining the dimensions of community capacity to provide a basis for measurement. *Health Education and Behavior, 25*(3), 258–278.

Greber, C., Ziviani, J., & Rodger, S. (2011). Clinical utility of the four-quadrant model of facilitated learning: perspectives of experienced occupational therapists. *Australian Occupational Therapy Journal, 58*(3),187–94. DOI: 10.1111/j.1440-1630.2010.00901.x.

Green, L. W., & Kreuter, M. W. (2005). *Health program planning: An educational and ecological approach.* (4th ed.). New York: McGraw-Hill.

Greenberg, J. S. (2003). *Health education: Learner-centered instructional strategies* (5th ed.). New York: McGraw-Hill.

Gronfeldt, S., & Strother, J. B. (2006). Service leadership: The quest for the competitive advantage. Newbury Park, CA: Sage.

Guo, J. (2015, September 11). Where refugees go in America. *The Washington Post.* Retrieved from https://www.washingtonpost.com/news/wonk/wp/2015/09/11/where-refugees-go-in-america/?utm_term=.b222c9f23edb

Graffunder, C., & Sakurada, B. (2016, April 6). *Preparing health care and public health professionals for team performance: The community as classroom.* Retrieved from https://nam.edu/preparing-health-care-and-public-health-professionals-for-team-performance-the-community-as-classroom/

Green, L. W., & Kreuter, M. W. (1999). *Health promotion planning: An educational and ecological approach* (3rd ed.). Mountain View, CA: Mayfield.

Green, L. W., & Kreuter, M. W. (2005). *Health program planning: An educational and ecological approach* (4th ed.). Boston: McGraw-Hill.

Grootaert, C., Narayan, D., Jones, V. N., & Woolcock, M. (2004). *Measuring social capital: An integrated questionnaire.* Washington, DC: The World Bank.

Haile, S., Emmanuel, T., & Dzathor, A. (2013). Barriers and challenges confronting women for leadership and management positions: Review and analysis. *International Journal of Business & Public Administration, 13*(1), 36-51.

Hajar, R. (2016, Apr–Jun). Framingham Contribution to Cardiovascular Disease. *Heart Views, 17*(2): 78–81. Retrieved from http://dx.doi:10.4103/1995-705X.185130

Harvard School of Public Health. (n.d.). *Center for health communication.* Retrieved from http://www.hsph.harvard.edu/chc

Health Resources and Services Administration. (2018). *About HRSA.* Retrieved from https://www.hrsa.gov/about/index.html

Henderson, D. A. (2006). Vaccines and the eradication of smallpox. In B. A. DeBuono (Ed.), *Milestones in public health: Accomplishments in public health over the last 100 years* (pp. 5–20). New York: Pfizer Global Pharmaceuticals.

Henry, J., & Ward, S. E. (1999). The art and science of health education. Unpublished paper.

Herman, M. (2005). *How to use Wiki.* Retrieved at http://www.openspaceworld.org/cgi/netwiki.cgi?HowToUseWiki

Heron, M. P., Hoyert, D. L., Murphy, S. L., Xu, J., Kochanek, K. D., & Tejada-Vera, B. (2009, April). Deaths: Final data for 2006. *National Vital Statistics Reports, 57*(14). Retrieved from http://www.cdc.gov/nchs/data/nvsr/nvsr57/nvsr57_14.pdf

Hettler, B. (1976). *The six dimensions of wellness model.* Stevens Point, WI: National Wellness Institute. Retrieved from http://www.nationalwellness.org/?page=Six_Dimensions

Hill, J., Nielsen, M., & Fox, M. H. (2013). Understanding the social factors that contribute to diabetes: A means to informing health care and social policies for the chronically ill. *Permanente Journal, 17*(2), 67–72.

Hochbaum, G. M. (1958). *Public participation in medical screening programs: A sociopsychological study.* PHS Publication No. 572. Washington, DC: U.S. Government Printing Office.

Hodge, D. R., Zidan, T., & Husain, A. (2016). Depression among Muslims in the United States: Examining the role of discrimination and spirituality as risk and protective factors. *Social Work, 61*(1), 45–52.

Hofstede, G. (2001). *Culture's consequences: Comparing values, behaviors, institutions and organizations across nations* (2nd ed.). Thousand Oaks, CA: Sage.

Holland, J. (2003). *Applying complexity science to health and healthcare.* Minneapolis: Center for the Study of Health Care Management, University of Minnesota.

Holtby, A., Klein, K., Cook, K., & Travers, R. (2015). To be seen or not to be seen: Photovoice, queer and trans youth, and the dilemma of representation. *Action Research, 13,* 317–335. DOI: 1476750314566414.

Hook, J. N., Davis, D. E., Owen, J., Worthington, E. L., & Utsey, S. O. (2013). Cultural humility: Measuring openness to culturally diverse clients. *Journal of Counseling Psychology, 60*(3), 353–366.

Hoyert, D. L. (2012, March). *75 years of mortality in the United States, 1935–2010.* NCHS data brief, no 88. Hyattsville, MD: National Center for Health Statistics. Retrieved from http://www.cdc.gov/nchs/data/databriefs/db88.htm#x2013;2010</a>

Hukkelberg S. S., Hagtvet K. A., & Kovac, V. B. (2014). Latent interaction effects in the theory of planned behaviour applied to quitting smoking. *British Journal of Health Psychology, 19*(1), 83–100. DOI: 10.1111/bjhp.12034

Ibrahim, M. A. (1985). *Epidemiology and health policy.* Rockville, MD: Aspen.

Idaho State Epidemiological Outcomes Work Group. (2015). *Substance abuse prevention needs assessment.* Retrieved from https://odp.idaho.gov/wp-content/uploads/sites/40/2016/12/2015SPFSIGNeedsAssessment_Final.pdf

Igielnik, R., & Krogstad, J. M. (2017, February 3). Where refugees to the U.S. come from. *FactTank: News in the numbers.* Retrieved from http://www.pewresearch.org/fact-tank/2017/02/03/where-refugees-to-the-u-s-come-from/

Ingram, P. D., Dorsey, M. H., & Smith, S. (2004). Tips for Designing Publications for Underrepresented Audiences. *Journal of Extension, 24*(4). Retrieved from https://joe.org/joe/2004august/tt2.php

Infed Search. (2008). *Naturalistic intelligence.* Retrieved from http://www.edwebproject.org/edref.mi.th8.html

Insel, P. M., & Roth, W. T. (1994, 2000). *Core concepts in health.* Mountain View, CA: Mayfield.

Institute of Medicine. (1972). *Educating for the health team.* Washington, DC: National Academy of Sciences.

Institute of Medicine. (2000). *Promoting health: Intervention strategies from social and behavioral research.* B. D. Smedley & S. L. Syme (Eds.). Washington, DC: National Academies Press.

Institute of Medicine. (2002). *The future of the public's health in the 21st century.* Washington, DC: National Academies Press.

Institute of Medicine. (2003). *Who will keep the public healthy? Educating public health professionals for the 21st century.* Washington, DC: National Academies Press.

Institute of Medicine. (2007, June). *Training physicians for public health careers* [Report brief]. Washington, DC: National Academies Press.

Institute of Medicine. (2012). *Primary care and public health: Exploring integration to improve population health.* Washington, DC: The National Academies Press.

Institute of Medicine. (2013). *Partnering with patients to drive shared decisions, better value, and care improvement: Workshop proceedings.* Washington, DC: The National Academies Press.

Institute of Medicine & National Research Council. (2014). *Investing in the health and well-being of young adults.* Washington, DC: The National Academies Press. Retrieved from http://www.iom.edu/Reports/2014/Investing-in-the-Health-and-Well-Being-of-Young-Adults.aspx

International Union for Health Promotion and Education. (2007). *Shaping the future of health promotion: Priorities for action.* Retrieved from https://www.ncbi.nlm.nih.gov/pubmed/18024422

Interprofessional Education Collaborative Expert Panel. (2011). *Core competencies for interprofessional collaborative practice: Report of an expert panel.* Washington, DC: Interprofessional Education Collaborative. Retrieved from http://www.aacn.nche.edu/education-resources/IPECReport.pdf

Interprofessional Education Collaborative. (2016). *Core competencies for interprofessional collaborative practice: 2016 update.* Washington, DC: Interprofessional Education Collaborative. Retrieved from https://www.ipecollaborative.org/resources.html

Ireland, J. D. (1999, June). *Udana VI.4, Tittha Sutta, various sectarians (1).* Buddhist publication society. Retrieved from http://www.world.std.com/~metta/canon/khuddaka/udana/ud6–4.html

ITU Telecom World. (2011). *The world in 2011: ICT facts and figures.* Retrieved from http://www.itu.int/ITU-D/ict/facts/2011/material/ictfactsfigures2011.pdf

Johnson, C., & Wannemacher, P. (2011). *Mobile channel strategy: An overview.* Cambridge, MA: Forrester Research, Inc.

Joint Committee on Terminology for Health Education and Promotion. (2012). Report of the 2011 Joint Committee on Health Education and Promotion Terminology. *American Journal of Health Education, 43*(2), 9–103.

Jost, K. (2006, November 3). Understanding Islam. *CQ Researcher, 16,* 913–936. Retrieved from http://library.cqpress.com/cqresearcher/document.php?id=cqresrre2006110300

Jones, P. S., Lee, J. W., Phillips, L. R., Zhang, X. E., & Jaceldo, K. B. (2001). An adaptation of Brislin's translation model for cross-cultural research. *Nursing Research, 50*(5), 300–304.

Kaplan, A. M., & Haenlein, M. (2010). Users of the world, unite! The challenges and opportunities of social media. *Business Horizons, 53*(1), 59–68.

Keck, C. W. (2006). U.S. public health infrastructure. In B. A. DeBuono (Ed.), *Milestones in public health: Accomplishments in public health over the last 100 years* (pp. 213–226). New York: Pfizer Global Pharmaceuticals.

Keller, C., Fleury, J., Perez, A., Ainsworth, B., & Vaughn, L. (2008). Using visual methods to uncover context. *Qualitative Health Research, 18*(3), 428–436.

Kennedy, A. J. (1999). *The Internet: The rough guide 2000.* New York: Rough Guide.

Kishi, K. (2017, November 15). Assaults against Muslims in U.S. surpass 2001 level. *Fact tank: News in the numbers.* Retrieved from http://www.pewresearch.org/fact-tank/2017/11/15/assaults-against-muslims-in-u-s-surpass-2001-level/

Kitano, M. K. (1997). A rationale and framework for course change. In A. I. Morey & M. K. Kitano (Eds.), *Multicultural course transformation in higher education: A broader truth* (pp. 1–17). Boston: Allyn & Bacon.

Kotler, P., & Zaltman, G. (1971). Social marketing: An approach to social change. *Journal of Marketing, 35*(3), 3–12.

Krogstad, J. M., & Radford, J. (2017, January 30). Key facts about refugees to the U.S. *Fact tank: News in the Numbers.* Retrieved from at http://www.pewresearch.org/fact-tank/2017/01/30/key-facts-about-refugees-to-the-u-s

KU Work Group for Community Health and Development. (2018a). *Coalition building I: Starting a coalition* (chap. 5, sec. 5). Lawrence: University of Kansas. Retrieved from http://www.ctb.ku.edu/en/tablecontents/section_1057.htm

KU Work Group for Community Health and Development. (2018b). *Communications to promote interest* (chap.6). Lawrence: University of Kansas. Retrieved from https://ctb.ku.edu/en/table-of-contents/participation/promoting-interest

KU Work Group for Community Health and Development. (2018c). *Developing a logic model or theory of change* (chap. 2, sec. 1). Lawrence: University of Kansas. Retrieved from http://ctb.ku.edu/en/table-of-contents/overview/models-for-community-health-and-development/logic-model-development/main

KU Work Group for Community Health and Development. (2018d). *Participatory approaches to planning community interventions* (chap. 18, sec. 2). Lawrence: University of Kansas. Retrieved from http://ctb.ku.edu/en/table-of-contents/analyze/where-to-start/participatory-approaches/main

KU Work Group for Community Health and Development. (2018e). *Principles of advocacy* (chap. 30). Lawrence: University of Kansas. Retrieved from http://www.ctb.ku.edu/tools

KU Work Group for Community Health and Development. (2018f). *SWOT Analysis: Strengths, weaknesses, opportunities, threats* (chap. 3, sec. 14). Lawrence: University of Kansas. Retrieved from http://ctb.ku.edu/en/table-of-contents/assessment/assessing-community-needs-and-resources/swot-analysis/main

Kumar, S., & Preetha, G. (2012). Health promotion: An effective tool for global health. *Indian Journal of Community Medicine: Official Publication of Indian Association of Preventive & Social Medicine, 37*(1), 5–12. Retrieved from http://doi.org/10.4103/0970-0218.94009

Lalonde, M. (1974). *A new perspective on the health of Canadians: A working document.* Ottawa, Canada: Minister of Health.

Lee, B. X., Kjaerulf, F., Turner, S., Cohen, L., Donnelly, P. D., Muggah, R., . . . Gilligan, J. (2016). Transforming our world: Implementing the 2030 agenda through Sustainable Development Goal indicators. *Journal of Public Health Policy, 37*(1), 13.

Lee, C. J., & Kim, D. (2013, March). A comparative analysis of the validity of US state- and county-level social capital measures and their associations with population health. *Social Indicators Research, 111*(1), 307–326. DOI: 10.1007/s11205-012-0007-y

Lenhart, A., & Fox, S. (2006). *Bloggers: A portrait of the internet's new storyteller* [Special Report]. Washington, DC: Pew Internet and American Life Project. Retrieved from http://www.pewinternet.org/PPF/r/186/report_display.asp

Liburd, L. C., & Sniezek, J. E. (2007). Changing times: New possibilities for community health and well-being. *Preventing Chronic Disease, 4*(3), 1–5.

Liubarets, T. (2016). Top blogging statistics: 45 reasons to blog. *Yahoo Small Business.* Retrieved from https://smallbusiness.yahoo.com/advisor/top-blogging-statistics-45-reasons-blog-180101993.html

Lopez, C. E. (2014). Addressing health disparities in refugees. *Master's Projects and Capstones, 58.* Retrieved from https://repository.usfca.edu/capstone/58

Lopez, E. D., Eng, E., Randall-David, E., & Robinson, N. (2005). Quality of life concerns of African American breast cancer survivors within rural North Carolina: Blending the techniques of Photovoice and grounded theory. *Qualitative Health Research, 15*(1), 99–115.

Losh, S. C. (2012). Age, generation, education, and change in the American public understanding of science, 1979–2006. In R. S. Bauer & N. Allum (Eds.), *The culture of science: How the public relates to science across the globe*. New York: Routledge.

March of Dimes. (1999). *March of Dimes*. Retrieved from http://www.marchofdimes.org

March of Dimes. (2017). *Low birth weight*. From http://www.marchofdimes.org/complications/low-birthweight.aspx

Martínez-Pérez, B., de la Torre-Díez, I., Candelas-Plasencia, S., & López-Coronado, M. (2013). Development and evaluation of tools for measuring the quality of experience (QoE) in mHealth applications. *Journal of Medical Systems, 37*(5): 9976. DOI: 10.1007/s10916-013-9976

Maslow, A. (1954). *Motivation and personality*. New York: Harper & Row.

Massachusetts Department of Public Health. (2018). *National healthy community principles*. Retrieved from http://www.mass.gov/eohhs/gov/departments/dph/programs/admin/comm-office/chna/healthy-community-principles.html

Matocha, L. K. (1998). Chinese-Americans. In L. D. Purnell and B. J. Paulanka (Eds.), *Transcultural health care: A culturally competent approach* (pp. 163–188). Philadelphia: F. A. Davis.

Mattessich, P. W., & Rausch, E. J. (2014). Cross-sector collaboration to improve community health: A view of the current landscape. *Health Affairs, 33*(11), 1968–1974.

Marmot, M., & Wilkinson, R. G. (2006). *Social determinants of health*. Oxford: Oxford University Press.

McDermott, R. J., & Sarvella, P. D. (1999). *Health education evaluation and measurement: A practitioner's perspective* (2nd ed.). Boston: McGraw-Hill.

McKenzie, J. F., Neiger, B. L, & Thackeray, R. (2013). *Planning, implementing, and evaluating health promotion programs: A primer* (6th ed.). Boston: Pearson.

McKenzie, J. F., Neiger, B. L., and Thackeray, R. (2017). *Planning, implementing, and evaluating health promotion programs: A primer* (7th ed.). Boston, MA: Pearson.

McLaughlin, G. (1969). SMOG grading—A new readability formula. *Journal of Reading, 12*(May), 639–646.

McLeroy, K. R., Bibeau, D., Steckler, A., & Glanz, K. (1988). An ecological perspective on health promotion programs. *Health Education and Behavior, 15*(4), 351–377.

McManus, A. (2013). Health promotion innovation in primary health care. *Australasian Medical Journal, 6*(1), 15–18.

Melancon, J., Oomen-Early, J., & del Rincon, L. (2009). Using the PEN-3 Model to assess knowledge, attitudes, and beliefs about diabetes type 2 among Mexican American and Mexican Native men and women in North Texas. *International Electronic Journal of Health Education, 12*, 203–221.

Merriam-Webster's Online. (2008). *Merriam-Webster's online dictionary*. Retrieved from http://www.merriam-webster.com/dictionary/cooperation

Metzler, M. M., Higgins, D. L., Beeker, C. G., Freudenberg, N., Lantz, P. M., Senturia, K. D., . . . Softley, D. (2003). Abstract: Addressing urban health in Detroit, New York City, and Seattle through community-based participatory research partnerships. *American Journal of Public Health, 93*(5), 803–811. Retrieved from http://www.ajph.org/cgi/content/abstract/93/5/803

Ministry of Social Development. (2008). *Physical environment: Desired outcomes. The social report 2008*. Wellington, New Zealand: Author.

Ministry of Social Development. (2016). Social connectedness. *The Social Report 2016*. Wellington, New Zealand: Author. Retrieved from http://socialreport.msd.govt.nz/social-connectedness.html

Minkler, M. (2004). Ethical challenges for the "outside" researcher in community-based participatory research. *Health Education & Behavior, 31*(6), 684–697.

Minkler, M. (Ed.). (2012). *Community organizing and community building for health* (3rd ed.). New Brunswick, NJ: Rutgers University Press.

Minkler, M., Blackwell, A. G., Thompson, M., & Tamir, H. (2003). Community-based participatory research: Implications for public health funding. *American Journal of Public Health, 93*(8), 1210–1213. Retrieved from http://www.ajph.org/cgi/reprint/93/8/1210.pdf

Mohamed, B. (2016, January 6). A new estimate of the U.S. Muslim population. *Fact Tank: News in the Numbers.* Washington, DC: Pew Research Center. Retrieved from http://www.pewresearch.org/fact-tank/2016/01/06/a-new-estimate-of-the-u-s-muslim-population/

Mohnen, S. M., Völker, B., Flap, H., Subramanian, S. V., & Groenewegen, P. P. (2013). You have to be there to enjoy it? Neighbourhood social capital and health. *European Journal of Public Health, 3*(1), 33–39. DOI: https://doi.org/10.1093/eurpub/cks039

Mora, M. (2015, September). The increasing importance of Hispanics to the U.S. workforce. *Monthly Labor Review,* U.S. Bureau of Labor Statistics. Retrieved from https://doi.org/10.21916/mlr.2015.33

Morris, J. N. (1975). *Uses of epidemiology* (3rd ed.). Edinburgh: Churchill Livingstone.

Murray J. L., Lopez, A. D., Mathers, C. D., & Stein, C. (2001*). The global burden of disease: 2000 project aims, methods, and data sources* [Global programme on evidence for health policy discussion paper no. 36]. Geneva, Switzerland: World Health Organization.

Nardi, D. A., & Petr, J. M. (2003). *Community health and wellness needs assessment: A step by step guide.* Thomson: New York.

National Academies of Sciences, Engineering, and Medicine. (2017). *Communities in action: Pathways to health equity.* Washington, DC: The National Academies Press. DOI: 10.17226/24624.

National Association of County and City Health Officials. (2006, July). *2005 national profile of local health departments.* Washington, DC: Author.

National Association of County and City Health Officials. (2016). *Public health communications toolkit: The role of local health departments.* Retrieved from http://www.naccho.org/advocacy/marketing/toolkit/factsheets.cfm

National Association of County and City Health Officials. (2017). *Mobilizing for action through planning and partnerships (MAPP).* Retrieved from http://www.naccho.org/programs/public-health-infrastructure/mapp

National Board of Public Health Examiners. (2016). *CPH: Certified in public health.* Washington DC: Author. Retrieved from http://www.nbphe.org/

National Cancer Institute. (2008). *Making health communication programs work.* U.S. Dept. of Health and Human Services. Retrieved from https://www.cancer.gov/publications/health-communication/pink-book.pdf

National Cancer Institute. (2018). *Cancer statistics.* Retrieved from https://www.cancer.gov/about-cancer/understanding/statistics

National Center for Environmental Health. (2008). *Healthy community design.* Retrieved from http://www.cdc.gov/healthyplaces/factsheets/healthy_community_design_factsheet_final.pdf

National Center for Health Statistics. (2016a, May). *Health, United States, 2015: With special feature on racial and ethnic health disparities.* Hyattsville, MD: USDHHS. Retrieved from http://www.cdc.gov/nchs/data/hus/hus15.pdf#019

National Center for Health Statistics. (2016b, April 27). Older person's health. *Faststats.* Retrieved from http://www.cdc.gov/nchs/fastats/older-american-health.htm

National Commission for Health Education Credentialing. (n.d.). *Responsibilities and competencies for health education specialists.* Retrieved from http://www.nchec.org/responsibilities-and-competencies

National Commission for Health Education Credentialing. (2015). *Areas of responsibilities, competencies, and sub-competencies for health education specialists.* Retrieved from https://www.speakcdn.com/assets/2251/hespa_competencies_and_sub-competencies.pdf

National Institute of Allergy and Infectious Diseases. (2014, July 25). *Emerging and reemerging microbes.* Retrieved from http://www.niaid.nih.gov/topics/microbes/Pages/Emerging.aspx

National Institute of Allergy and Infectious Diseases, (2015, August 7). *Emerging infectious diseases/pathogens research.* Retrieved from http://www.niaid.nih.gov/topics/emerging/Pages/default.aspx

National Institutes of Health. (1999). *NIH overview.* Retrieved from http://www.nih.gov/welcome/nihnew.htm

National Institutes of Health (2018, April). *What we do: Budget.* Retrieved from https://www.nih.gov/about-nih/what-we-do/budget

National Library of Medicine. (n.d.). *Quick guide to health literacy: Fact sheet.* Retrieved from http://www.health.gov/communication/literacy/quickguide/factsbasic.htm

National Library of Medicine and National Institutes of Health. (2006). *Panel 2: NLM health information for underserved and diverse populations in the 21st century.* Retrieved from http://www.nlm.nih.gov/pubs/plan/lrp06/panel2report.doc

National Library of Medicine and National Institutes of Health. (2007). *Director's comments transcript: Health literacy 3/30/07.* Retrieved from http://www.nlm.nih.gov/medlineplus/podcast/transcript033007.html

National Prevention Council. (2011). *National prevention strategy.* Washington, DC: United States Department of Health and Human Services, Office of the Surgeon General. Retrieved from http://www.surgeongeneral.gov/priorities/prevention/strategy/report.pdf

National Science Board. (2004). Science and technology: Public attitudes and understanding. In *Science and Engineering Indicators 2004.* Retrieved from http://www.nsf.gov/statistics/seind04/pdf/c07.pdf

National Science Foundation. (1997). *User friendly handbook for missed method evaluation.* Retrieved http://www.her.nsf.gov/HER/REC/pubs/NSF97–1531/start/htm

Navarro, A. M., Voetsch, K. P., Liburd, L. C., Giles, H. W., & Collins, J. L. (2007, July). Charting the future of community health promotion: Recommendations from the national expert panel on community health promotion. *Prevention of Chronic Disease, 4*(3), Retrieved from http://www.cdc.gov/pcd/issues/2007/jul/07_0013.htm

Nielsen. (2012). *State of the media: The social media report 2012.* Retrieved from http://www.nielsen.com/content/corporate/us/en/reports/2012/state-of-the-media-the-social-media-report-2012.html.

Nieuwenhuijsen, E. R., Zemper, E., Miner, K. R., & Epstein, M. (2006). Health behavior change models and theories: Contributions to rehabilitation. *Disability & Rehabilitation, 28*(5), 245–256.

Nishii, L. H. (2013). *The benefits of climate for inclusion for gender diverse groups.* New York: Cornell University. Retrieved from https://digitalcommons.ilr.cornell.edu/cgi/viewcontent.cgi?article=2226&context=articles

Office of Adolescent Health. (2016, November 1). The changing face of America's adolescents. *America's Adolescents.* Washington, DC: U.S. Department of Health and Human Services. Retrieved from http://www.hhs.gov/ash/oah/adolescent-health-topics/americas-adolescents/changing-face.html

Office of Minority Health. (2001). *National standards for culturally and linguistically appropriate services in health care.* Washington, DC: U.S. Department of Health and Human Services.

Office of Minority Health. (2017). *National Minority Health Month 2017: Learn more.* Retrieved from https://minorityhealth.hhs.gov/NMHM17/

Office of Women's Health. (2014, June 26). *BodyWorks.* Retrieved from http://www.womenshealth.gov/bodyworks/

Oliffe, J. L., & Bottorff, J. L. (2007). Further than the eye can see? Photo elicitation and research with men. *Qualitative Health Research, 17*(6), 850–858.

Online NewsHour. (1999, July–December). *Patients' Bill of Rights: A health spotlight report.* Retrieved from http://www.pbs.org/newshour/health/patientsrights/index.html

Oomen-Early, J., & Burke, S. (2007). Entering the Blogosphere: Blogs as teaching and learning tools in health education. *The International Electronic Journal of Health Education, 10,* 186–196.

O'Reilly, T. (2005, September 3). What is 2.0? *O'Reilly.* Retrieved at http://www.oreilly.com/pub/a/web2/archive/what-is-web-20.html

Padela, A. I. (2015, Spring). American Muslim health disparities: The state of the Medline Literature. *Journal of Health Disparities Research and Practice, 8*(1), 1–9. Retrieved from http://digitalscholarship.unlv.edu/jhdrp/

Parker, E. A., Eng, E., Laraia, B., Ammerman, A., Dodds, J., Margolis, L., & Cross, A. (1998). Coalition building for prevention. In R. C. Brownson, E. A. Baker, & L. F. Novick (Eds.), *Community-based prevention: Programs that work.* Gaithersburg, MD: Aspen.

Parker, R. C. (1997). *Web design and desktop publishing for dummies* (2nd ed.). Hoboken, NJ: Hungry Minds.

Partnership for Prevention. (2008). *The community health promotion handbook: Action guides to improve community health.* Washington, DC: Author.

Partnership for Prevention. (2009). *Healthy workforce 2010 and beyond.* Washington, DC: Author. Retrieved from http://www.prevent.org/data/files/topics/healthyworkforce2010andbeyond.pdf

Patton, E. (2016, July 1). Racial, gender wage gaps persist in U.S. despite some progress. *Fact Tank: News in the Numbers.* Retrieved from http://www.pewresearch.org/fact-tank/2016/07/01/racial-gender-wage-gaps-persist-in-u-s-despite-some-progress/

Payne, C. A. (1999). The challenges of employing performance monitoring in public health community-based efforts. *Journal of Community Health, 24*(2), 159–170.

PCMag.com. (n.d.). "Podcast." Retrieved from http://www.pcmag.com/encyclopedia_term/0,2542,t=podcast&i=49433,00.asp

Penner, L. A., & Finkelstein, M. A. (1998). Dispositional and structural determinants of volunteerism. *Journal of Personality and Social Psychology, 74*(2), 525–537.

Perlino, C. M. (2006, September). *The public health workforce shortage: Left unchecked, will we be protected?* [American public health association issue brief]. Retrieved from http://www.apha.org/NR/rdonlyres/8B9EBDF5-8BE8-482D-A779-7F637456A7C3/0/workforcebrief.pdf

Pertschuk, M. (2012, August 15). *Grassroots public health and preemption.* Retrieved from http://www.rwjf.org/en/culture-of-health/2012/08/mark_pertschuk_gras.html

Peterson, L. E., Phillips, R. L., Puffer, J. C., Bazemore, A., & Petterson, S. (2013). Most family physicians work routinely with nurse practitioners, physician assistants, or certified nurse midwives. *Journal of the American Board of Family Medicine, 26*(3), 244–245.

Pew Research Center. (2016, October 18). *Who votes, who doesn't, and why.* Retrieved from http://www.people-press.org/2006/10/18/who-votes-who-doesnt-and-why/

Prochaska, J. O., Redding, C. A., & Evers, K. E. (1997). The transtheoretical model and stages of change. In K. Glanz, F. M. Lewis, and B. K. Rimer (Eds.), *Health behavior and health education: Theory, research, and practice* (2nd ed., pp. 60–84). San Francisco: Jossey-Bass.

Putnam, R. D. (1995). Bowling alone: America's declining social capital. *Journal of Democracy, 6*(1), 65–78.

Radius, S. M., Galer-Unti, R. A., & Tappe, M. K. (2009). Educating for advocacy: recommendations for professional preparation and development based on a needs and capacity assessment of health education faculty. *Health Promotion Practice, 10*(1), 83–91.

Raskin, M. S. (1994). The Delphi Study in field instruction revisited: Expert consensus on issues and research priorities. *Journal of Social Work Education, 3*(1), 75–89.

Reardon, T. R. (1999, September 23). *Pass Norwood-Dingell patient protection bill.* American Medical Association (Released statement). Retrieved from http://www.ama-assn.org/advocacy/statemnt/990923.htm

Reeves, S., Perrier, L., Goldman, J., Freeth, D., & Zwarenstein, M. (2013). Interprofessional education: Effects on professional practice and healthcare outcomes (update). *Cochrane Database of Systematic Reviews 2013,*(3), DOI: 10.1002/14651858.CD002213.pub3

Reid, M. (2011). Behind the Glasgow effect. *Bulletin of the World Health Organization, 89,* 706–707.

Rescue Organization. (2017). *Resettlement: Refugees in America.* Retrieved from https://www.rescue.org/topic/refugees-america

Renzuli, J. S., & Dai, D. Y. (2001). Abilities, interests, and styles as aptitudes for learning: A person-situation-interaction perspective. In R. J. Sternberg & L. Zhang (Eds.), *Perspectives on thinking, learning, and cognitive styles* (pp. 23–46). Mahwah, NJ: Lawrence Erlbaum.

Rodman, J., Weill, K., Driscoll, M., Fenton, T., Hill, A., Salem-Schatz, S., & Palfrey, J. (1999). A nationwide survey of financing health-related services for special education students. *Journal of School Health, 69*(4), 133–139.

Robert Wood Johnson Foundation. (2017). *About RWJF.* Retrieved from http://www.rwjf.org/en/about-rwjf.html

Romm, J. (2011, June 8). *"The Earth Is Full": Tom Friedman on "The Great Disruption"* http://thinkprogress.org/climate/2011/06/08/240372/tom-friedman-the-great-disruption/

Rosenstock, I. M., Strecher, V. J., & Becker, M. H. (1988). Social learning theory and the health belief model. *Health Education & Behavior, 15*(2), 175–183.

Roser, M., & Ritchie, H. (2018a). Burden of disease. *Our World In Data.* Retrieved from https://ourworldindata.org/burden-of-disease

Roser, M., & Ritchie, H. (2018b). HIV/AIDS. *Our World In Data.* Retrieved from https://ourworldindata.org/hiv-aids_

Ryan, D. (2014). *Understanding digital marketing* (3rd ed.). London, England: Kogan Page Publishers. Retrieved from http://proquest.safaribooksonline.com.ezproxy.library.tamu.edu

Ryan, C. L., & Bauman, K. (2016, March). Educational attainment in the United States: 2015, population characteristics. *U.S. Census Bureau, Current Population Reports,* P20–578. Retrieved from https://www.census.gov/content/dam/Census/library/publications/2016/demo/p20-578.pdf

Safe Kids Worldwide. (2013). *Safe kids day coalition toolkit.* Retrieved from https://www.safekids.org/safe-kids-day-coalition-toolkit

Schaffhauser, Dian. (2012, September 19). OCAD University deploys Guardly campus safety app. *Campus Technology.* Retrieved from https://campustechnology.com/articles/2012/09/19/ocad-university-deploys-guardly-campus-safety-app.aspx

Schaller, E. K., Woodall, K. A., Lemus, H., Proctor, S. P., Russell, D. W., & Crum-Cianflone, N. F. (2014). A longitudinal comparison of posttraumatic stress disorder and depression among military service components. *Military Psychology, 26*(2), 77–87. Retrieved from http://dx.doi.org/10.1037/mil0000034

Schneider, C., Milat, A. J., & Moore, G. (2016). Barriers and facilitators to evaluation of health policies and programs: Policymaker and researcher perspectives. *Evaluation and Program Planning, 5,* 208–215. Retrieved from https://doi.org/10.1016/j.evalprogplan.2016.06.011

Seelye, H. N., & Seelye-James, A. (1996). *Culture clash: Managing in a multicultural world.* Lincolnwood, IL: NTC.

Semega, J., Fontenot, K., & Kollar, M. (2017, September 12). *Income and poverty in the United States: 2016.* Retrieved from https://www.census.gov/library/publications/2017/demo/p60-259.html

Silver H., Strong R., & Perini, M. (1997). Integrating Learning Styles and Multiple Intelligences. *Teaching for Multiple Intelligences, 55*(1), 22–27.

Skolnik, R. (2008). *Essentials of global health.* Sudbury, MA: Jones & Bartlett.

Smith, G. I. (2005). On construct validity: Issues of method and measurement. *Psychological Assessment, 17*(4), 396–408.

Smith, K. C., & Wakefield, M. (2005). Textual analysis of tobacco editorials: How key are media gatekeepers for framing the issues? *American Journal of Health Promotion, 19*(5), 472–480.

Smith, K. R., Woodward, A., Campbell-Lendrum, D., Chadee, D. D., Honda, Y., Liu, Q., Olwoch, J. M., . . . Sauerborn, R. (2014). Human health: Impacts, adaptation, and co-benefits. In *Climate change 2014: Impacts, adaptation, and vulnerability. Part A: Global and sectoral aspects. Contribution of Working Group II to the Fifth Assessment Report of the Intergovernmental Panel on Climate Change* [C. B., Field, V. R. Barros, D. J. Dokken, K. J. Mach, M. D. Mastrandrea, T. E. Bilir, M. Chatterjee, K. L. Ebi, Y. O. Estrada, R. C. Genova, B. Girma, E. S. Kissel, A. N. Levy, S. MacCracken, P. R. Mastrandrea, & L. L. White (eds.), pp. 709–754]. Cambridge, UK: Cambridge University Press.

Spector, R. E. (1996). *Cultural diversity in health and illness* (4th ed.). Norwalk, CT: Appleton and Lange.

Spector, R. E. (2013). *Cultural diversity in health and illness* (8th ed.). Upper Saddle River, NJ: Pearson Education.

Statista. (2018). *Share of search queries handled by leading U.S. search engine providers as of April 2018.* Retrieved from https://www.statista.com/statistics/267161/market-share-of-search-engines-in-the-united-states/

Steptoe, A., & Wardle, J. (2001). Locus of control and health behaviour revisited: A multivariate analysis of young adults from 18 countries. *British Journal of Psychology, 92*(4), 659–672.

Strack, R. W., Magill, C., & McDonagh, K. (2003). Engaging youth through Photovoice. *Health Promotion Practice, 5*(1), 49–58.

Strecher, V. J., & Rosenstock, I. M. (1997). The health belief model. In K. Glanz, F. M. Lewis, & B. K. Rimer (Eds.), *Health behavior and health education: Theory, research, and practice* (2nd ed., pp. 41–59). San Francisco: Jossey-Bass.

Sullivan, D. (2005, January 28). Search engine sizes. *Search Engine Watch.* Retrieved from http://www.searchenginewatch.com/2156481

Synique. (2008). *Transformational leadership.* Retrieved from http://www.changingminds.org/disciplines/leadership/styles/transformational_leadership.htm

Tarrass, F., & Benjelloun, M. (2012). The effects of water shortages on health and human development. *Perspectives in Public Health, 132*(5), 240–244. Retrieved from http://search.proquest.com/docview/1086347634?accountid=14872

Tervalon, M., & Murray-Garcia, J. (1998). Cultural humility versus cultural competence: A critical distinction in defining physician training outcomes in multicultural education. *Journal of Health Care for the Poor and Undeserved, 9,* 117–125

The Henry J. Kaiser Family Foundation. (2004). *Health insurance coverage in America, 2003 data update.* Retrieved from http://www.kff.org/uninsured/7153.cfm

The Henry J. Kaiser Family Foundation. (2018). *Summary of the Affordable Care Act.* Retrieved from http://www.kff.org/health-reform/fact-sheet/summary-of-the-affordable-care-act/

The Nemours Foundation. (2016). *Going to college.* Retrieved from http://kidshealth.org/en/teens/college.html

The Trevor Project. (2017, June 12). *Pulse shooting day of remembrance brings together LGBTQ, Muslim, and Latinx communities.* Retrieved from https://www.thetrevorproject.org/2017/06/12/pulse-shooting-day-of-remembrance-brings-together-lgbtq-muslim-and-latinx-communities/#sm.001helnmikcvels11531nafleq7dm

Tonkin, E. (2006). Making the case for a Wiki. *Ariadne, 42*(12), 43–44.

Tsingos, C., Bosnic-Anticevich, S., & Smith, L. (2014). Reflective practice and its implications for pharmacy education. *American Journal of Pharmacy Education, 78*(1), 18–25. Retrieved from https://www.ncbi.nlm.nih.gov/pmc/articles/PMC3930242/

Tysiac, K. (2016). Getting creative in fundraising. *Journal of Accountancy*. Retrieved from https://www.journalofaccountancy.com/issues/2016/jul/creative-fundraising-ideas.html

Ueno, K. (2005). Sexual orientation and psychological distress in adolescence: examining interpersonal stressors and social support processes. *Social Psychology Quarterly, 68,* 258–277.

United Health Foundation. (2017). Poor mental health days–United States. *America's Health Rankings*. Retrieved from http://www.americashealthrankings.org/ALL/Overall

United Nations. (2009). *World population prospects: The 2008 revision.* New York: Author. Retrieved from http://www.un.org/esa/population/

United Nations. (2011, March 9). *Investing in women, girls—especially education—drives development, makes good economic sense, Deputy Secretary-General tells International Women's Day forum meetings.* Retrieved from http://www.un.org/press/en/2011/dsgsm541.doc.htm

United Nations. (2012a, April). *Population Facts. Population ageing and non-communicable diseases* (p. 1). Retrieved from http://www.un.org/esa/population/publications/popfacts/popfacts__2012-1.pdf

United Nations. (2012b). *Social indicators.* Geneva, Switzerland: Author. Retrieved from http://unstats.un.org/unsd/demographic/products/socind

United Nations. (2015). *World population prospects: The 2015 revision, key findings and advance tables.* Working Paper No. ESA/P/WP/241.

United Nations. (2017). *World population prospects: The 2017 revision, key findings and advance tables.* Working Paper No. ESA/P/WP/248.

United Nations Development Programme. (2010). *Human development report 2010. The real wealth of nations: Pathways to human development.* Retrieved from http://hdr.undp.org/en/content/human-development-report-2010

United Nations Development Programme. (2013). *Human development report 2013. The rise of the South: Human progress in a diverse world* [Press Release]. Retrieved from http://hdr.undp.org/sites/default/files/pr1-main-2013hdr-eng_0.pdf

United Nations Development Programme. (2016). *Sustainable development goals.* Retrieved from http://www.undp.org/content/dam/undp/library/corporate/brochure/SDGs_Booklet_Web_En.pdf

United Nations General Assembly. (2013, July 26). *A life of dignity for all: accelerating progress towards the Millennium Development Goals and advancing the United Nations development agenda beyond 2015.* Report of the Secretary-General.

United Nations Population Fund. (2013a, October 30). *More than 7 million girls in poor countries give birth before 18 each year, finds new UNFPA report.* Retrieved from https://www.unfpa.org/press/more-7-million-girls-poor-countries-give-birth-18-each-year-finds-new-unfpa-report

United Nations Population Fund. (2013b). *Motherhood in childhood: facing the challenge of adolescent pregnancy: State of world population report 2013.* Retrieved from https://www.unfpa.org/sites/default/files/pub-pdf/EN-SWOP2013-final.pdf

United Nations Population Fund. (2017). *State of the world population report 2016.* Retrieved from https://www.unfpa.org/sites/default/files/sowp/downloads/The_State_of_World_Population_2016_-_English.pdf

U.S. Administration on Aging. (2008). *Media advocacy toolkit.* Retrieved from http://www.aoa.gov/press/more/media_advocacy/media_advocacy.aspx

U.S. Cancer Statistics Working Group. (2017). *United States cancer statistics: 1999–2014 incidence and mortality Web-based report.* Atlanta: U.S. Department of Health and Human Services, Centers for Disease Control and Prevention and National Cancer Institute. Retrieved from www.cdc.gov/uscs

U.S. Department of Agriculture. (2007). *OH firm recalls frozen pizza meats.* Retrieved from https://www.fsis.usda.gov/wps/portal/fsis/topics/recalls-and-public-health-alerts/recall-case-archive/recalls-case-archive-2007/

U.S. Department of Health and Human Services (n.d.). *About HHS*. Retrieved from http://www.hhs.gov/about

U.S. Department of Health and Human Services. (1980). *Promoting health/preventing disease: Objectives for the nation*. Washington, DC: U.S. Government Printing Office.

U.S. Department of Health and Human Services. (1990). *Healthy people 2000: National health promotion disease prevention objectives*. Washington, DC: U.S. Government Printing Office.

U.S. Department of Health and Human Services. (1998). *Report to the vice president of the United States: Status of implementation of the Consumer Bill of Rights and responsibilities in the Department of Health and Human Services*. Retrieved from http://aspe.os.dhhs.gov/health/vpreport.htm

U.S. Department of Health and Human Services. (2000, November). *Healthy people 2010: Understanding and improving health*. Washington, DC: U.S. Government Printing Office.

U.S. Department of Health and Human Services. (2004). *Successful strategies for recruiting, training, and utilizing volunteers: A guide for faith and community-based service providers* [Manual]. Retrieved from http://www.ncadistore.samhsa.gov/catalog/

U.S. Department of Health and Human Services. (2010). *Healthy people 2020*. Retrieved from www.healthypeople.gov.

U.S. Department of Health and Human Services. (2011). *Principles of community engagement* (2nd Ed.). Retrieved from https://www.atsdr.cdc.gov/communityengagement/pdf/PCE_Report_508_FINAL.pdf

U.S. Department of Health and Human Services. (2014a). *Healthy People 2020: About Healthy People*. Retrieved from http://www.healthypeople.gov/2020/About-Healthy-People

U.S. Department of Health and Human Services. (2014b). *Healthy People 2020: Disparities*. Retrieved from https://www.healthypeople.gov/2020/about/foundation-health-measures/Disparities

U.S. Department of Health and Human Services. (2014c). *Healthy People 2020: Educational and community-based programs*. Retrieved from http://www.healthypeople.gov/2020/topics-objectives/topic/educational-and-community-based-programs

U.S. Department of Health and Human Services. (2014d). *Healthy People 2020: Leading health indicators*. Retrieved from https://www.healthypeople.gov/2020/Leading-Health-Indicators

U.S. Department of Health and Human Services. (2014e). *Healthy People 2020: Program planning*. Retrieved from https://www.healthypeople.gov/2020/tools-and-resources/Program-Planning

U.S. Department of Health and Human Services. (2014f). *MAP-IT: A guide to using Healthy People 2020 in your community*. Retrieved from https://www.healthypeople.gov/2020/tools-and-resources/Program-Planning

U.S. Department of Health and Human Services. (2015a, May). *Health, United States, 2014*. Retrieved from http://www.cdc.gov/nchs/data/hus/hus14.pdf#016

U.S. Department of Health and Human Services. (2015b, October 18*). HHS initiative on multiple chronic conditions*. Retrieved from http://www.hhs.gov/ash/about-ash/multiple-chronic-conditions/index.html

U.S. Department of Health and Human Services. (2017a, June 19). *Healthy People 2020: Adolescent health*. Retrieved from https://www.healthypeople.gov/2020/topics-objectives/topic/Adolescent-Health

U.S. Department of Health and Human Services. (2017b, June 19). *Healthy People 2020: Early and middle childhood*. Retrieve from https://www.healthypeople.gov/2020/topics-objectives/topic/early-and-middle-childhood

U.S. Department of Health and Human Services. (2017c, February 11). *Healthy People 2020: Health-related quality of life and well-being*. Retrieved from http://www.healthypeople.gov/2020/about/QoLWBabout.aspx

U.S. Food and Drug Administration. (2007). *Experimental study of health claims on food packages.* Retrieved from http://www.cfsan.fda.gov/~comm/crnutri4.html

U.S. Health Resources and Services Administration. (n.d.). *Medically underserved areas/populations: Guidelines for MUA and MUP designation.* Retrieved from http://www.hrsa.gov/shortage/mua/index.html

U.S. National Library of Medicine. (2017, June 13). College health. *MedlinePlus.* Retrieved from https://www.nlm.nih.gov/medlineplus/collegehealth.html

U.S. Public Health Service. (1979). *Healthy people: The surgeon general's report on health promotion and disease prevention.* Washington, DC: U.S. Government Printing Office.

Vega, W. A., Rodriguez, M. A., & Gruskin, E. (2009). Health disparities in the Latino population. *Epidemiol Rev. 2009*(31), 99–112. DOI:10.1093/epirev/mxp008

Ventola, C. L. (2014). Mobile devices and apps for healthcare professionals: uses and benefits. *Pharmacy and Therapeutics, 39*(5): 356-364.

Walker, A., & Early, J. (2010). We have to do something for ourselves: Using Photovoice and participatory action research to assess the barriers to caregiving for abandoned and orphaned children in Sierra Leone. *Global Journal of Health Education and Promotion, 13*(1).

Wallerstein, N., Minkler, M., Carter-Edwards, L., Avila, M., & Sanchez, V. (2015). Improving health through community engagement, community organization, and community building. In K. Glanz, B. K. Rimer, & K. Viswanath (Eds.), *Health behavior and health education: Theory, research and practice* (5th ed., pp. 277–300). San Francisco: Jossey-Bass.

Wang, C. C., & Burris, M. (1997). Photovoice: Concept, methodology, and use for participatory needs assessment. *Health Education and Behavior, 24*(3), 369–387.

Wang, W. L., Lee, H. L., & Fetzer, S. J. (2006). Challenges and strategies of instrument translation. *Western Journal of Nursing Research, 28*(3), 310–321.

Ward, M. (1998, March). Embracing volunteerism. *School Foodservices and Nutrition, 52*(3), 24–31.

Ward, S. E., & Koontz, N. (1999). Putting advocacy into action. *Eta Sigma Gamma Monograph, 17*(2), 36–40.

Waters, A., & Asbill, L. (2013). Reflections on cultural humility. *CYF News, American Psychological Association.* Retrieved from http://www.apa.org/pi/families/resources/newsletter/2013/08/cultural-humility.aspx

Webster's New Millennium Dictionary of English. (2007). "Blog." Retrieved from http://www.dictionary.reference.com/browse/blog

Weiner, J., Aguirre, A., Ravenell, K., Kovath, K., McDevit, L., Murphy, J., Asch, D. A., & Shea, J. (2004). Designing an illustrated patient satisfaction instrument for low-literacy populations. *American Journal of Managed Care, 10*(part 2), 853–860.

Weinreich Communications. (1999). *What is social marketing?* Retrieved from http://www.socialmarketing.com/whatis.html

Weinstein, N. D., & Sandman, P. M. (1992). A model of precaution adoption process: Evidence from home radon testing. *Health Psychology 11*(3), 170–180.

Westerinen, A. (2003). *What is policy and what can it be?* Retrieved from http://www.policy-workshop.org/2003/web/policy2003/common/AndreaPresentation.pdf

W. K. Kellogg Foundation. (n.d.). *Who we are.* Retrieved from http://www.wkkf.org/who-we-are/overview

W. K. Kellogg Foundation. (2006, February). *Logic model development guide.* Battle Creek, MI: Author. Retrieved from http://www.wkkf.org/resource-directory/resource/2006/02/wk-kellogg-foundation-logic-model-development-guide

Woodhouse, L. D., Auld, M. E., Livingood, W. C., & Mulligan, L. A. (2006). Survey of accredited master of public health (MPH) programs with health education concentrations: A resource for strengthening the public health workforce. *Health Promotion Practice, 7*(2), 258–265.

World Bank. (2014). *Millennium Development Goal 1. Eradicate extreme poverty and hunger by 2015.* Retrieved from http://www.worldbank.org/mdgs/poverty_hunger.html

World Bank. (2015). *World Bank forecasts global poverty to fall below 10% for first time; Major hurdles remain in goal to end poverty by 2030.* Retrieved from http://www.worldbank.org/en/news/press-release/2015/10/04/world-bank-forecasts-global-poverty-to-fall-below-10-for-first-time-major-hurdles-remain-in-goal-to-end-poverty-by-2030

World Bank. (2017). *Community-driven development overview.* Retrieved from http://www.worldbank.org/en/topic/communitydrivendevelopment

World Bank. (2018, April 11). *Understanding poverty.* Retrieved from http://www.worldbank.org/en/topic/poverty/overview

World Health Organization. (n.d.). *Social determinants of health.* Retrieved from http://www.who.int/social-determinants/en/

World Health Organization. (1947). Constitution of the World Health Organization. *Chronicle of the World Health Organization, 1,* 1–2.

World Health Organization. (1999). *Health for all.* Retrieved from http://www.who.org/aboutwho/en/healthforall.htm

World Health Organization. (2004). *Global health and infectious disease: Tropics disease report.* Retrieved from http://www.who.int/tdr/topics/social-research/globalization.htm

World Health Organization. (2005). The World Health Organization Quality of Life Assessment (WHOQOL): Position paper from the World Health Organization. *Social Science Medicine, 41*(10), 1403–1409.

World Health Organization. (2006a, April). *Migration of health workers* [Fact sheet No. 301]. Retrieved from http://www.who.int/mediacentre/factsheets/fs301/en/ index.html

World Health Organization. (2006b). *Working together for health: World health report 2006.* Geneva, Switzerland: Author.

World Health Organization. (2008a). *Global burden of disease: 2004 update.* Retrieved from http://www.who.int/healthinfo/global_burden_disease/2004_report_update/en/

World Health Organization. (2008b). *Millennium development goals.* Retrieved from http://www.who.int/topics/millennium_development_goals/en/

World Health Organization. (2008c). *Strengthening health systems through primary health care.* Retrieved from http://www.who.int/healthsystems/en/index.html

World Health Organization. (2010). *Framework for Action on Interprofessional Education & Collaborative Practice.* Geneva: Author. Retrieved from http://whqlibdoc.who.int/hq/2010/WHO_HRH_HPN_10.3_eng.pdf

World Health Organization. (2011, June 7). mHealth: New horizons for health through mobile technologies. *Global Observatory for eHealth Series. Volume 3.* Retrieved from http://www.who.int/goe/publications/ehealth_series_vol3/en/index.html

World Health Organization. (2012a). *Global report for infectious disease and poverty.* Retrieved from http://www.who.int/tdr/publications/global_report/en/

World Health Organization. (2012b). *World conference on social determinants of health: Meeting report.* Geneva, Switzerland: Author.

World Health Organization. (2013). *World health statistics 2013.* Retrieved from http://www.who.int/gho/publications/world_health_statistics/2013/en/

World Health Organization. (2017a). *About WHO: Leadership priorities.* Retrieved from http://www.who.int/about/agenda/en/

World Health Organization. (2017b). *Health promotion.* Retrieved from http://www.who.int/healthpromotion/about/en/

World Health Organization. (2017c). *Social determinants of health.* Retrieved from http://www.who.int/social_determinants/thecommission/finalreport/key_concepts/en/

World Health Organization. (2018, February 18). *HIV/AIDS* [WHO Fact Sheets]. Retrieved from http://www.who.int/en/news-room/fact-sheets/detail/hiv-aids

Wright, K. B. (2005). Researching Internet-based populations: Advantages and disadvantages of online survey research, online questionnaire authoring software packages, and web survey services. *Journal of Computer-Mediated Communication, 10*(3), article 11. Retrieved from http://www.jcmc.indiana.edu/vol10/issue3/wright.html

Yan, H. (2015, December 9). The truth about Muslims in America. *CNN.* Retrieved from https://www.cnn.com/2015/12/08/us/muslims-in-america-shattering-misperception/index.html

Zeng, Q., Eunjung, K., & Tse, T. (n.d.). *A text corporal-based estimation of the familiarity of health terminology.* Retrieved from http://www.lhncbc.nlm.nih.gov/lhc/docs/published/2005/pub2005041.pdf

Index